Sleep and Cardiorespiratory Control

Sommeil et contrôle cardio-respiratoire

Colloques **INSERM**
ISSN 0768-3154

Other *Colloques* published as co-editions by John Libbey Eurotext and INSERM

133 Cardiovascular and Respiratory Physiology in the Fetus and Neonate. *Physiologie Cardiovasculaire et Respiratoire du Fœtus et du Nouveau-né.*
Scientific Committee : P. Karlberg,
A. Minkowski, W. Oh and L. Stern;
Managing Editor : M. Monset-Couchard.
ISBN : John Libbey Eurotext 0 86196 125 0
INSERM 2 85598 340 1

134 Porphyrins and Porphyrias. *Porphyrines et Porphyries.*
Edited by Y. Nordmann.
ISBN : John Libbey Eurotext 0 86196 087 4
INSERM 2 85598 281 2

137 Neo-Adjuvant Chemotherapy. *Chimiothérapie Néo-Adjuvante.*
Edited by C. Jacquillat, M. Weil and D. Khayat.
ISBN : John Libbey Eurotext 0 86196 125 0
INSERM 2 85598 340 1

139 Hormones and Cell Regulation (10th European Symposium). *Hormones et Régulation Cellulaire (10e Symposium Européen).*
Edited by J. Nunez, J.E. Dumont and R.J.B. King.
ISBN : John Libbey Eurotext 0 86196 125 0X
INSERM 2 85598 340 1

147 Modern Trends in Aging Research. *Nouvelles Perspectives de la Recherche sur le Vieillissement.*
Edited by Y. Courtois, B. Faucheux, B. Forette,
D.L. Knook and J.A. Tréton.
ISBN : John Libbey Eurotext 0 86196 126 0X
INSERM 2 85598 340 1

149 Binding Proteins of Steroid Hormones. *Protéines de liaison des Hormones Stéroïdes.*
Edited by M.G. Forest and M. Pugeat.
ISBN : John Libbey Eurotext 0 86196 125 0
INSERM 2 85598 340 1X

151 Control and Management of Parturition. *La Maîtrise de la Parturition.*
Edited by C. Sureau, P. Blot, D. Cabrol, F. Cavaillé and G. Germain.
ISBN : John Libbey Eurotext 0 86196 125 0
INSERM 2 85598 340 1

Suite page 273

Sleep and Cardiorespiratory Control

Sommeil et contrôle cardio-respiratoire

Proceedings of the Symposium on Sleep and Cardiorespiratory Control held in Kremlin-Bicêtre (France), September 12-13, 1991

Supported by the Institut National de la Santé et de la Recherche Médicale, the Association des Physiologistes, the Délégation à la Recherche Clinique de l'Assistance Publique - Hôpitaux de Paris and the Fondation de France

Edited by

C. Gaultier
P. Escourrou
L. Curzi-Dascalova

LES EDITIONS
INSERM

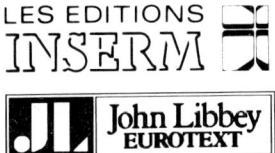

British Library Cataloguing in Publication Data

Sleep and cardiorespiratory control.
 I. Title. Gaultier, Cl. II. Escourrou, P.
 III. Dascalova, L. Curzi, IV. Series
 606.2

ISBN 0-86196-307 5
ISSN 0768-3154

First published in 1991 by

Editions John Libbey Eurotext
6 rue Blanche, 92120 Montrouge, France. (1) 47 35 85 52
ISBN 0 86196 307 5

John Libbey and Company Ltd
13 Smiths Yard, Summerley Street, London SW18 4HR,
England.
(1) 947 27 77

Institut National de la Santé et de la Recherche Médicale
101 rue de Tolbiac, 75654 Paris Cedex 13, France.
(1) 44 23 60 00
ISBN 2 85598 484 X

ISSN 0768-3154

© 1991 Colloques INSERM/John Libbey Eurotext Ltd,
All rights reserved
Unauthorized publication contravenes applicable laws

Foreword

In the last decade, description of the pathophysiology of breathing disorders during sleep has become increasingly important for physicians and research teams. With improvement of our knowledge, the issue of cardiorespiratory interactions during sleep has emerged. We have learned that relationships between cardiovascular and respiratory systems may be usefully considered at the level of central control mechanisms as well as at the effectors.

Our goal for this Symposium is to bring together a broad range of specialists in cardiorespiratory physiology and pathophysiology in infants and adults to take stock of the different aspects of sleep and cardiorespiratory control. The first session concerns recent research in the physiology of cardiorespiratory control and states of alertness including the developing process of cardiorespiratory interactions. The second session of the Symposium focuses on new methods of testing the autonomic system especially during sleep studies. Clinical and diagnostic aspects of the pathology of cardiorespiratory control will be considered in the third session. An important part of this session will be a focus on cardiorespiratory adaptation during sleep in infants and its relationship with sudden infant death. Finally the last session is devoted to interactions between hemodynamics and treatment of sleep apnea syndrome.

We wish to thank our colleagues from many different countries for their participation by lectures, abstracts and discussions. The organizers are grateful to the Institut National de la Santé et de la Recherche Médicale, the Association des Physiologistes, the Délégation à la Recherche Clinique de l'Assistance Publique-Hôpitaux de Paris and the Fondation de France for support of this Symposium.

Claude Gaultier

Acknowledgements / *Remerciements*

We wish to thank the following corporations for their support :
Nous remercions les sociétés suivantes pour leur concours :

    Ambulatory Monitoring Inc.
    A.B.S. - Synectics
    Bayer Pharma
    Compagnie Française des Produits Oxygénés
    De Vilbiss Medical France SA
    Gould
    Institut de Recherche Servier
    MSR
    PPG Hellige
    SEFAM
    Synthelabo, Département Egic-Joullié

Avant-propos

Les dix dernières années ont été marquées par un intérêt croissant des médecins et des équipes de recherche pour la physiologie et la physiopathologie respiratoires du sommeil. L'amélioration de nos connaissances a fait apparaître l'importance des interactions cardio-respiratoires. Nous avons appris à les prendre en considération au niveau du contrôle central comme au niveau des effecteurs.

Le but de ce Symposium est de réunir un large éventail de spécialistes en physiologie et physiopathologie respiratoires du nourrisson et de l'adulte pour faire le point sur les différents aspects du contrôle cardio-respiratoire au cours du sommeil. La première session concerne les recherches récentes sur la physiologie du contrôle cardio-respiratoire et des états de vigilance en incluant le développement des interactions cardio-respiratoires. La seconde session du Symposium est consacrée aux nouvelles méthodes d'investigation du système nerveux autonome, en particulier au cours du sommeil. Les aspects cliniques et diagnostiques de la pathologie du contrôle cardio-respiratoire seront débattus au cours de la troisième session. Une partie de celle-ci concernera l'adaptation cardio-respiratoire du nourrisson au cours du sommeil et ses relations avec la mort subite. La dernière session est réservée aux interactions entre hémodynamique et traitement du syndrome d'apnées du sommeil.

Nous voulons remercier les collègues de nombreux pays qui ont accepté de donner une conférence, présenter des résultats personnels et participer à la discussion. Les organisateurs expriment leurs remerciements, pour le soutien de ce Symposium, à l'Institut National de la Santé et de la Recherche Médicale, à l'Association des Physiologistes, à la Délégation à la Recherche Clinique de l'Assistance Publique - Hôpitaux de Paris et à la Fondation de France.

Claude Gaultier

List and address of contributors
Liste et adresse des conférenciers

Bradley T., Sleep Disorders Clinic, Toronto General Hospital, RM 212 10 EN, 200 Elizabeth St, Toronto M5G ON, Canada

Cherniack N., School of Medicine, Case Western Reserve University, 2074 Abington Road, Cleveland, OH 44106, États-Unis

Curzi-Dascalova L., Laboratoire de Physiologie, INSERM CJF 8909, Hôpital Antoine Béclère 92141 Clamart, France

Elghozi J.L., Service de Pharmacologie Clinique, Association Claude Bernard, Faculté de Médecine Necker-Enfants Malades, 156 rue de Vaugirard, 75015 Paris, France

Escourrou P., Laboratoire de Physiologie, INSERM CJF 8909, Hôpital Antoine-Béclère 92141 Clamart, France

Gaultier C., Laboratoire de Physiologie, INSERM CJF 8909, Hôpital Antoine-Béclère, 92141, Clamart, France

Goldman M., Sleep Disorders Center, The Medical College of Pennsylvania, Philadelphia, États-Unis

Guilleminault C., Sleep Disorders Clinic, Stanford University Medical College, Stanford CA 94305, États-Unis

Haddad G.G., Yale University, Department of Pediatrics, Section of Respiratory Medicine, School of Medicine, 333 Cedar street, New Haven, Connecticut 06520-8064, États-Unis

Harper R.M., Department of Anatomy, University of California, Los Angeles CA 90024, États-Unis

Johnson P., Nuffield Department of Obstetrics and Gynaecology, John Radcliffe Hospital, Maternity Department, Headington, Oxford OX3 9DU, Royaume-Uni

Kahn A., Hôpital Universitaire des Enfants Reine Fabiola, Avenue J.J. Crocq, 15, 1020 Bruxelles, Belgique

Kauffmann F., Laboratoire de Mathématiques, Faculté des Sciences, Université de Caen, 14032 Caen, France

Krieger J., Laboratoire de Neurophysiologie, Centre Hospitalier Régional et Universitaire, BP 426, 67091 Strasbourg Cedex, France

Laguzzi R., INSERM U 288, Neurobiologie cellulaire et fonctionnelle, CHU Pitié-Salpêtrière, 91 boulevard de l'Hôpital, 75634 Paris Cedex 13, France

Mirmiran M., Netherlands Institute for Brain Research, Meibergdreef 33, 1105 AZ Amsterdam 20, Pays-Bas

Penzel T., Klinikum der Philipps-Universität Marburg, Postfach 2360, Baldingerstrasse, 3550 Marburg/Lahn, Allemagne

Podszus T., Klinikum der Philipps-Universität Marburg, Postfach 2360, Baldingerstrasse, 3550 Marburg/Lahn, Allemagne

Ramet J., Hôpital Académique, Vrije Universiteit Bruxelles, 101, Laarbeeklaan, B1090 Bruxelles, Belgique

Spyer K.M., Department of Physiology, Royal Free Hospital, Rowland Hill street, London NW3 2 PF, Royaume-Uni

Shepard J.W.Jr., Mayo Sleep Disorders Center, Mayo Clinic, 200 First Street SW, Rochester, Minnesota 55905, États-Unis

Stradling J., Sleep Clinic, The Churchill Hospital Headington, Oxford, OX37LJ, Royaume-Uni

Välimäki I., Department of Paediatrics, University of Turku, SF 20 250 Turku, Finlande

Wallin B.G., Department of Clinical Neurophysiology, University of Göteborg, Sahlgren's Hospital, Göteborg, Suède

Weitzenblum E., Service de Pneumologie, Centre Hospitalier Régional et Universitaire, Hospices Civils de Strasbourg, BP 426, 67091 Strasbourg, France

Contents
Sommaire

V   Foreword
VI Acknowledgements
    Remerciements
VII *Avant-propos*
IX List and address of contributors
    Liste et adresse des conférenciers

    I. PHYSIOLOGY OF CARDIORESPIRATORY CONTROL AND STATES OF ALERTNESS
    I. PHYSIOLOGIE DU CONTRÔLE CARDIO-RESPIRATOIRE ET ÉTATS DE VIGILANCE

3   **K.M. Spyer**
    Functional organization of cardiorespiratory control
    Organisation fonctionnelle du contrôle cardio-respiratoire

9   **R. Laguzzi**
    Cardiovascular changes during the sleep-wake cycle
    Modifications cardio-vasculaires au cours du cycle veille-sommeil

15 **N.S. Cherniack**
    Periodic breathing
    Respiration périodique

23 **J.L. Elghozi, D. Laude, A. Girard**
    Heart rate and blood pressure oscillations related to respiration
    Oscillations de la fréquence cardiaque et de la pression artérielle liées à la respiration

35 **D.F. Donnelly, G.G. Haddad**
    Carotid chemotransduction : mechanisms and development
    Chémotransduction carotidienne : mécanismes et développement

45 P. Johnson, D.C. Andrews
The role of thermometabolism on cardiorespiratory function in postnatal life
Rôle du métabolisme thermique sur la fonction respiratoire dans la vie post-natale

55 R.M. Harper
Brain mechanisms underlying cardiorespiratory control during sleep
Mécanismes centraux du contrôle cardio-respiratoire au cours du sommeil

II. PATHOPHYSIOLOGY OF CARDIORESPIRATORY CONTROL
II. PHYSIOPATHOLOGIE DU CONTRÔLE CARDIO-RESPIRATOIRE

63 J.W. Shepard Jr.
Gas exchange during apnea : effects on lung and blood oxygen stores
Echanges gazeux pendant l'apnée : effet sur les réserves pulmonaires et sanguines d'oxygène

73 B.G. Wallin
Human sympathetic nerve activity during normal sleep and in sleep apnoea
Activité nerveuse sympathique chez l'homme pendant le sommeil normal et le syndrome d'apnées

79 T. Penzel, J.H. Peter, P. von Wichert
Spectral analysis of heart rate and blood pressure in sleep apnea syndrome
Analyse spectrale de la fréquence cardiaque et de la pression artérielle dans le syndrome d'apnées du sommeil

87 M.D. Goldman, K.R. Casey, C.R. Jones
Cardiorespiratory autonomic reflex behaviour during sleep
Réflexes autonomes cardio-respiratoires pendant le sommeil

95 C. Guilleminault, T. Shiomi, R. Stoohs, I. Schnittger
Echocardiographic studies in adults and children presenting with obstructive sleep apnea or heavy snoring
Etude échocardiographique chez l'adulte et l'enfant avec apnées obstructives du sommeil ou un ronflement important

105 **F. Kauffmann, B. Cauchemez**
Extraction of cardiorespiratory parameters
Extraction des paramètres cardio-respiratoires

III. PATHOPHYSIOLOGY OF CARDIORESPIRATORY CONTROL. CLINICAL AND DIAGNOSTIC ASPECTS
III. PHYSIOPATHOLOGIE DU CONTRÔLE CARDIO-RESPIRATOIRE. ASPECTS CLINIQUES ET DIAGNOSTIQUES

115 **J. Stradling**
Systemic hypertension and sleep apnoea
Hypertension artérielle systémique et syndrome d'apnées du sommeil

123 **J. Krieger**
Regulation of body fluid compartments in obstructive sleep apnea syndrome
Régulation des compartiments liquidiens dans le syndrome d'apnées du sommeil

133 **A. Kahn, E. Rebuffat, M. Sottiaux, J.J. Grosswasser, D. Michel**
Cardiorespiratory mechanisms implicated in sudden infant death syndrome : a possible role for the autonomic nervous system
Mécanismes cardio-respiratoires impliqués dans la mort subite du nourrisson : rôle possible du système nerveux autonome

145 **J. Ramet, M. Dehan, C. Gaultier**
Cardiac and respiratory vagal reactivity in infants
Réactivité vagale cardio-respiratoire du nourrisson

155 **L. Curzi-Dascalova, J. Clairambault, F. Kauffmann, C. Médigue, P. Peirano**
Cardiorespiratory variability and development of sleep state organization
Variabilité cardio-respiratoire et développement de l'organisation du sommeil

165 **M. Mirmiran, Y. Maas, J. Kok**
Circadian rhythms of cardiorespiratory controls in preterm infants
Rythmes circadiens du contrôle cardio-respiratoire chez les nourrissons prématurés

169 **I. Välimäki, J. Jalonen, T. Äärimaa**
Postnatal organization of cardiorespiratory interaction in neonates during quiet sleep
Organisation post-natale de l'interaction cardio-respiratoire des nouveau-nés en sommeil calme

IV. PATHOPHYSIOLOGY OF CARDIORESPIRATORY CONTROL. CLINICAL ASPECTS AND TREATMENT
IV. PHYSIOPATHOLOGIE DU CONTRÔLE CARDIORESPIRATOIRE. ASPECTS CLINIQUES ET THÉRAPEUTIQUES

177 **T. Podszus, O. Feddersen, J.H. Peter, P. von Wichert**
Cardiovascular risk in sleep related breathing disorders
Le risque cardio-vasculaire dans les anomalies respiratoires du sommeil

187 **E. Weitzenblum, J. Krieger, M. Oswald, M. Apprill**
Pulmonary hemodynamics and sleep apnea syndrome
Hémodynamique pulmonaire et syndrome d'apnées du sommeil

193 **P. Escourrou, V. Le Gros, C. Gaultier**
Baroreflex control of heart rate in sleep apnea patients. Comparison of normotensive and hypertensive patients and effect of CPAP therapy
Contrôle baroréflexe de la fréquence cardiaque dans le syndrome d'apnées du sommeil. Comparaison des patients normotendus et hypertendus et effet de la PPNC

203 **T.D. Bradley, Y. Takasaki, R. Rutherford**
Effects of CPAP on Cheyne-Stokes respiration and cardiac function in heart failure
Effets de la PPNC sur la respiration de type Cheyne-Stokes et la fonction cardiaque dans l'insuffisance cardiaque

ABSTRACTS
RÉSUMÉS

I. Sleep apnea syndrome : mechanisms
I. Syndrome d'apnées du sommeil : mécanismes

217 **F. Series, I. Series, L. Atton, A. Blouin**
Influence of airway resistance on periodic breathing (PB)

218 **K. Gleeson, L.W. Sweer, C.W. Zwillich**
Hyperventilation due to experimental asphyxic blood gases is sometimes followed by apnea during sleep but not during wakefulness

II. SAS : diagnosis and complications
II. SAS : évaluation diagnostique et conséquences

221 **R.J.O. Davies, K.B. Vardi-Visy, J.R. Stradling**
Systolic blood pressure profiles in sleep and breathing disorders

222 **M.R. Bonsignore, O. Marrone, S. Romano**
Beat-by-beat estimate of right ventricular stroke volume (RVSV) in obstructive sleep apnea (OSA)

223 **V. Le Gros, P. Escourrou, H. Nedelcoux, C. Gaultier**
Arterial chemoreflex and baroreflex control of heart rate in normotensive and hypertensive sleep apnea patients

224 **D. Veale, J.L. Pepin, C. Bonnet, J.P. Siché, P. Lévy**
Autonomic stress tests in the obstructive sleep apnoea syndrome

225 **P. Parchi, E. Sforza, P. Cortelli, G. Pierangeli, E. Lugaresi**
Cardiovascular reflexes in obstructive sleep apnea syndrome

226 **K. Ehlenz, P. Herzog, P. von Wichert, H. Kaffarnik, J.H. Peter**
Renal excretion of endothelin in obstructive sleep apnea syndrome

227 F. Barbe, J.J. Kiladjian, R. Patte, F. Daniel, B. Fleury
Sodium renal excretion in heavy snorers and obstructive sleep apnea syndrome

228 M. Pradella, D.O. Rodenstein, G. Aubert-Tulkens
Breathing frequency in patients with sleep related respiratory disturbances (SRRD)

229 H. Encabo, M. Nogués
Respiratory abnormalities during sleep in syringomyelia and syringobulbia

III. SAS : effects of treatment
III. SAS : effets du traitement

233 O. Marrone, V. Bellia, A. Salvaggio, C. Macaluso, G. Bonsignore
Transmural pulmonary artery pressure and oxygen administration in obstructive apneas

234 P. Kozev, S. Slavchev
Nasal CPAP and pulmonary haemodynamics in OSA patients

235 E. Sforza, E. Lugaresi
Hemodynamic effects of short-term nasal continuous positive airway pressure in obstructive sleep apnea syndrome

236 T. Perez, A. Didier, C. Puel, M. Tiberge, P. Leophonte, J.P. Besombes
Improvement in daytime ventilatory responses to CO_2 with or without inspiratory load after CPAP therapy for obstructive sleep apnea syndrome (OSAS)

237 F. Series, I. Series, Y. Cormier
Effects of the enhancement of slow wave sleep (SWS) by gamma hydroxybutyrate (γ-OH) on obstructive sleep apnea (OSA)

238 M. Rey, F. Philip-Joet, M. Reynaud-Gaubert, C. Delpuech, M. Saadjian, A. Arnaud
CPAP effect on EEG spectral analysis in sleep apnea syndrome

239 V. Jounieaux, T. Toris, P. Levi-Valensi
Appropriated therapy for overlap syndrome (COPD and SAS) : the point at issue

IV. Sleep and cardiovascular system (physiology, pathology)
IV. Sommeil et système cardio-vasculaire (physiologie, pathologie)

243 **R.J.O. Davies, P. Belt, N.J. Ali, J.R. Stradling**
Effects of minor arousal stimuli on blood pressure in normal sleeping man

244 **J.E. Fewell, C.S. Kondo, V. Dascalu**
Influence of sleep state on coronary hemodynamics in young lambs

245 **E. Dreizzen, Y. Shabtai-Musih, N. Gavriely**
Step reduction of alveolar PCO_2 causes ECG abnormalities

246 **R.J.O. Davies, K.J. Harrington, J.R. Stradling**
Placebo controlled trial of nocturnal continuous positive airway pressure in chronic heart failure with sleep disordered breathing

247 **A. Braghiroli, F. De Vito, C. Sacco, M. Erbetta, V. Ruga, S. Magnaghi, A. Giordano, C.F. Donner**
Nocturnal periodic breathing in patients with stable chronic heart failure : effects of oxygen versus placebo

248 **F. De Vito, A. Braghiroli, C. Sacco, S. Magnaghi, M. Erbetta, C.F. Donner, A. Giordano**
Sleep respiratory disorders in patients with stable chronic heart failure : a polysomnographic study

249 **D. Auge**
Sleep apnea and myocardial ischemia

250 **H.A.M. Middelkoop, M. Bootsma, B. Kemp, C.A. Swenne, H.A.C. Kamphuisen, A.V.G. Bruschke**
Sleep apnea syndrome and ischemic heart disease

251 **C. Rostykus, J.C. Meurice, J. Mergy, P. Dore, J. Paquereau, F. Patte**
Atrial vulnerability revealed by nasal CPAP

252 **M. Benachouba, J.C. Roy**
Effects of autonomic blockade on heart rate responses to pyramidal tract stimulation

V. Sleep and cardio-respiratory adaptations in infants
V. Sommeil et adaptations cardio-respiratoires du nourrisson

255 E. Girin, M. Bellet, Y. Grossi, J. Le Bot, M.D. Donnou, C. Cabelguen, D. Alix
Ventilatory pattern, occlusion pressure and sudden infant death syndrome (SIDS)

256 M.F. Vecchierini-Blineau, B. Nogues
Respiratory and cardiac rates in 2-month-old normal infants : nycthemeral changes

257 B. Nogues, M.F. Vecchierini-Blineau
Spontaneous awakenings during sleep in two-month-old infants : influence on respiratory and cardiac rates

258 A. de Broca, A. Mahomedaly, F. Kochert, N. Kalach, M. Vural, B. Risbourg
Infants' vagal reactivity disclosed during a standardized ocular compression test and a 12 hours cardio-respiratory monitoring

259 D. Lagarde, O. Mouterde, E. Mallet
Atropin test : a new test to appreciate vagal tone in children during sleep

260 M.E. Schläfke, T. Schäfer
Sleep-phase related tc PCO_2 in infants under closed and open loop conditions of the central pH/PCO_2 control system

261 M.A. Woo, M.S. Woo, W. Brendle Glomb, D. Bautista, S.L. Davidson Ward
Heart rate variability in infants at increased risk for sudden infant death syndrome

262 M.A. Woo, M.S. Woo, D. Gozal, T.G. Keens
R-R interval Poincaré plots in normal children and in children with congenital central hypoventilation syndrome

263 M. Eiselt, L. Curzi-Dascalova, U. Zwiener
Correlation between event related heart rate changes and mean heart rate in newborns during sleep

264 M. Eiselt, J. Clairambault, C. Médigue, C. Leffler, L. Curzi-Dascalova
Heart rate variability during sleep in prematures of 39 weeks postconceptional age

265 M. Rother, H. Witte, M. Eiselt
Heart rate fluctuation analysis in newborns. A review on possibilities, limitations and possibilities of misinterpretation

266 M. Rother, U. Koschel, M. Eiselt, B. Clausner
Cardiorespirography improves the prognostic value of EEG in neonates

VI. Sleep and altitude
VI. Sommeil et altitude

269 O. Marrone, S. Romano, S. Carollo, R. Milazzo, S. Porcu
Heart rate during sleep at high altitude : effect of acclimatization

270 H. Normand, J. Bordachar, J. Raynaud, E. Vargas, O. Benoit
Arterial O_2 saturation during sleep at high altitude in normal and polycythemic highlanders

271 Author index
Index des auteurs

I. Physiology of cardiorespiratory control and states of alterness

I. Physiologie du contrôle cardio-respiratoire et états de vigilance

Functional organization of cardiorespiratory control

K.M. Spyer

Department of Physiology, Royal Free Hospital, School of Medicine, Rowland Hill Street, London NW3 2PF, UK

INTRODUCTION
The supply of oxygen to the tissues of vertebrates demands the coordination of the cardiovascular and respiratory systems. To achieve such "cardio-respiratory" homeostasis it appears that the central nervous system has retained an evolutionary simple mode of control that involves a unified reticular neural network that generates activity in the motor outflows to the two systems (Richter & Spyer, 1990). Further, the reflex mechanisms that provide a feedback control of the two systems operate, at least in part, through this shared neural substrate and so have simultaneous effects on both systems. A consequence of these interactions is seen in the respiratory variations in heart rate and blood pressure, which result from the marked respiratory related discharge patterns of the autonomic innervation of the cardiovascular system (Anrep et al, 1936 a,b). The purpose of this review is to describe the features of the brainstem cardiorespiratory network that generates these patterns of activity and to demonstrate the physiological significance of its operation. In addition, attempts will be made to identify the effects of the disruption of this control on both physiological responses to changing circumstances and their potential pathological consequences.

Central generation of rhythmic discharge in cardio-respiratory outputs.
The primary area involved in the generation of this cardio-respiratory rhythm is the medulla oblongata (Feldman, 1987). The medulla contains the vagal preganglionic neurones that control heart rate and several populations of neurones that send their axons down the spinal cord to innervate the sympathetic preganglionic neurones of the intermediolateral cell columns of the thoracolumbar spinal cord which number amongst their functions vasomotor and cardiac control (Spyer 1981). The respiratory motoneurones - phrenic and intercostal - are also innervated by bulbospinal neurones that arise from two major areas of the medulla. The first is the dorsal respiratory group of inspiratory neurones localised in the vicinity of the nucleus tractus solitarius (NTS); the second a highly differentiated column of cells in the lateral medulla associated with the nucleus ambiguus-

retroambigualis (NA/NRA, the ventral group). For convenience, the pattern of activity of the different components of the network will be described separately prior to outlining the basis for their interactions.

Respiratory neurones

The pattern of respiratory activity is determined by the discharge of a network of neurones located in the medulla oblongata (Richter, 1982). Traditionally, it has been assumed that two broad and heterogenous groups of neurones - 'inspiratory' and 'expiratory', together with some diverse 'phase-spanning' neurones interact to produce the pattern of activity of the respiratory motoneurones (Feldman, 1987 for review). With the recognition that the respiratory cycle is divisible into a three-phase process, largely as a consequence of the work of Richter and his colleagues (Richter, 1982; Richter et al, 1986), a much simpler classification has become possible. Respiratory neurones are defined on the basis of the temporal relationships between membrane potential or discharge and the activity recorded in the phrenic nerve. In this way, several distinctive categories of respiratory neurone have been identified (see Fig. 1) which show manifestations of the three-phase cycle that have been engendered through mutual synaptic interactions. Two groups in particular, post-inspiratory neurones (PI) that are active in the first stage of expiration (Stage I), and early inspiratory neurones (eI), that fire at the onset of inspiration with a declining discharge, are of extreme importance in the timing and shaping of the rhythm. These are "interneurones" as they do not relay beyond the brainstem in either the cranial nerves or with axons descending down the spinal cord to innervate the respiratory motoneurones. Their influence is, however, profound being seen throughout the respiratory and accessory respiratory (e.g., laryngeal, pharyngeal, etc.) and, as we will see in the cardiovascular networks.

Recent modelling studies have indicated that the respiratory neurones indicated in Fig. 1 could not, through their interactions, generate a suitable respiratory rhythm. These studies indicated the requirement for an additional class of neurone (Pack et al, 1991). These would fire just preceding the onset of inspiration and results from several laboratories have now identified such a category of cell, their discharge peaks at the onset of inspiration declining rapidly thereafter. They appear to have a restricted localisation in the more rostral extreme of the NA/NRA complex in the vicinity of the Bötzinger group of respiratory neurones. The detailed physiological properties of these neurones remain to be resolved.

Cardiac vagal motoneurones

Cardiac vagal motoneurones provide the major regulation of moment by moment heart rate (Spyer, 1981). The preganglionic neurones are located primarily in the NA although, in some species they are also found in the DVN. These vagal neurones receive a direct innervation from the NTS in both cat and rat, and are also innervated by 5-hydroxytryptamine (5-HT) containing terminals that appear to originate from perikarya localised within the raphe obscuras and magnus. Their discharge is characterised by both respiratory modulation and a powerful baroreceptor control (Spyer, 1990 for review). They tend to be silent during inspiration, but are active in Stage I expiration and have variable activity in Stage II expiration. This centrally determined firing pattern is the primary cause of sinus arrhythmia, ensuring a relative bradycardia during expiration. Studies in this laboratory have established that this firing pattern is induced by a

FIG. 1

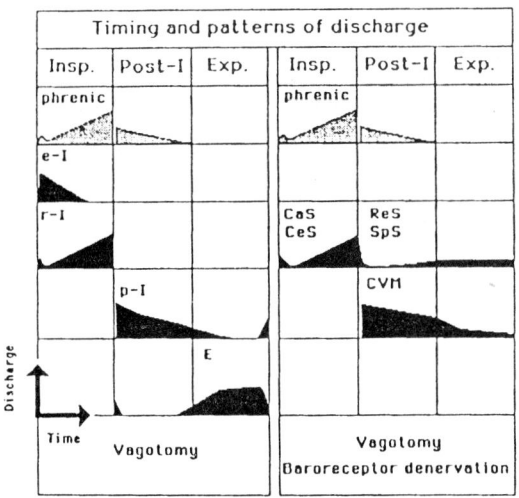

Timing and patterns of discharge of respiratory and cardiovascular neurons. The time frequency profile of the discharge of early (e-I), ramp (r-I), late (l-I), and post-inspiratory (p-I) as well as stage 2 expiratory (E) neurons is illustrated schematically in the left panel and that of the cardiac (CaS), cervical (CeS), renal (ReS), and splanchnic (SpS) sympathetic neurons as well as vagal cardiomotor (CVM) neurons of the cat in the right panel. These activity patterns are related to the inspiratory, postinspiratory, and stage 2 expiratory phase of the respiratory cycle as indicated by the phrenic nerve discharge (PN). The illustration refers to the descriptions given by Bainton et al (1985), Cohen and Gootman (1970), and Numao et al (1987). (Reproduced from Richter and Spyer, 1990).

FIG. 2

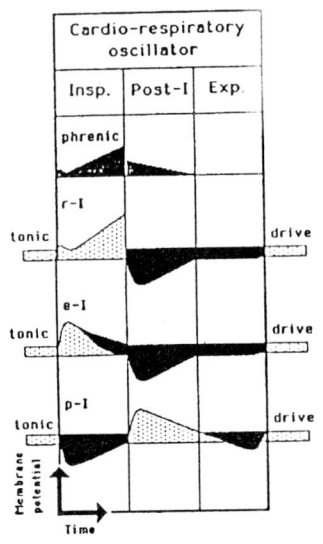

A common cardiorespiratory oscillator? The three - ramp (r-I), early (e-I), and postinspiratory (p-I) - subsystems of the cardiorespiratory network are suggested to constitute a common "cardiorespiratory oscillator". These components convert the excitatory, tonic drive from the activating reticular formation into rhythmic activity with alternating periods of rebound and synaptic excitation (dotted areas) and synaptic inhibition (black areas). For further explanation see text. (Reproduced from Richter and Spyer, 1990).

Cl⁻-dependent hyperpolarisation of CVMs during inspiration that is mediated by a muscarinic cholinergic synapse (Gilbey et al,1984). This effectively suppresses the normal excitatory input from the arterial baroreceptors whose input is the main excitatory determinant of their activity. In this regard, the reflex inputs associated with lung inflation must exert their influence at some stage in the reflex pathway of the baroreceptor reflex within the medulla, since no direct effect on the membrane of CVMs has been revealed. Equally, there does not appear to be an interaction between these afferent inputs at the level of the nucleus tractus solitarius (NTS).

"Premotor" sympathetic neurones

Sympathetic preganglionic neurones (SPNs) receive a direct innervation from several cell groups localised within the lower brainstem (Loewy, 1990). There is particularly detailed evidence that raphe-spinal neurones originating in both the raphe obscurus and magnus make monosynaptic contacts onto SPNs as do neurones located within the ventromedial medulla (Bacon et al, 1990; Zagon & Bacon, 1990). A potentially important role in vasomotor control has been suggested for neurones in the rostroventrolateral medulla (RVLM) that, again, innervate the IML (Guyenet, 1990 for review). These neurones are located in close proximity in both the rat and cat to the CVMs described above and, similarly, are powerfully influenced by baroreceptor inputs, although these are invariably inhibitory. Further, they are also modulated in phase with respiration but exhibit an inspiratory modulated discharge (McAllen, 1987). There is much less well defined information on the basis of this rhythm, with some indications that it might depend on afferent feedback from pulmonary receptors, whilst other suggestions indicate a centrally generated phenomenon.

Sympathetic preganglionic neurones

There is an expansive literature that describes the respiratory modulation of the discharge of both pre- and post-ganglionic sympathetic nerves (Jänig, 1985). This generalised modulation can be seen in the discharge of individual neurones, and it is from an analysis of this phenomenon in the case of individual SPNs recorded with microelectrodes that a detailed assessment of the factors generating these patterns can be made (Gilbey et al, 1986; Dembowsky, 1990). In the rat, both upper thoracic and a proportion of thoraco-lumbar SPNs show marked respiratory patterns of discharge that accord to the three phase respiratory cycle defined in the cat and rat. Indeed, in the cat a detailed intracellular analysis of SPN activity in relation to the respiratory cycle has revealed that excitatory but not inhibitory influences can be identified, suggesting that the pattern of discharge is imprinted from a medullary source(s) through bulbospinal connections (Dembowsky, 1990). In essence, the phases of apparent inhibition represent disfacilitation. However, any change in central respiratory drive will lead to a concomitant change in sympathetic activity and, hence, vasomotor tone and heart rate.

The marked heterogeneity of respiratory rhythm in SPNs and post-ganglionic discharge may have functional significance, but this has yet to be fully documented. It would appear to be a particular key to the physiological control of those sympathetic neurones that have a role in cardiovascular control.

Factors influencing the performance of the cardio-respiratory network

The clear evidence that shared rhythms exist in the motor pathways for both cardiovascular and respiratory control allows speculations to be made with regard to the physiological significance of this coupling and the ways in which this network is regulated by both central and reflex inputs. In Fig. 2 the network is shown to be dependent on a tonic input from the reticular formation to drive the network into operation. Such a connection can explain many of the state-dependent changes that occur in cardio-respiratory control during the sleep-wake cycle and its various substates. Similarly, activating the hypothalamic defence in anaesthetised animals has parallel effects on both systems, and the effects observed are clear examples of the underlying interactions described so far. This is shown by the hyperpnoea accompanied by tachycardia, with particularly marked alterations occurring in expiration, and especially Stage I (Ballantyne et al, 1988). Presumably, the changes that occur during temperature regulatory mechanisms manifest a similar modification of the network operation.

These processes will also result in considerable afferent feedback from a wide range of peripheral receptors. In the main, these receptors operate to influence both systems, and for afferents with endings in the cardiovascular and respiratory systems themselves, this is particularly clear (Richter & Spyer, 1990). However, these potent interactions do not prevent a level of specialisation of reflex input. For example, arterial baroreceptors elicit particularly powerful effects on autonomic outflows but have less marked effects on respiratory medullary neurones, and phrenic and intercostal motoneurones; they also affect the excitability of a wide range of other motoneurones, including hypoglossal and even limb motoneurones. The changes induced in respiratory activity will, of course, be generated through actions on the shared network, but some access may be directed more powerfully to the output neurones to the two systems.

In these processes the timing of an input becomes important. There are numerous examples of the variation of effectiveness of reflex inputs altering with the timing of their delivery with respect to the respiratory cycle. The most effective period for the cardiac effects of the baroreceptors, laryngeal and many other afferent inputs is if they are delivered during Stage I of expiration. Equally, this is the crucial timing for inputs of central origin to have their most dramatic effects on the pattern of the respiratory cycle. Accordingly, pathological states in which prolonged periods of apnoea are induced, which is largely a consequence of Stage I, or post-inspiratory activity -renders the cardiovascular systems susceptible to heightened reflex and central inputs, with an emphasis on eliciting bradycardia. This is a potential mechanism for explaining sudden, and unexplained, cardiac death and may have implications for SIDS.

Acknowledgements
Original studies by the author were funded by grants from the Medical Research Council and the British Heart Foundation.

References

Anrep, G.V., Pascual, W. and Rössler, R. (1936a): Respiratory variations of the heart rate. I. The reflex mechanism of the sinus arrhythmia. Proc. Roy. Soc. Lond, Series B 119, 191-217.

Anrep, G.V., Pascual, W. and Rössler, R. (1936b): Respiratory variations of the heart rate. II. The central mechanism of the sinus arrhythmia and the inter-relationships between central and reflex mechanisms. Proc. Roy. Soc. Lond, Series B 119, 218-230.

Bacon, S.J., Zagon, A. and Smith, A.D. (1990): Electron microscopic evidence of a monosynaptic pathway between cells in the caudal raphe nuclei and sympathetic preganglionic neurons in the rat spinal cord. Ex. Brain Res, **79**, 589-602.

Ballantyne, D., Jordan, D., Spyer, K.M. and Wood, L.M. (1988): Synaptic rhythm of caudal medullary expiratory neurones during stimulation of the hypothalamic defence area of the cat. Physiol, **405**, 527-546.

Dembowsky, K.. (1990): Spinal integration of the cardio-respiratory outflow. Proc. 13th Ann. Meeting ENA, Stockholm, 1990.

Feldman, J.L. (1987): Neurophysiology of breathing in mammals. **In:** Handbook of Physiology: The nervous system, Vol. IV, F.E. Bloom (Ed), American Physiological Society, Bethesda, MD, pp 463-524.

Gilbey, M.P., Jordan, D., Richter, D.W. and Spyer, K.M. (1984). Synaptic mechanisms involved in the inspiratory modulation of the vagal cardioinhibitory neurones in the cat. J. Physiol. **356**, 65-78.

Gilbey, M.P., Yoshinobu, N. and Spyer, K.M. (1986): Discharge patterns of cervical sympathetic preganglionic neurones:related to central respiratory drive in the rat. J. Physiol. **378**, 253-266.

Guyenet, P.G. (1990): Role of the ventral medulla oblongata in blood pressure regulation. **In:** Central Regulation of Autonomic Functions, Edits. A.D. Loewy and K.M. Spyer, OUP (NY), pp145-167.

Jänig, W. (1985): Organisation of the lumbar sympathetic outflow to skeletal muscle and skin of the cat hindlimb and tail. Rev. Physiol, Biochem and Pharmacol, **102**, 119-213.

McAllen, R.M. (1987): Central respiratory modulation of subretrofacial bulbospinal neurones in the cat. J. Physiol. **388**, 533-545.

Pack, A.I., Galante, R.J., Walker, R.E., Kubin, L.K. and Fishman, A.P. (1991): Comparative approach to neural control of respiration. **In:** Central and peripheral mechanisms in the control of breathing, Eds. D.F. Speck, M.S. Dekin, W.R. Revelette and D.T. Frazier, Univ. Press of Kentucky (In Press).

Richter, D.W. (1982): Generation and maintenance of the respiratory rhythm. J. Exp. Biol., **100**, 93-107.

Richter, D.W., Ballantyne, D. and Remmers, J.E. (1986). Respiratory rhythm generation: a model. News in Physiol. Sci. **1**, 109-112.

Richter, D.W. and Spyer, K.M. (1990): Cardiorespiratory control. In: Central Regulation of Autonomic Functions, Edits A.D.Loewy and K.M. Spyer, OUP (NY), 189-207.

Spyer, K.M. (1981): Neural organisation and control of the baroreceptor reflex. Rev. Physiol, Biochem and Pharmacol., **88**, 23-124.

Spyer, K.M. (1990): The central nervous organisation of reflex circulatory control. **In:** Central regulation of autonomic functions, Edits. A.D. Loewy and K.M. Spyer, OUP (NY), pp168-188.

Zagon, A. and Bacon, S.J. (1991). Evidence of a monosynaptic pathway between cells of the ventromedial medulla and the motoneuron pool of the thoracic spinal cord in rat: electron miscroscopic analysis of synaptic contacts. The Europ. J. Neurosci. **3**, No. 1, 55-65.

Cardiovascular changes during the sleep-wake cycle

Raùl Laguzzi

Unité de Neurobiologie Cellulaire et Fonctionnelle, INSERM U288, Faculté de Médecine Pitié-Salpêtrière, 91, boulevard de l'Hôpital, 75634 Paris Cedex 13, France

In terms of observable somatic behaviours, there are two behavioral states of the organism : wakefulness and sleep. The study of the mechanisms which control arterial pressure throughout the sleep-wake cycle shows that there are no qualitative modifications in these mechanisms during the transition quiet wakefulness - slow wave sleep (SWS). However, during sleep, SWS is the gateway to another state with a physiology of its own : paradoxyxal sleep (PS). PS is characterised by an inhibition of both sympathic tone and of the central mechanisms of homeostatic regulation of physiological functions. These modifications brought about by PS are the basis for the cardiovascular events seen during the transition SWS-PS. Detailed analysis of these events, as well as of the mechanisms which determine them, therefore appears to be of undeniable physiological and physiopathological importance.

If one records blood pressure (BP) and heart rate (HR) every second during a period of wakefulness (W) and during the following period of slow wave sleep (SWS), one observes that the mean values are higher in W than in SWS. For most animal species cardiovascular (CV) parameters decrease during sleep (Mancia and Zanchetti, 1980). However, W is not a uniform state. It is necessary to differentiate at least active W from quiet W. During active W, in particular during instinctive or voluntary behaviours, physiological parameters are modified and become very variable. Some of these modifications are essential for the effective performance of behaviours. For example, during aggressive and defensive behaviours, the organisms needs to maintain CV parameters at a higher level than during quiet W. Therefore it is necessary to interrupt briefly the homeostatic control mechanisms of these parameters. This fact explains the partial inhibition of the baroreceptor reflex observed during the defense reaction (Hilton and Redferm, 1986). Thanks to this reflex, if the BP rises above a certain threshold, there is an immediate, compensatory hypotension and bradycardia. This response prevents the organism from mounting an effective defence reaction. We can thus understand why the baroreceptor reflex is inhibited during this behaviour. However, this reflex is not totally blocked during active W, it can become operational at any moment if it is necessary for the organism's survival. Claude Bernard and Cannon's principle for the homeostatic regulation of physiological functions is valid for active and quiet W. This principle is also valid for SWS. In fact, as regards CV control, there does not seem to be a qualitative difference between quiet W and SWS. At the beginning of SWS, some fluctuations in BP and HR may be observed, but later on deep SWS is characterised by a pronounced stability of CV parameters and by a very slight decrease in BP (Mancia and Zanchetti, 1980; Lacombe et al., 1988). The fluctuations in these parameters at the beginning of SWS are, according to Parmaggiani (1982), due to the progressive inactivation of voluntary (cortical) mechanisms; autonomic mechanisms have to adjust the activity of effector structures to the new state of reduced energy expenditure.

Studies carried out in the cat show that there is no reduction in total peripheral resistance (TPR) during SWS (Mancia et al., 1971). The small decrease in BP observed in most animal species therefore appears to be the result of the slight reduction in HR which is also a characteristic feature of this state (Mancia and Zanchetti, 1980; Lacombe et al., 1988). During SWS the organism is in a state which can be described as "vegetative". However, in the sleep-wake cycle, this state is the gateway to another state which is far from being "vegetative": the state named (with justification) paradoxical sleep (PS). The transition from SWS to PS completely alters the organism's physiology. All the studies carried out in different animal species concur in showing great variation in BP and HR during PS. In contrast, depending on the species examined, the mean BP level can increase, decrease or remain unchanged, with regard to SWS (Mancia and Zanchetti, 1980; Lacombe et al., 1988). The evolution of BP during sleep therefore differs among animal species. One of the factors determining this difference could be the intensity of phasic activity which characterises PS, because this activity influences BP. Thus, detailed studies in the cat have shown two types of influence of PS on BP (Guazzi and Zanchetti, 1965). There is a tonic influence, which produces a progressive decrease in BP during the length of the PS episode, and a phasic influence which results in frequent and abrupt changes in the tonic reduction of BP. The inter-species variations in this phasic influence could therefore explain the differences in the level of mean BP during PS between different animal species.

While the slight reduction in BP oberved during SWS is the consequence of a decrease in HR, the tonic and phasic modifications in BP produced by PS are basically due to modifications in TPR. Thus PS fundamentally influences sympathetic tone. In fact; it has been shown that, during PS, TPR is always the results of a compromise between generalised vasodilatation (reduction in sympathetic tone) with a central origin and vasoconstriction at the skeletal muscle level with a spinal origin (Mancia et Zanchetti, 1980; Mancia et al., 1971; Bacelli et al., 1974). The tonic decrease in TPR and as a result in BP, is due to the fact that generalised vasodilatation predominates over skeletal vasoconstriction. During phasic activity, BP increases because the vasoconstriction at the level of the red skeletal muscles increases and predominates over the generalised vasodiliatation.

The CV changes observed during the transition between SWS and PS therefore shown a qualitative difference in the central mechanisms which control CV activity during these two sleep states.

We will now return to the factors which determine that the change in BP produced between SWS and PS is not the same in different animal species. In the cat BP decreases during PS, while it increases in the rat. Thus one must ask oneself if the reduction in sympathic tone seen in the cat during PS is also seen in the rat. An attempt to answer this question, by experiments using sino-aortic denervation (SAD), resulted in the discovery of an important factor which determines the evolution of BP between SWS and PS. It is known that SAD produces an increase in BP. However, this denervation also alters the BP changes during the sleep-wake cycle. Thus, after SAD, the evolution of BP during sleep in the rat, is similar to that seen in normal cats : a decrease rather than an increase in BP is observed in the SWS-PS transition (Junqueira and Kreiger, 1986). This is a very important finding as it shows that sino-aortic reflexes are one the factors which determine the evolution of BP during sleep. In addition, it also shows that in the rat, as in the cat, PS is accompanied by a decrease in sympathetic tone and that the difference between these two species lies in the efficacity of the sino-aortic reflexes to compensate for the sympathetic inhibition.

In the cat SAD accentuates the decrease in BP which is normally seen in this species between SWS and PS. Furthermore, this decrease reaches values which are sometimes incompatible with a normal cerebral circulation (Mancia and Zanchetti, 1980). This shows that the sympathetic reduction during PS is very important and that the homeostatic regulation of BP during this state is fundamentally maintained by sino-aortic reflexes. Therefore, PS appears to be a state characterised by the inactivation of central homeostatic regulation of BP. Studies which analysed the influence of PS on respiration and body temperature regulation drew the same conclusions (Parmeggiani et al., 1971; Phillipson and Sullivan, 1978).

PS is controlled by a neural system localised in the pontine and bulbar structures (Sakai, 1988). In the same way that SWS is characterised by the inactivation of cortical mechanisms, PS is characterised by the inactivation of hypothalamic mechanisms (Parmeggiani, 1982). This hypothalamic inactivation would produce the loss of homeostatic regulation of most of the major physiological systems, but would be particulary marked for systems where the principal control mechanisms are located in the hypothalamus. Cardiovascular control is therefore less affected than thermoregulation as the former posseses a certain degree of auto-regulation and reflex regulation. Therefore Claude Bernard and Cannon's principle of homeostatic regulation cannot be applied to the PS state. Based on this evidence Parmeggiani (1985) described the SWS-PS transition as a "functional crisis".

The reduction in the efficacity of the homeostatic mechanisms which operates during PS provides an explanation for results which suggest that certain visceral receptors send messages to the SNC capable of inhibiting PS. Thus, it has been shown in the rat that aortic denervation significantly increases the daily amount of PS (Orer et al., 1991). Furthermore, other experiments appear to show that these PS-inhibitory messages arrive at the nucleus tractus solitarius by serotonergic afferents (Nosjean et al., 1990; Orer et al., 1991). These results also suggest that there is a functional interaction, at the level of the medula oblongata, between neurons controlling sympathetic tone (Guyenet et al., 1989) and the executive PS neurons (Sakai, 1988). This interaction could explain the appearance of direct transitions between W and PS ("experimental narcolepsy") which have been observed in the rat after aortic denervation or after destruction of the serotonergic afferents which arrive at the nucleus tractus solitarius from the nodose ganglia (Orer et al., 1991).

In summary, the study of CV modifications, and of physiological modifications in general, which operate during the whole of the sleep-wake cycle, is clearly of multidisciplinary importance. These modifications provide evidence for qualitative changes in the central mechanisms which control physiologycal functions between states. This evidence shows the need to perform experiments during sleep if one wants to define fully the hemodynamic profile during everyday life. This knowledge is clearly needed to explain the pathophysiology of some CV events that seem to occur with particular frequency during sleep.

In terms of observable somatic behaviours, there are two behavioral states of the organisms : wakefulness and sleep. However, if the recording of electrical parameters, such as the EEG, has shown the existence of another state, PS, the study of physiological modifications during sleep, has, in its turn, shown that each state of sleep (SWS and PS) has its own physiology which differs from one to another. This evidence provides new perspectives for research designed to investigate the central mechanisms controlling sleep states.

REFERENCES

BACELLI, G., ALBERTINI, R., MANCIA, G. and ZANCHETTI, A. (1974): Central and reflex regulation of sympathetic vasoconstrictor activity of limb muscle during desynchronized sleep in the cat. Cir. Res., 35: 625-635.

GUAZZI, M. and ZANCHETTI, A. (1965): Blood pressure and heart during natural sleep of the cat and their regulation by carotid sinus and aortic reflexes. Arch. Ital. Biol., 103: 789-817.

GUYENET, P., HASELTON, J. and SUN, M-K. (1989): Sympathoexcitatory neurons of the rostroventrolateral medulla and origin of the sympathetic vasomotor tone. Prog. Brain Res., 81: 105-116.

HILTON, S.M. and REDFERM, W.S. (1986): A search for brain stem cell groups integrations the defence reaction in the cat. J. Physiol. (London). 150: 114-133.

JUNQUEIRA, L.F. and KRIEGER, E.M. (1976): Blood pressure and sleep in the rat in normotension and in neurogenic hypertension. J. Physiol. (London), 259: 725-735.

LACOMBE, J., NOSJEAN, A., MEUNIER, J.M. and LAGUZZI, R. (1988): Computer analysis of cardiovascular changes during the sleep-wake cycle in Sprague-Dawley rats. Am. J. Physiol., 254: H217-H222.

MANCIA, G., BACELLI, G., ADAMS, D.B. and ZANCHETTI, A. (1971): Vasomotor regulation during sleep in the cat. Am. J. Physiol., 220: 1086-1093.

MANCIA, G. and ZANCHETTI, A. (1980): Cardiovascular regulation during sleep. In: Physiology in sleep, eds J. Orem and C. Barnes, pp.1-55, New York: Academic Press.

NOSJEAN, A., COMPOINT, C., BUISSERET-DELMAS, C., ORER, H.S., MERAHI, N., PUIZILLOUT, J.J. and LAGUZZI, R. (1990): Serotonergic projections from the nodose ganglia to the nucleus tractus solitarius. An immunohistochemical and double labeling study in the rat. Neurosci. Lett., 114: 22-26.

ORER, H., MERAHI, N., NOSJEAN, A., GOZLAN, H. and LAGUZZI, R. (1991): Sleep changes induced by the local application of the 5,7-dihydroxytryptamine into the nodose ganglia and aortic denervation in the rat. Pflügers Arch. (In press).

PARMEGGIANI, P.L. (1982): Regulation of physiological functions during sleep. Experientia, 38: 1405-1408.

PARMEGGIANI, P.L. (1985): Homeostatic regulation during sleep: facts and hypotheses. In: Brain mechanisms of sleep. eds D. McGinty, R. Drucker-Colin, A. Morrison and P. Parmeggiani, pp.385-397. New York: Raven Press.

PARMEGGIANI, P.L., FRANZINI, C., LENZI, P. and CIANCI, T. (1971): Inguinal subcutaneous temperature changes in cats sleeping at different environmental temperatures. Brain Res., 33: 397-404.

PHILLIPSON, E.A. and SULLIVAN, C.E. (1978): Respiratory control mechanisms during NREM and REM sleep. In: Sleep apnea syndromes. eds C. Guilleminault and W.C. Dement, pp.47-64. New York: Alan R. Liss.

SAKAI, K. (1988): Executive mechanisms of paradoxical sleep. Arch. Ital. Biol., 126: 239-257.

Résumé

Du point de vue comportemental on peut différencier deux états de l'organisme: l'éveil et le sommeil. L'analyse des mécanismes qui contrôlent la pression artérielle tout au long du cycle veille-sommeil montre qu'il n'existe pas de modifications qualitatives de ces mécanismes lors de la transition éveil calme-sommeil lent (SL). Cependant, à l'intérieur du sommeil, le SL est la porte d'entrée d'un autre état: le sommeil paradoxal (SP), qui présente une physiologie qui lui est propre. Le SP se caractérise par une inhibition à la fois du tonus sympathique et des mécanismes centraux de régulation homéostatique des fonctions physiologiques. Ces modifications apportées par le SP sont à la base des événements cardiovasculaires qui s'observent dans la transition SL-SP. L'analyse détaillée de ces événements, ainsi que des mécanismes qui les déterminent, apparaît donc d'une importance physiologique et physiopathologique indéniable.

Periodic breathing

Neil S. Cherniack

School of Medicine, Case Western Reserve University, Cleveland, Ohio 44106-4915, USA

By traditional standards "periodic breathing" and "normal breathing" stand in sharp contrast. Normal breathing is regular and stereotyped and is by definition a sign of health; while periodic breathing is characterized by waxing and waning of both tidal volume and breathing frequency, including apnea, and has been considered a sign of disease (Longobardo et al., 1989; Dowell et al., 1971).

Over the years it has been recognized that normal breathing is not strictly regular and that variations in tidal volume and breathing frequency of 20% are far from unusual. Also, it is now appreciated that periodic breathing is not an indication of life-threatening damage to the heart or brain but can occur normally to a degree during sleep. Periodic breathing when it appears often disappears spontaneously. Moreover, apnea is not an essential feature of periodic breathing. In addition, in some normal people even while awake, sophisticated mathematical techniques reveal periodicities in breathing.

Apneas when they occur can be central, obstructive, or mixed. In central apneas all respiratory movements cease. In obstructive apneas, only airflow at the mouth stops because upper airway blockade periodically renders breathing efforts ineffectual. Mixed apneas frequently begin with a central apnea and terminate with an obstructive component. All three types of apnea can occur in the same individual (Phillipson, 1977; Cherniack, 1984).

Periodic breathing is often accompanied by fluctuations in blood pressure, heart rate, consciousness, sympathetic and vagal activity, and pupillary size, that occur with the same cycle length as breathing (Dowell et al., 1971).

In this paper we will discuss three possible mechanisms of periodic breathing; instabilities in the feedback control of respiration; normally occurring oscillations in breathing which are obscured usually but become more evident or stronger in certain circumstances; and breathing swings which result from instabilities or oscillations in other physiological systems which are linked to respiration.

INSTABILITIES IN FEEDBACK CONTROL OF BREATHING

The output of the respiratory system, regulated in part through feedback of information of receptors, seems to behave so as to keep arterial PCO_2 and PO_2 within acceptable limits (Cherniack & Longobardo, 1986).

This control system like control systems seen in industry, can be thought of as consisting of a controller and a controlled system (also called the plant). The controller consists of the central and peripheral chemoreceptors, and the respiratory neurons which generate and shape the respiratory output. The plant consists of the respiratory muscles, the lung, and the chest wall, and the O_2 and CO_2 in physical solution and chemically combined which are stored in the body tissues. Changes in ventilation are produced as a result of transmission over neural pathways of signals from chemoreceptors to the respiratory muscles. The effect of ventilation on arterial tension of PO_2 and PCO_2 are transmitted to the chemoreceptors by the blood as it is pumped from the lungs to the body tissues. Transmittal through the blood (equivalent to the circulation time) is appreciably longer than signal transmission over nerves (see Fig. 1). Mathematical models of the respiratory system have been developed to explore the factors causing instability (Longobardo et al., 1989; Khoo et al., 1982).

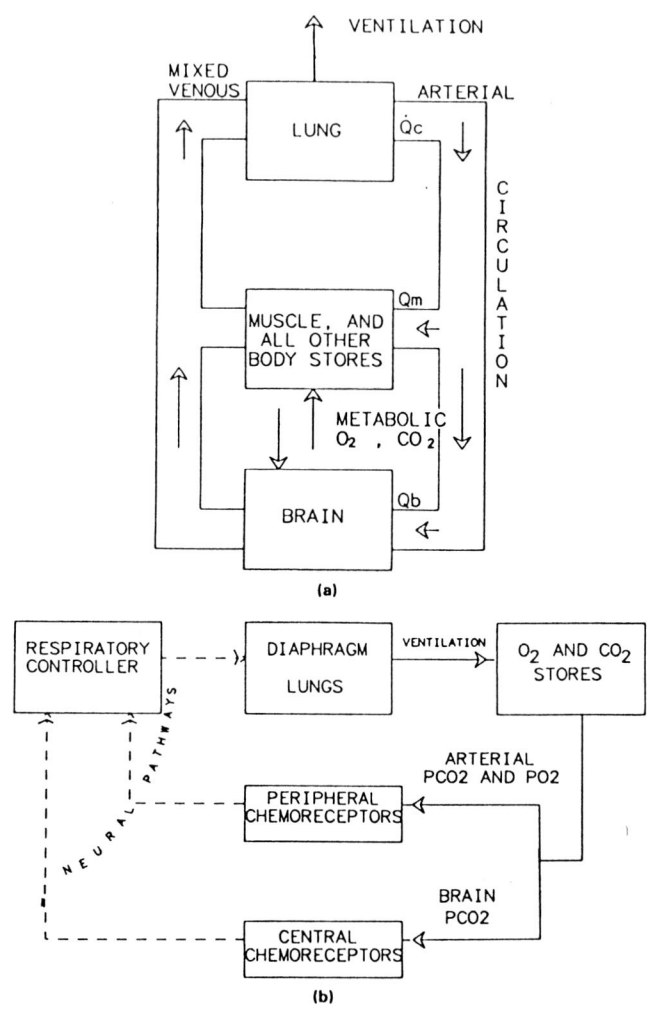

Fig. 1. Schematic of the model of the respiratory control system. (a) As shown in the upper panel, CO_2 and O_2 storage pools are divided into parallel compartments connected by the circulation. Each compartment, an arterial, brain, and a muscle and "all other" compartment, is assigned its own blood flow, metabolic rate, and tissue dissociation slope for CO_2. (b) Shown in the lower panel are the information flow paths in the respiratory system. Dotted lines indicate neural pathways. The output of the peripheral and central receptors drive the

diaphragm and lungs via the respiratory controller. The resulting ventilation changes alter the carbon dioxide and oxygen content of the body, changing the excitation of the chemoreceptors, and readjusting the ventilation. (Longobardo et al., 1989)

FACTORS PROMOTING INSTABILITY

Physiological feedback systems, like mechanical feedback control systems, can react to a disturbance by a transient oscillation in output. Whether or not the oscillation occurs and how long it will persist depends on the "damping" of the system. In general, though, in the underdamped system, the larger the disturbance, the greater the amplitude and duration of the oscillation (Fig. 2).

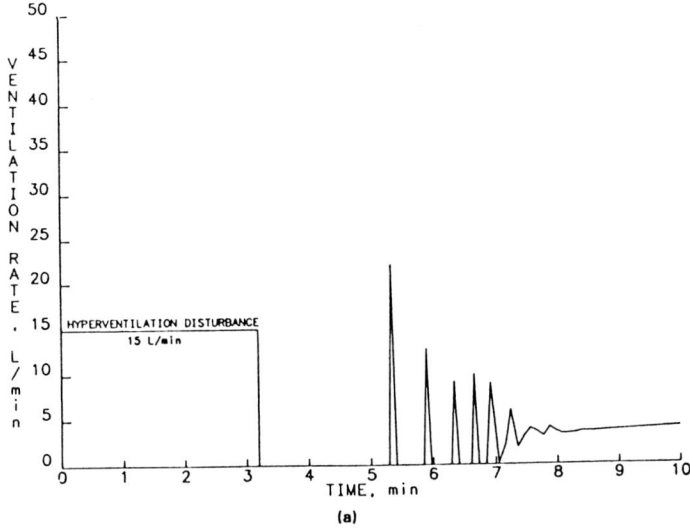

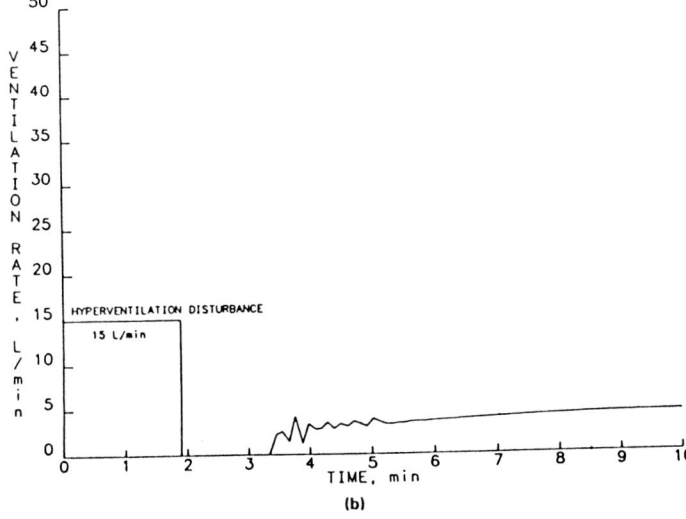

Fig. 2. (a) The upper panel shows a model simulation following hyperventilation which reduces arterial carbon dioxide tension from 40 mm Hg to 15 mm Hg, as compared

to panel (b) which shows a simulation when hyperventilation is less severe; arterial PCO_2 is reduced only to 20 mm Hg. The greater the disturbance, the more oscillatory is the response, and the greater the number of apneas. (Longobardo et al., 1989)

The greater the time required for information transfer in the system (for all practical purposes the circulation time in the respiratory system), the more likely the occurrence of oscillation. With sufficiently long circulation time, even small disturbances to ventilation can produce permanent oscillations (Longobardo et al., 1989).

"High loop gain" is another factor that promotes the occurrence of periodic breathing. High loop gains can be produced by high controller gain, i.e., the ratio $\Delta V/\Delta PCO_2$ or $\Delta V/\Delta PO_2$ becomes larger. The effects of increases in CO_2 or O_2 controller gain are not exactly identical. The peripheral chemoreceptors respond more rapidly to changes in CO_2 than to the central chemoreceptors. Peripheral chemoreceptor denervation tends to make breathing more stable even if total controller gain ($O_2 + CO_2$) is somehow maintained (Fig. 3). The O_2 and CO_2 controllers act in a multiplicative manner so that a given change in PCO_2 causes a larger change in ventilation during hypoxia than during hyperoxia. In addition to hypoxia in experimental animals overall controller gain can be increased by experimental interventions, such as decortication and by stimulation of muscle spindles (Cherniack & Longobardo, 1986).

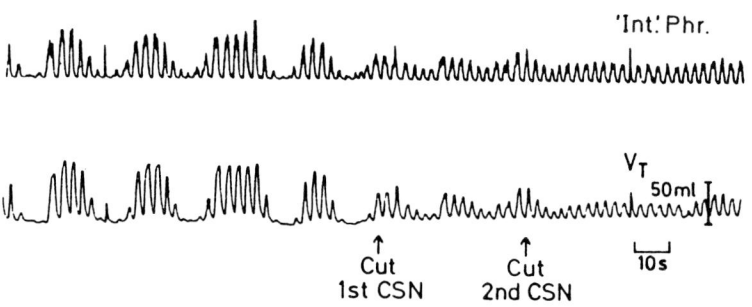

Fig. 3. Effect of carotid sinus nerve (CNS) section on periodic breathing in a cat (Cherniack et al., 1979).

Loop gain also can be increased and instability caused by an increase in plant gain measured as the change in PO_2 or PCO_2 caused by a given change in ventilation, i.e., the ratio $\Delta PCO_2/\Delta V$ or $\Delta PO_2/\Delta V$. Plant gain can be elevated by decreases in the amount of O_2 stored in the body. O_2 is stored mainly in the lungs and in combination with hemoglobin. Hence, changes in functional residual capacity or hypoxia tend to increase plant gain. Increases in resting PCO_2 augment the volume of CO_2 that can be removed from the body stores by a given ventilation level and, hence, also augment plant gain (Cherniack & Longobardo, 1986).

Most of the CO_2 contained in the body is in the form of bicarbonate and is formed by the buffering action of proteins in the blood and tissues as CO_2 changes. The less the tissue volume available for buffering, the greater the plant gain. Because the processes involved in CO_2 buffering require time, particularly to allow all tissue CO_2 stores to equilibrate with each other, only a small portion of the body's buffering capacity is available for CO_2 storage immediately after a ventilatory disturbance (Cherniack & Longobardo, 1970). Hence, alterations in cardiac output and its distribution can affect plant gain. As the volume of tissue available for buffering CO_2 is reduced, plant gain rises. Changes in perfusion rates to tissues where chemoreceptors are located, like the brain, are particularly important in their effects on stability of breathing.

A number of changes occurring during sleep affect loop gain. It has been suggested that in REM sleep brain perfusion can increase so much so that brain tissue PCO_2 is lowered below the threshold levels required to produce ventilation and causes apnea. More important, during sleep resting PCO_2 increases so that for a given increase in ventilation more CO_2 is removed from the body. On the other hand, inhalation of CO_2 interferes with the ability of the body to alter CO_2 tensions by increases in ventilation (Longobardo et al., 1982).

EFFECTS OF HYPOCAPNIA

A critical issue that still needs resolution in connection with periodic breathing is the relation between PCO_2 and ventilation when PCO_2 is low. Acute passive hypervention in sleeping humans can produce apnea even though arterial PCO_2 is reduced just a few millimeters. Much greater hyperventilation is needed in conscious subjects, indicating that some stimulus associated with wakefulness acts to maintain ventilation even when chemical drives are severely lowered (Cherniack & Longobardo, 1986).

Apnea is even harder to produce in conscious subjects by voluntary hyperventilation than by passive means; and when voluntary hyperventilation is stopped, the increased levels of ventilation seem to decline quite slowly to baseline levels. This slow decline which has been termed "after discharge" is another factor that helps prevent apneas in awake subjects. Hence, the appearance of apnea during breathing indicates that the subject is not fully alert and is in some state where after-discharge is eliminated (Eldridge, 1974).

A number of experimental observations support the idea that in many instances periodic breathing results from an instability in feedback control (Cherniack et al., 1979). In man and animals the hyperventilatory cycle is accompanied by higher levels of PCO_2 and lower levels of PaO_2 than during hypoventilation or apnea as predicted by theory. CO_2 inhalations, as predicted, frequently eliminate periodic breathing. In experiments in animals lengthening of circulation time produces periodic breathing, while in animals and in man increases in loop gain also cause breathing to become periodic (Chapman et al., 1988).

INTRINSIC OSCILLATIONS

Some reports of periodic breathing are, however, difficult to explain simply on the basis of instability. For example, we have observed the occurrence of periodic breathing in peripherally chemodenervated anesthetized animals exposed to hypoxia. While drastic elevations in PCO_2 with hypoxia or the occurrence of oscillations in some other system linked to respiration could explain these findings, this does not seem likely. In addition, experiments in anesthetized animals have demonstrated that periodic breathing can be made to occur by hemorrhage even after all known feedback loops in both the respiratory and circulatory systems were cut. This has led to the idea that cyclic fluctuations in respiratory activity are normally always present but are usually obscured (Preiss et al., 1975; Pack et al., 1988; Chapman et al., 1988).

The normal circadian rhythm is an example of natural oscillation that produces long cycles in breathing. The obstructive apneas observed in REM sleep could be another example of spontaneous oscillation in the nervous system (PGO waves) which can cause periodicities in the respiratory system.

In healthy persons, particularly the elderly, mathematical analysis of ventilation reveals periodicities in wakefulness which can become obvious to observers during sleep (Pack et al., 1988; Chapman et al., 1988).

PERIODIC BREATHING RESULTING FROM INTERACTIONS WITH OTHER PHYSIOLOGICAL SYSTEMS

Because of heavy interlinkages, respiratory oscillations are frequently accompanied by oscillations in other systems. These connections arise because the respiratory system shares receptors with other systems, as well as by direct and indirect connections among respiratory and non-respiratory neurons.

Obstructive apneas may occur because of these connections (Cherniack & Longobardo, 1986). The cranial nerves that innervate upper airway muscle display a respiratory rhythm which may play a role in preventing obstructive apneas during sleep. Contractions of the diaphragm and other inspiratory muscles produce a negative pressure in the pharynx. Obstruction can occur then because of compression of the compliant soft tissue walls of the pharynx or because the mobile structures within the pharynx are displaced by the suction of inspiration so that the upper airway is occluded.

However, this collapsing tendency is offset by the dilating action of some muscle of the pharynx, such as the genioglossus and the laryngeal abductor which also contract during inspiration. It seems that to be maximally effective it is important that these upper airway muscles contract slightly before the thoracic muscles.

Oscillations in arterial gas tensions in periodic breathing alter the activity of both sets of muscles. However, in this dynamic state, differences in either the timing or amplitude of the response to the two muscle sets can temporarily affect the balance of forces that allow free air flow and cause obstruction even though respiratory activity continues.

EEG changes suggesting arousal are frequently associated with the termination of obstructive and sometimes central apneas (Phillipson, 1977). Since in the awake state upper airway muscle activity is much greater than during sleep, arousal can interrupt the obstruction. One might even argue that periodic breathing itself might result from instability in a system that regulates state of consciousness. Arousal seems to occur when chemical drive of the muscular forces they produce exceed a certain level. Sleep occurs when arousal inputs fall below this threshold. Sleep itself elevates resting PCO_2 and decreases the effect of chemical drives on ventilation. PCO_2 may rise too high causing arousal and increasing ventilation allowing sleep to occur once again. If the arousal system is too sensitive to changes in PCO_2 or PO_2 there could be cyclic changes in arousal which indirectly produce periodic breathing.

Changes in blood pressure acting via the baroreceptors can alter ventilation (Fig. 4). Increased gain in the feedback system that regulates blood pressure could produce periodic breathing. More commonly, the blood pressure oscillations observed in conjunction with periodic breathing are the result rather than the cause of the breathing pattern.

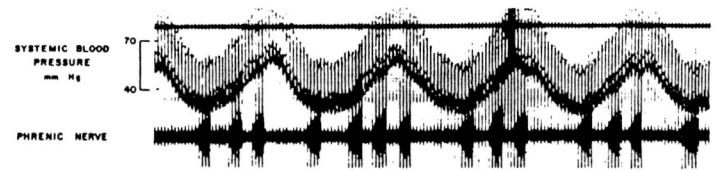

Fig. 4. Periodic breathing associated with systemic blood pressure oscillations in an anesthetized dog.

PATTERNS OF PERIODIC BREATHING

Periodic breathing can arise in several different ways. But once having occurred tends to bring about simultaneous oscillations in many important physiological variables which, in turn, can affect ventilation. Since physiological systems are non-linear, the oscillations interact complexly with each other; and the pattern of periodic breathing can vary considerably even with relatively minor physiological changes as can the length of increased and decreased ventilation within a cycle. While, in general, longer circulation times cause greater total cycle length, it is difficult to determine the etiology of periodic breathing just from its pattern.

REFERENCES

Chapman, K.R., Bruce, E.N., Gothe, B., and Cherniack, N.S. (1988): Possible mechanisms of periodic breathing during sleep. *J. Appl. Physiol.* 64: 1000-1008.
Cherniack, N.S., and Longobardo, G.S. (1970): Oxygen and carbon dioxide stores of the body. *Physiol. Rev. 50*: 196-243.
Cherniack, N.S., Euler, C.von, Homma, I., and Kao, F.F. (1979): Experimentally induced Cheyne-Stokes breathing. *Respir. Physiol.* 37: 185-200.
Cherniack, N.S. (1984): Sleep apnea and its causes. *J. Clin. Invest. 73*: 1501-1506.
Cherniack, N.S. and Longobardo, G.S. (1986): Abnormalities in respiratory rhythm. In *The Handbook of Physiology, The Respiratory System, Vol. II, Control of Breathing*, ed N.S. Cherniack and J.G. Widdicombe, pp. 729-750. Bethesda: American Physiological Society.

Dowell, A.R., Buckley, C.E. III, Cohen, R., Whalen, R.E., and Seikes, H.O. (1971): Cheyne-Stokes respiration: a review of clinical manifestations and critique of physiological mechanisms. *Arch. Intern. Med. 127*: 712-726.

Eldridge, F.T. (1974): Central neural respiratory stimulating effect of active respiration. *J. Appl. Physiol. 37*: 723-735.

Khoo, M.C.K., Kronauer, R.E., Strohl, K.P., and Slutsky, A.S. (1982): Factors inducing periodic breathing in humans: a general model. *J. Appl. Physiol. 53*: 644-659.

Longobardo, G.S., Gothe, B., Goldman, M.D., and Cherniack, N.S. (1982): Sleep apnea as a control system instability. *Respir. Physiol. 50*: 311-333.

Longobardo, G.S., Cherniack, N.S., and Gothe, B. (1989): Factors affecting respiratory system stability. *Annals Biomed. Engrg. 17*: 377-396.

Pack, A.I., Silage, D.A., Millman, R.P., Knight, H., Shore, E.T., and Chung D-C. (1988): Spectral analysis of ventilation in elderly subjects awake and asleep. *J. Appl. Physiol. 64*: 1257-1267.

Phillipson, E.A. (1977): Regulation of breathing during sleep. *Am. Rev. Respir. Dis. 115 (Suppl. 6)*: 217-224.

Preiss, G., Iscoe, S., and Polossa, C. (1975): Analysis of periodic breathing patterns associated with Mayer waves. *Am. J. Physiol. 228*: 768-774.

Heart rate and blood pressure oscillations related to respiration

Jean-Luc Elghozi*, Dominique Laude and Arlette Girard

Service de Pharmacologie Clinique, Association Claude Bernard, Faculté de Médecine Necker-Enfants Malades, 156 rue de Vaugirard, 75015 Paris, France
*Author for correspondence

SUMMARY

We combined non-invasive continuous finger blood pressure (BP) measurement and a spectral technique based on the fast Fourier transform (FFT) to quantify short-term fluctuations in hemodynamic variables.

BP recordings combined low frequency plus high frequency (respiratory) oscillations. The presence of high frequency oscillations of systolic blood pressure (SBP) probably reflects fluctuations in cardiac output. Heart rate (HR) also exhibited a combination of low and high frequency (respiratory) oscillations. The HR oscillation synchronized with the respiration is called the respiratory sinus arrhythmia (RSA). The vagus nerve mediates the efferent control of RSA.

The corresponding spectra illustrate these observations. The high frequency (respiratory) oscillation corresponded to one peak easily detected on the spectrum of SBP and/or HR. Slow waves were detected in a 4-129 mHz range and divided into a 4-66 mHz low frequency region and a 66-129 mHz mid frequency region (Mayer waves).

The effect of changing the breathing frequency on HR and BP was illustrated with tracings and the corresponding spectra. A low breathing frequency was associated with ample HR and BP fluctuations of long periods while a rapid breathing determined fast HR and BP fluctuations of small amplitude.

SBP and HR spectra documented these changes. The high frequency (respiratory) peaks were shifted to the corresponding breathing frequency and the modulus reflected the amplitude of the corresponding respiratory oscillation.

This study illustrates the applicability of this clinical and engineering approach to estimate the respiratory control of cardiovascular oscillations.

This study was supported by a grant "Coeur et hypertension artérielle" from Département Dausse, Laboratoires Synthélabo.

Quantitative description of the structure of short-term blood pressure (BP) and heart rate (HR) waves can result in important information concerning circulatory control processes (Monos and Szücs, 1978). Modern power spectrum analysis techniques are utilized for the description of periodicities in the BP and HR fluctuations by deconvolution of the BP or HR time series into sinusoidal functions of different frequencies.

Using these methods it is possible to partition the total BP and HR variabilities into their various constituents. Discrete power spectrum analysis techniques have revealed that these fluctuations can be divided according to their frequency into three main wavebands. One is at respiration frequency (0.25 Hz), another at 0.1 Hz (Mayer waves) and the third in a lower frequency region of 0.05 Hz. The amplitude of these wave components can vary with functional states of the organism.

The variability of R-R interval is well documented since the electrocardiogram is by far the most accessible and reliable. It is for these rather practical reasons that for the last decades methods to extract information about the activity of cardiovascular regulatory processes from this signal have been developed (Hyndman, 1980).

Respiration has a marked effect on HR at rest. The HR increases on inspiration and decreases on expiration. This phenomenon is called the respiratory sinus arrhythmia (RSA). Many investigators have studied the separate effects of breathing frequency, tidal volume, and static lung volume on the RSA amplitude and wave form or phase angle (Hellman and Stacy, 1976; Hirsch and Bishop, 1981; Weise and Heydenreich, 1989). Parasympathetic nervous system mediates the efferent control of RSA via the vagal nerve, and is responsible for rapid changes in the HR (Pomeranz et al., 1985; Weise et al., 1987; Japundzic et al. 1990). There are several factors contributory to the production of RSA, including reflexes with afferents in the lungs, baroreceptor responses to arterial pressure variations produced by respiratory movements, reflexes with afferents in the right heart, and direct modulation of vagal centers by the respiratory centers. The end result of operation of these factors is a rhythmic variation of vagal activity to the heart, synchronized with the respiratory movements. The integrity of the parasympathetic activity in quadriplegic humans explains why RSA is unaffected in those patients with interrupted descending sympathetic pathways (Inoue et al., 1990). Finally, intrinsic HR responses to wall stress may contribute to a minor degree to RSA (Bernardi et al., 1989).

In contrast, relatively few studies on the influence of the respiration on BP have been made in man since invasive ie intraarterial BP recording was necessary to characterize the short-term components of BP variability. It was observed that BP shows a small decline with inspiration and a rise during expiration. An increased net pressure of the filled right ventricle was observed during inspiration of moderately increased depth, as a result of an increased venous return (Lauson et al., 1946). Then, the stroke volume of the right ventricle increased with inspiration (Lauson et al., 1946; Caplin et al., 1989). Although the respiratory fluctuations in the output of the two ventricles appear to be almost exactly in phase, careful examination indicated that the right ventricular changes preceded

the left ventricular fluctuations by one cardiac cycle in most instances (Franklin et al., 1962). If it may be assumed that the peripheral resistance is constant during the respiratory cycle, the small variations in the net arterial pressures may be attributed to variation in stroke volume from the left ventricle. The necessity of using noninvasive measurements for proper investigation of cardiovascular function in patients has been repeatedly stressed. The Finapres device, by which arterial pressure is measured non-invasively in the finger, provides an alternative to intrabrachial artery recording for continuous BP measurement (Imholz et al., 1991). Besides differences in BP related to the site of measurement, differences in BP may be introduced by changes in vasomotor tone, since these may have a greater impact on the pressure in the finger than on the pressure in the brachial artery. However, the responses of BP obtained by the Finapres device do not differ substantially from the information obtained by invasive measurements (Imholz et al., 1991).
The instrument follows the method of Peñaz (1973), using the principle of the unloaded vascular wall. A transducer comprising a photoelectric plethysmograph and inflatable cuff is fitted to the finger. The plethysmographic signal is used to operate an air valve which controls the pressure in the cuff so that the plethysmographic signal is clamped to a pre-set value. If this value is made to correspond to the unloaded region of the finger arteries diameter, the cuff pressure will follow the instantaneous pressure in those arteries.
We recently combined non-invasive continuous finger blood pressure measurement and a spectral technique based on the fast Fourier transform (FFT) to quantify spontaneous fluctuations in hemodynamic (BP and HR) variables (Elghozi et al., 1991b). This clinical and engineering approach might be used to estimate autonomic control of cardiovascular oscillations.
Subjects were studied in standing and supine position. Finger pressure was measured by a Finapres device (model 2300, Ohmeda, Maurepas, France). All subjects were instructed to keep the cuffed finger in the midaxillary position at heart level. The analog output from the Finapres was connected to an A/D converter to permit data acquisition, storage and analysis using a Dynamit PC computer. The BP signal was digitized using a 12-bit A/D converter at a rate of 500 Hz and processed by an algorithm based on feature extraction to detect and measure the characteristics of a BP cycle with its maximum in a 1 s window (Anapres 2.3, Notocord Systems, Igny). This systolic blood pressure (SBP), the preceding diastolic blood pressure (minimum), integrated Mean Blood Pressure and HR calculated as 60,000/ heart period ms (measured from the systolic pressure present in the 1 s window and the preceding peak) were stored on floppy disk. This 1 Hz sampling suited to patients beating usually in a 55-85 bpm range. The resultant file consisted of 300 lines of 4 values each. The evenly spaced (equidistant) sampling allowed a direct spectral analysis of each distribution using a FFT algorithm on 256 point time series. This corresponded to a 4 min 16 s period at this 1 Hz sampling rate. Thus each spectral component (band)

CONTROLLED BREATHING

150 mHz = 9 cycles/min

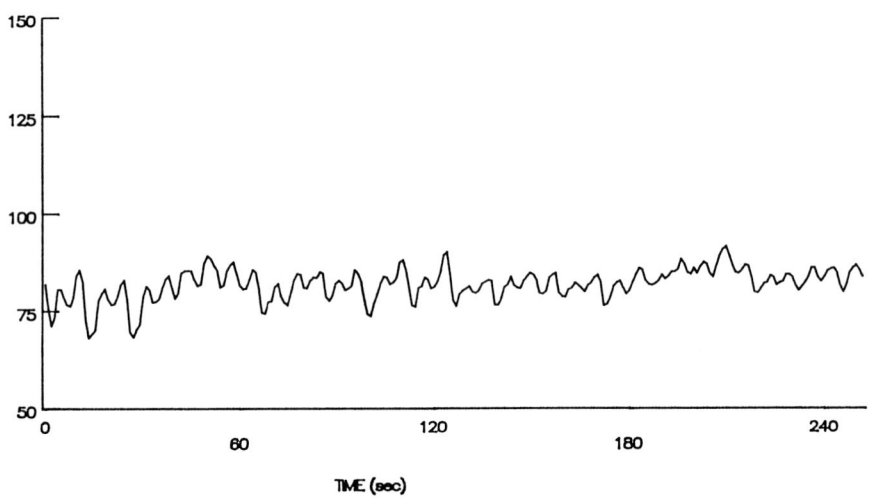

300 mHz = 18 cycles/min

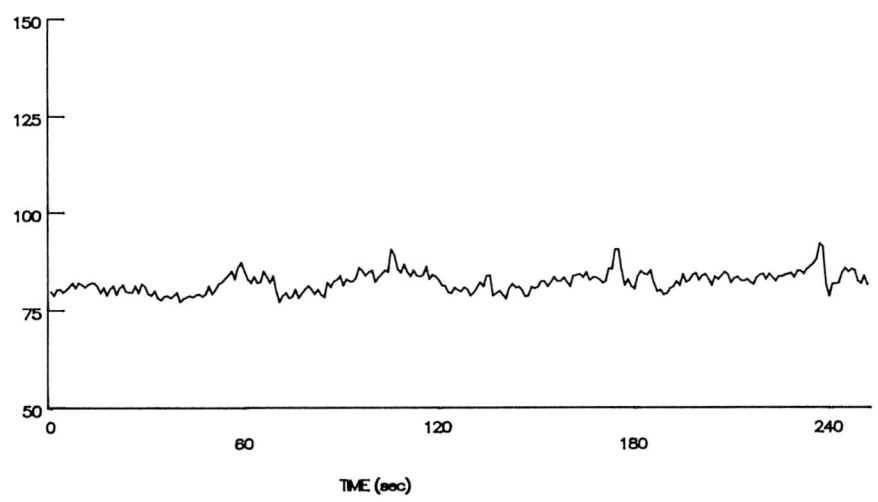

Fig. 1.
Digitized HR recordings obtained during a slow (150 mHz) and a fast (300 mHz) controlled breathing.

HEART RATE SPECTRA
150 mHz = 9 cycles/min

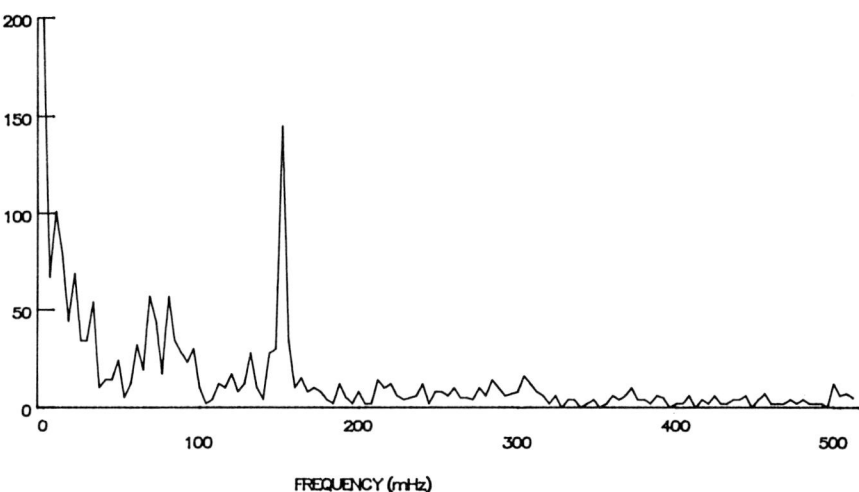

300 mHz = 18 cycles/min

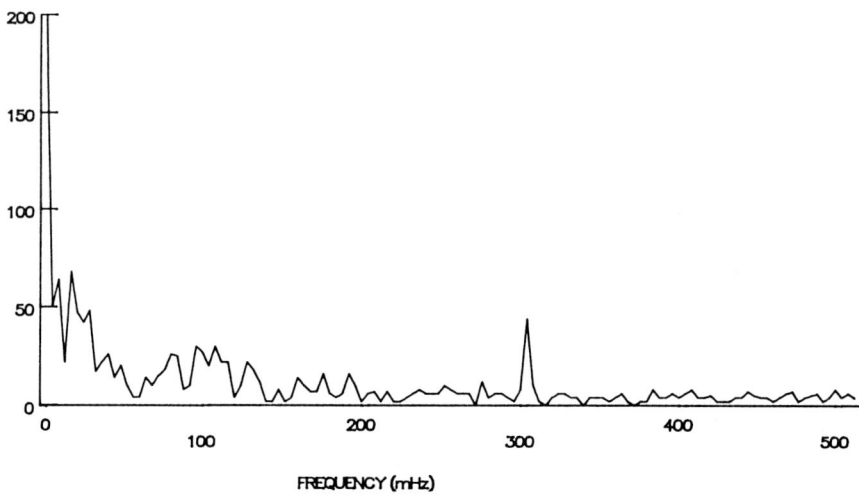

Fig. 2.
Spectra of the HR obtained from the slow (150 mHz) and the fast (300 mHz) controlled breathing HR time series.

CONTROLLED BREATHING
150 mHz = 9 cycles/min

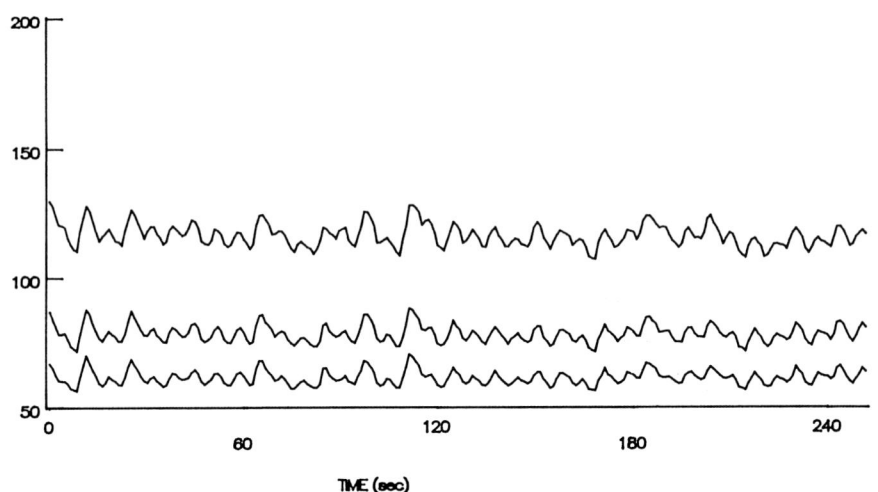

300 mHz = 18 cycles/min

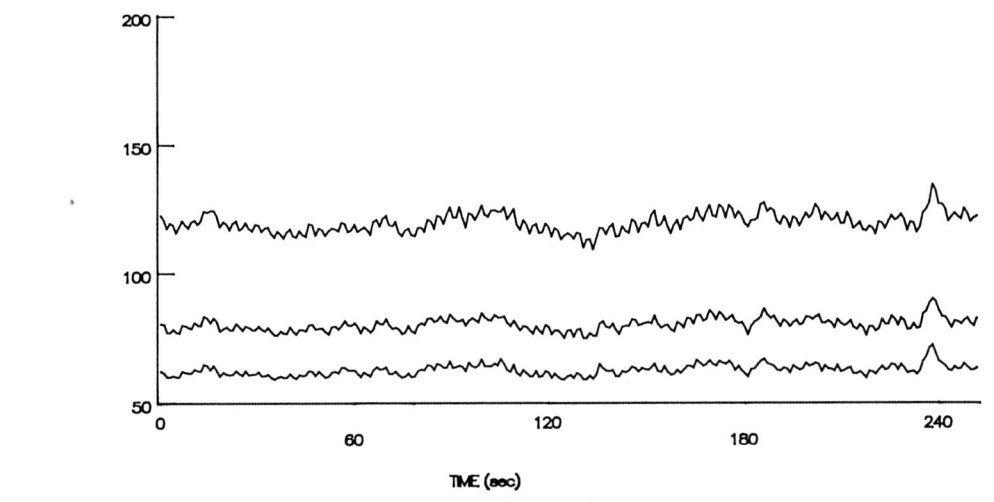

Fig. 3.
Digitized BP recordings obtained during a slow (150 mHz) and a fast (300 mHz) controlled breathing.

SYSTOLIC PRESSURE SPECTRA

150 mHz = 9 cycles/min

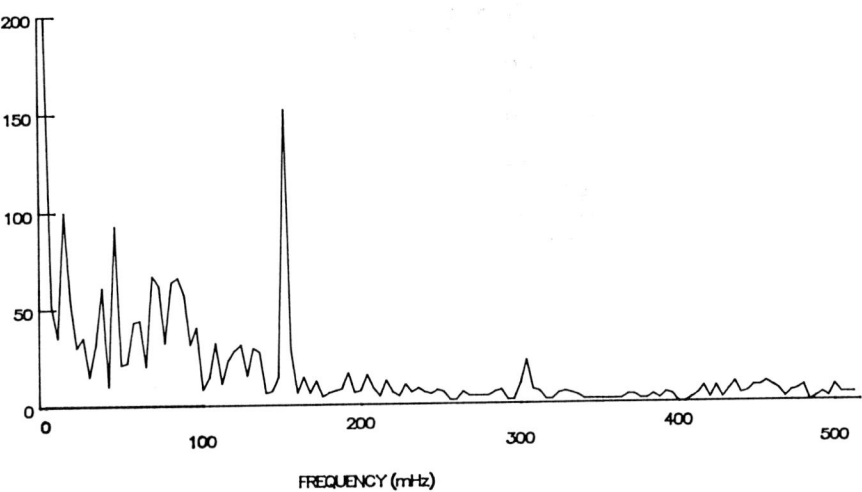

300 mHz = 18 cycles/min

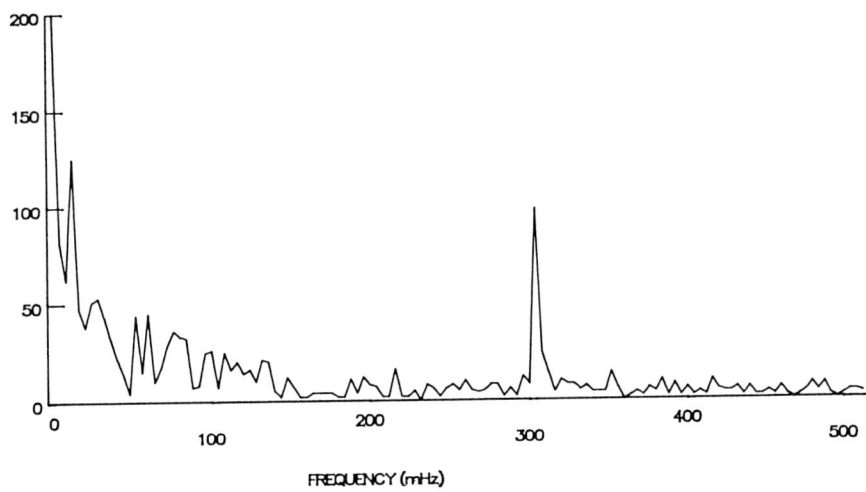

Fig. 4.
Spectra of the SBP obtained from the slow (150 mHz) and the fast (300 mHz) controlled breathing SBP time series.

corresponded to an harmonic of 1000/256 mHz ie 3.91 mHz. The first spectral component (0-3.91 mHz) corresponded to the baseline. The frequency of oscillation scale (abscissa) was analyzed up to 500 mHz. Modulus of the HR or BP spectrum (ordinates) had units of $bpm.Hz^{-1/2}$ or $mmHg.Hz^{-1/2}$.

The subject taken as an example was instructed to control breathing frequency with a electronic metronome.

HR recordings obtained at 2 different breathing frequencies are shown in **Fig. 1**. **Figure 2** represents the corresponding HR spectra. It is noticeable that mean levels of HR were unaffected. The effect of changing the breathing frequency on HR was limited to HR fluctuations around the mean level. A low frequency was associated with ample HR fluctuations of long periods while a rapid breathing determined fast HR fluctuations of small amplitude. HR spectra illustrate these changes. As expected the HR oscillated at the exact controlled breathing frequency of 150 mHz (9 cycles/min) and 300 mHz (18 cycles/min). In addition the modulus of this respiratory HR oscillation (RSA) was minored when the subject was breathing at a high frequency of 18 cycles/min, reflecting the reduced amplitude of this oscillation. In this supine position the low frequency (100 mHz, Mayer waves) HR oscillation was relatively small when compared to the marked low frequency observed in standing position (Girard et al., 1991).

The present tracings illustrate the dependency of RSA upon the breathing frequency. An increased depth of breathing at the low breathing frequency probably contributed to amplify the respiratory waves. Hirsch and Bishop (1981) quantified RSA and demonstrated that the mean RSA may be predicted for any given combination of depth and frequency of breathing. The variation in beat-to-beat interval, which occurs during a respiratory cycle, has been extensively studied since the electrocardiogram is easily accessible. We here developed an alternative for estimating HR fluctuations which also permits a study of BP oscillations.

BP recordings from the same subject are shown in **Fig. 3**. **Figure 4** represents the corresponding SBP spectra. It is again noticeable that mean levels were unaffected. The effect of changing the breathing frequency on BP was limited to BP fluctuations around the average values. A low frequency was associated with ample BP fluctuations of long periods while a rapid breathing determined fast BP fluctuations of small amplitude. SBP spectra illustrate these changes. As expected the SBP oscillated at the exact controlled breathing frequency of 150 mHz (9 cycles/min) and 300 mHz (18 cycles/min). In addition the modulus of this respiratory SBP wave was minored when the subject was breathing at a high frequency of 18 cycles/min, reflecting the reduced amplitude of this oscillation. In this supine position the low frequency (100 mHz, Mayer waves) SBP oscillation was relatively small when compared to the marked low frequency observed in standing position (Girard et al., 1991).

The quantification of the oscillations constituting short-term variability of BP is recent. Spectral procedures have been successfully applied to the direct intraarterial signal (Monos and Szücs, 1978; Daniels et al., 1983; Akselrod et al., 1985; Pagani et al., 1986; Di Rienzo et al., 1989; Grichois et al., 1990; Japundzic et al., 1990; Turjanmaa et al., 1990). Ambulatory recording of direct intraarterial BP has made it possible to study short-term variability of BP and HR in man. Spectral techniques revealed that BP variability contains systematic oscillations concentrated in a limited number of spectral regions including breathing frequency (0.25 Hz in man, 1.5 Hz in rats) and Mayer waves (0.1 Hz in man, 0.4 Hz in rats). The magnitudes of the BP and pulse interval (PI) respiratory waves were studied throughout the 24 h period by Di Rienzo et al. (1989). These oscillations do not show any systematic difference during waking hours, but, on the contrary, they undergo marked systematic changes in relation to the day-night cycle. These changes consisted of the fact that the power of BP respiratory waves dropped at night, in contrast with the PI respiratory wave which was increased during the night. This implies that the relation between fast rhythmic oscillations of BP and HR is weak, suggesting that the mechanisms responsible for these phenomena are largely different. In addition, we have also shown that it is possible to dissociate BP from HR respiratory oscillations using atropine (Japundzic et al., 1990; Elghozi et al., 1991a). It is therefore excluded that the vagally-mediated HR oscillations associated with respiration generate the respiratory oscillations in BP. As discussed above, it is likely that the BP respiratory wave reflects the fluctuations in stroke volume. It has been generally assumed that increased depth and rate of respiration increases the "aspiratory" effect of the thorax and hence the inflow of blood to the right heart (Cahoon et al., 1941). The present findings confirm that the amplitude of BP respiratory oscillations depends on respiratory pattern. It would be interesting to control tidal volume and breathing frequency in order to quantify the BP respiratory oscillations, estimated from the BP power spectrum.

In conclusion the combination of a non invasive continuous BP measurement and a computer analysis of BP and HR variabilities in the frequency domain based on Fourier analysis appears useful to describe the effects of respiration on each hemodynamic variable. Quantification of HR and BP respiratory waves could be of interest to cardiopulmonary physiologists and to clinicians. One objective assessment of cardiac vagal dysfunction is the measurement of RSA as an indirect estimate of vagal activity. Examples of clinical applications of RSA measurement are the assessment of autonomic diabetic neuropathy (Pagani et al., 1988; Weise et al., 1988), the status of heart reinnervation following heart transplantation (Fallen et al., 1988) or the age-related decrease in RSA (Hellman and Stacy, 1976; Cinelli et al., 1987). The study of BP respiratory waves might also carry information useful for the elucidation of circulatory control mechanisms, and might promote further developments in clinical diagnostics. Our attempt to develop a non-invasive procedure for studying the short-term variability of BP should contribute to this research area.

REFERENCES

Akselrod, S., Gordon, D., Madwed, J.B., Snidman, N.C., Shannon,D.C. and Cohen, R.J. (1985): Hemodynamic regulation: investigation by spectral analysis. Am. J. Physiol. 249: H867-H875.

Bernardi, L., Keller, F., Sanders, M., Reddy, P.S., Griffith, B., Meno, F. and Pinsky, M.R. (1989): Respiratory sinus arrhythmia in the denervated human heart. Am. J. Physiol. 67: 1447-1455.

Cahoon, D.H., Michael, I.E. and Johnson, V. (1941): Respiratory modification of the cardiac output. Am. J. Physiol. 133: 642-650.

Caplin, J.L., Flatman, W.D., Dyke, L., Wiseman, M.N. and Dymond D.S. (1989): Influence of respiratory variations on right ventricular function. Brit. Heart J. 62: 253-259.

Cinelli, P., De Leonardis, V., De Scalzi, M., Becucci, A. and Grazzini, M. (1987): Effect of age on mean heart rate variability. Age 10: 146-148.

Daniels, F.H., Leonard, E.F. and Cortell, S. (1983): Spectral analysis of arterial blood pressure in the rat. IEEE Trans. Biomed. Eng. 30: 154-159.

Di Rienzo, M., Castiglioni, P., Mancia, G., Parati, G. and Pedotti, A. (1989): 24 h sequential spectral analysis of arterial blood pressure and pulse interval in free-moving subjects. IEEE Trans. Biomed. Engin. 36: 1066-1075.

Elghozi, J.L., Laude, D. and Girard, A. (1991a): La variabilité spontanée de la pression artérielle et de la fréquence cardiaque chez l'homme. J.E.P.U. in press

Elghozi, J.L., Laude, D. and Janvier, F. (1991b): Clonidine reduces blood pressure and heart rate oscillations in hypertensive patients. J. Cardiovasc. Pharmacol. 17: 000-000.

Fallen, E.L., Kamath, M.V., Ghista, D.N. and Fitchett, D. (1988): Spectral analysis of heart rate variability following human heart transplantation: evidence for functional reinnervation. J. Auton. Nerv. System 23: 199-206.

Franklin, D.L., Van Citters, R.L. and Rushmer, R.F. (1962): Balance between right and left ventricular output. Circ. Res. 10: 17-26.

Girard, A., Laude, D., Japundzic, N. and Elghozi, J.L. (1991): Effects of chronic beta-adrenoceptor blockade on blood pressure and heart rate variabilities : a non invasive spectral study. J. Hypertension in press

Grichois, M.L., Japundzic, N., Head, G.A. and Elghozi, J.L. (1990): Clonidine reduces blood pressure and heart rate oscillations in the conscious rat. J. Cardiovasc. Pharmacol. 16:449-454.

Hellman, J.B. and Stacy, R.W. (1976): Variation of respiratory sinus arrhythmia with age. J. Appl. Physiol. 41: 734-738.

Hirsch, J.A. and Bishop, B. (1981): Respiratory sinus arrhythmia in humans: how breathing pattern modulates heart rate. Am. J. Physiol. 241: H620-H629.

Hyndman, B.W. (1980): Cardiovascular recovery to psychological stress: a means to diagnose man and task? In The study of heart-rate variability, eds R.I. Kitney and O. Rompelman, pp. 191-224. Oxford: Clarendon Press.

Imholz, B.P.M., Wieling, W., Langewouters, G.J. and Van Montfrans, G.A. (1991): Continuous finger arterial pressure: utility in the cardiovascular laboratory. Clin. Auton. Res. 1: 43-53.

Inoue, K., Miyake, M., Kumashiro, M., Ogata, H. and Yoshimura, O. (1990): Power spectral analysis of heart rate variability in traumatic quadriplegic humans. Am. J. Physiol. 258: H1722-H1726.

Japundzic, N., Grichois, M.L., Zitoun, P., Laude, D. and Elghozi, J.L. (1990): Spectral analysis of blood pressure and heart rate in conscious rats : effects of autonomic blockers. J. Auton. Nerv. System 30: 91-100.

Lauson, H.D., Bloomfield, R.A. and Cournand, A. (1946): The influence of the respiration on the circulation in man. Am. J. Physiol. 1:315-336.

Monos, E. and Szücs, B. (1978): Effect of changes in mean arterial pressure on the structure of short-term blood pressure waves. Automedica 2: 149-160.

Pagani, M., Lombardi, F., Guzzetti, S., Rimoldi, O., Furlan, R., Pizzinelli, P., Sandrone, G., Malfatto, G., Dell'Orto, S., Piccaluga, E., Turiel, M., Baselli, G., Cerutti, S. and Malliani, A. (1986): Power spectral analysis of heart rate and arterial pressure variabilities as a marker of sympatho-vagal interaction in man and conscious dog. Circ. Res. 59: 178-193.

Pagani, M., Malfatto, G., Pierini, S., Casati, R., Masu, A.M., Poli, M., Guzzetti, S., Lombardi, F., Cerutti, S. and Malliani, A. (1988): Spectral analysis of heart rate variability in the assessment of autonomic diabetic neuropathy. J. Auton. Nerv. Syst. 23: 143-153.

Penaz, J. (1973): Photoelectric measurement of blood pressure, volume and flow in the finger. In Digest of the 10th International Conference on Medical and Biological Engineering. p.104. Dresden.

Pomeranz B., Macaulay, R.J.B., Caudill, M.A., Kutz, I., Adam, D., Gordon, D., Kilborn, K.M., Barger, A.C., Shannon, D.C., Cohen, R.J. and Benson, H. (1985): Assessment of autonomic function in humans by heart rate spectral analysis. Am. J. Physiol. 248: H151-H153.

Turjanmaa, V., Kalli, S., Sydänmaa, M. and Uusitalo, A. (1990): Short-term variability of systolic blood pressure and heart rate in normotensive subjects. Clin Physiol 10: 389-401.

Weise, F., Heydenreich, F. and Runge, U. (1987): Contribution of sympathetic and vagal mechanisms to the genesis of heart rate fluctuations during orthostatic load: a spectral analysis. J. Auton. Nerv. System 21: 127-134.

Weise, F., Heydenreich, F. and Runge, U. (1988): Heart rate fluctuations in diabetic patients with cardiac dysfunction: a spectral analysis. Diabetic Med.5: 324-327.

Weise, F. and Heydenreich, F. (1989): Effects of modified respiratory rhythm on heart rate variability during active orthostatic load. Biomed. Biochim. Acta 48: 549-556.

Résumé

Une mesure continue non invasive de pression artérielle (PA) au doigt et une technique spectrale reposant sur une décomposition en série de Fourier sont combinées pour quantifier la variabilité à court-terme des variables hémodynamiques.

Les fluctuations de PA associent des oscillations lentes et une oscillation rapide de nature respiratoire. Cette dernière reflète des oscillations de l'éjection cardiaque. La fréquence cardiaque (FC) associe également des oscillations lentes et une oscillation rapide respiratoire, connue sous le nom d'arythmie respiratoire. Celle-ci dépend du vague.

Les spectres de pression artérielle systolique (PAS) et de FC illustrent ces observations, avec un pic respiratoire nettement détaché des oscillations lentes divisibles en deux zones de 4-66 mHz et de 66-129 mHz (ondes de Mayer).

Les effets d'un changement de fréquence respiratoire sur la PA et la FC sont illustrés par les tracés et les spectres. Une respiration lente détermine des oscillations amples et lentes de PA et de FC alors qu'une respiration rapide accélère les oscillations de PA et de FC qui ont une amplitude réduite.

Les spectres illustrent ces faits. Les pics de haute fréquence se localisent au niveau de la fréquence respiratoire imposée. Leur module reflète l'amplitude de l'oscillation respiratoire.

Cette étude démontre que l'approche réunissant une méthodologie non invasive de mesure de la PA et une décomposition spectrale du signal en ses sinusoïdes constitutives est applicable à l'étude du contrôle respiratoire des oscillations cardio-vasculaires.

Carotid chemotransduction : mechanisms and development

David F. Donnelly and Gabriel G. Haddad

Section of Respiratory Medicine, Department of Pediatrics, Yale University School of Medicine, New Haven, Connecticut 06510, USA

ABSTRACT

The carotid bodies are the primary O_2 sensors in mammals. They play an important role in the respiratory control system but are also an integral element of cardiovascular and temperature regulation. Recently, we and others have demontrated their unique and critical role they play in early life regarding auto-resuscitation and survival. Although carotid hypoxic chemosensitivity has been described for several decades, the mechanisms underlying this sensitivity have been obscure until recently. A few working hypotheses and models have been put forth and these have been the results of newer experiments employing modern neurobiologic techniques including patch clamp recordings and optical methodologies. In spite of the fact that there are controversies, it seems that there are major alterations in certain membrane outward currents (K^+ currents) and marked changes in intracellular calcium with exposure to hypoxia. How these are related to each other and to the transduction and neurotransmitter release process is not clear. Similarly, for the first time, investigations aimed at understanding the maturational process of glomus cells and how they develop their ability to "taste" the level of PO_2 have been initiated.

Although the respiratory control system, as an entity, has been characterized in a general sense in the past several decades, there are still major gaps in our knowledge at the integrated level of the control system and certainly at the cellular mechanistic level. For example, we have recognized the fact that the carotid bodies are important regulatory elements of this control system but we do not know what the relative role of the carotid bodies is in determining the output of the central nervous system (CNS) in a variety of conditions or circumstances, especially when other elements of the control system are activated or when ventilatory needs are suppressed or enhanced. Over the past decade, however, we have made some tangible progress in our understanding of the respiratory control system at both integrated and cellular or subcellular level with respect to a number of its important elements, including the carotid bodies.

The respiratory control system is a negative feedback system, and like other such systems, is endowed with a number of sensors for error detection and correction. The carotid bodies, the laryngeal receptors, the central chemosensors and the chest mechanoreceptors are some of the important sensors of this control system. The fully mature carotid bodies, which are the primary O_2 sensors in mammals, characteristically increases its discharge when the bathing blood has a low PO_2 (< 50 Torr) or is acidic. Therefore, the carotid bodies are unique not only because they are the main O_2 sensors but because they differ from other sensors of this respiratory control system in a number of ways. Firstly, they provide a tonic excitatory discharge to the CNS to increase ventilation at rest. Hence the elimination of this input would lead to respiratory dysrhythmias and hypoventilation. This has been shown in adult animals and humans and methods of ablation of this excitatory input varied from benign such breathing 100% O_2 for a short period (few sec to min) to much more invasive such as carotid sinus nerve (CSN) section or crushing the carotid bodies themselves. Other sensors in the control system (e.g. laryngeal) may not have such a tonic discharge and elimination of these sensors may not be crucial for the tonic respiratory drive. Second, the sensor itself, as we presently understand the process of transduction, is not the nerve ending itself but the glomus cells in the carotid bodies which release neurotransmitters to stimulate or depress the petrosal neurons dendritic endings. This is very different from laryngeal nerve transduction, chest wall mechanoreception and possibly central chemoreception. Third, the blood supply and O_2 consumption of the carotids are probably the highest in the body per tissue weight; this observation would seem to be important and could be related to the transduction process. Fourth, the carotid bodies serve as a feedback sensor not only for respiration but also for cardiovascular function, metabolic rate, exercise and temperature regulation. Finally, the carotid bodies would seem to be important not only in regulating a number of integrated functions but might also be crucial for survival in early life in a number of mammalian species.

Reports appearing in the early 80's about the role of the carotid bodies in the generation of the first breath dampened the interest in the carotid bodies since these studies showed that the carotids played no role in inducing the first postnatal breath. Studies that had a similar effect regarding the importance of the carotid bodies in early life included investigations that showed that carotid denervation induces mild hypoventilation in the newborn, much like in the adult. However, the special role that the carotid bodies play in early life was not discovered till later with studies on lambs, rats and piglets (Donnelly 90). Investigations on the effect of carotid denervation in early life seemed to be very dependent on age postnatally. These studies have demonstrated that there is an early developmental window during which the carotid bodies play a major role in regulating cardiorespiratory function to the degree that very prolonged respiratory pauses occur in the young animal in the absence of the carotid bodies (Fig. 1). What was surprising to us is that there was a high probability of death in the denervated animals (as compared to sham) if the denervation was performed in early life but not later (Table 1). Although the reason for death is not clear, we have previously speculated that the cause is directly related to the role of the carotid bodies in early life. Because of the severity in outcome in mammals when deprived of carotids, we suspect that sublethal or severe cellular and subcellular changes could have taken place in the medulla with denervation. The intriguing idea that has not been tested yet regarding the relation between carotid input and respiratory dysrhythmia, apnea and death would be parallel to that of Hubel and Weisel regarding the development or mal-development of the visual cortex in response to enucleation or unilateral ablation of sensory visual input to the lateral geniculate bodies and occipital cortex. Pathologic changes have been reported in the visual system with sensory deprivation. Eye closure in cats and monkeys can induce marked neuronal changes, plasticity and rearrangement of synaptic connections, arrest of development and atrophy. It is therefore possible that a number of important brainstem and more rostral sites are affected by the total elimination of the carotid input in early life.

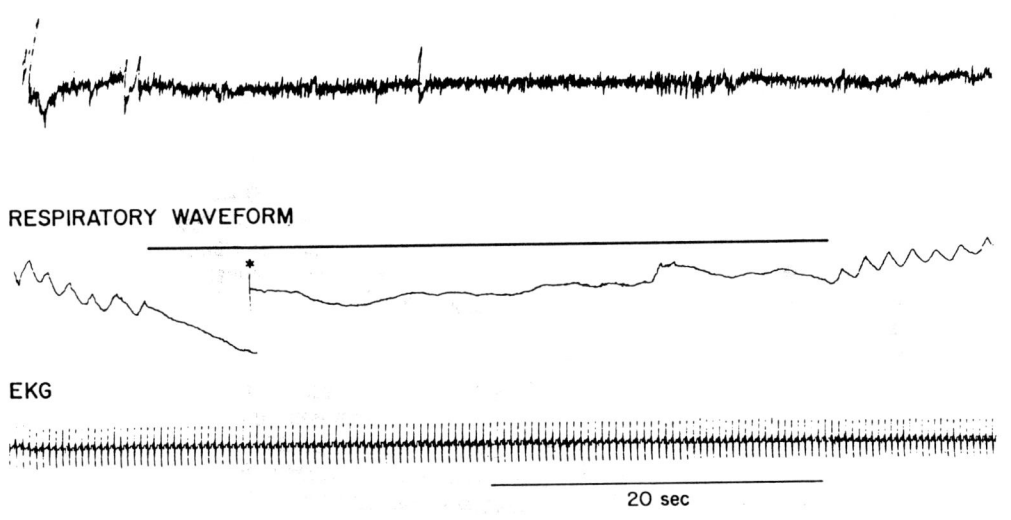

Figure 1. Original polygraph tracing obtained from a 10-day-old denervated piglet. Signals recorded were EEG (top), respiration (middle, inspiration upward), and ECG (bottom). Solid bar, spontaneous apnea lasting 42 s. * Addition of a direct-current offset to avoid saturating polygraph display.

TABLE 1

Measurements of metabolic, respiratory, and cardiovascular function in carotid denervated young piglets (CX, 1 wk) during normoxia.

	CX	SHAM
N	9	7
Age, days	7.1±1.1	6.3±0.8
T_{env}, °C	31.1±0.7	31.8±1.4
T_{body}, °C	38.9±0.6	39.2±0.2
Ap/h	8.0±3.0*	0
Ap dur, s	26±3*	0
PaO_2, Torr	78.8±7.2*	103.5±5.6
$PaCO_2$, Torr	47.1±2.6*	36.4±1.5
MAP, mm Hg	86±4	84±6
HR, beats/min	230±11	206±13
VE/kg, ml·min^{-1}·kg^{-1}	187±23*	372±48
F, breaths/min	32.6±6.4*	48.1±5.2
VT, ml	13.1±1.7*	17.8±1.7
Weight, kg	1.9±0.1	2.2±0.1
Died	5/9*	0/7

Values are means ± SE; N, no. of animals. T_{env}, environmental temperature; T_{body}, animal temperature; Ap/h, no. of apneas observed per Ap dur, apneic duration; PaO_2, arterial partial pressure of O_2; $PaCO_2$, arterial partial pressure of CO_2; MAP, mean arterial pressure; HR, rate; VE/kg, minute ventilation per kg body wt; F, respiratory frequency; VT, tidal volume; Weight, body weight. *Significant difference (0.05) from sham group.

It has been previously shown that the newborn mammal is less responsive to hypoxia than the mature one, and the ventilatory response of the newborn to hypoxia is characterized by an increase in ventilation followed by a gradual decrease (Haddad 82, 84, Eden 87a). It is unlikely that a central accommodation to carotid chemoreceptor input is the cause for the latter decrease in ventilation, because direct electrical stimulation of the sinus nerve (in the absence of hypoxia) results in a sustained hyperventilation (Lawson 84). Thus, the ventilatory depression is likely related to the central effects of hypoxia or to differences in the functioning of the newborn's chemoreceptors. There is evidence to support both theories; however, we will here focus on maturational differences at the chemoreceptor level.

The overall transduction process of the peripheral chemoreceptors has been assayed by recording from afferent axons which innervate the carotid organ. These recordings demonstrated that significant differences exist between the adult and newborn. In the adult, decreases in oxygen saturation (SaO_2) or increases in blood acidity cause a near linear increase in chemoreceptor discharge activity (Donnelly 81, Donnelly 82). However, attempts to perform this same type of experiment in the young were more difficult. Firstly, at the time of birth, chemoreceptor activity, in vivo, is difficult to find when probing the afferent nerve, suggesting that many chemoreceptor afferent axons are in a quiescent state (Jansen 80). When it is localized, the response curve to changes in SaO_2 are left shifted (less sensitive) from the adult. These differences from the adult diminish over time, such that maturation is complete by 2 weeks of age (Blanco 84, Kumar 89).

The maturational changes which account for the enhanced sensitivity are still unclear, but both vascular and cellular changes are implicated. As mentioned earlier, both the oxygen consumption and blood flow delivery for the organ are extremely high. Since the oxygen sensor is presumably exposed to tissue PO_2, changes in tissue blood flow around the time of birth may exert major changes at the sensor level. Experimental evidence shows this to be the case since the gradient between arterial PO_2 and tissue PO_2 increases dramatically in the post-natal period (Acker 80). Some of this gradient may be caused by increased sympathetic tone which occurs around the time of birth and has also been shown to enhance afferent chemoreceptor activity (Biscoe 67). In addition, the local release of neuromodulators, primarily dopamine, changes dramatically in the post-natal period. Dopamine release rate which is modulated by PO_2 (Gonzalez 77), increases after birth and then undergoes a gradual decrease (Hertzberg 90). It is only recently that the mechanism responsible for determining dopamine (and other neurotransmitters) release rate has been examined using cellular electrophysiologic and optical recording techniques.

Dopamine is localized to the carotid body glomus cell which contains catecholamines and other neurotransmitters in dense cored vesicles. Glomus cells also appear to be the chemosensor itself. Chemosensitivity is lost when they are destroyed by cooling (Verna 75) or when depleted of neurotransmitter by reserpine (Leitner 83). Furthermore, reestablishment of chemosensitivity following sinus nerve section is correlated with reestablishment of the synaptic relationship between sinus nerve endings and glomus cells (Ponte 89).

Exciting recent results have demonstrated that glomus cells respond electrically and chemically to decreases in PO_2 and that these changes are evoked at PO_2 levels that have little effect on other neurons. Whole cell patch clamp recordings have demonstrated changes in a voltage-activated outward current (K^+) in response to hypoxia and increased acidity (Biscoe 89a, Delpiano 89, Stea 91, Peers 90a, Peers 90b). Unfortunately, an experimental inconsistency exists among laboratories, and it is unclear whether K^+ current increases or decreases during hypoxia. Most investigators detected a <u>decrease</u> in K^+ current during hypoxia (Delpiano 89, Lopez-Barneo 88, Peers 90a, Peers 90b, Stea 91) and have postulated that a decrease in K^+ current leads to depolarization, activation of calcium channels and enhanced transmitter release secondary to increased calcium (Lopez-Barneo 88). In contrast, one investigative group observes an <u>increase</u> in K^+ current which they attribute to intracellular calcium release and activation of calcium-dependent K^+ channels (Biscoe 89b, Biscoe 90b, Biscoe 90c). In this latter scenario increased calcium leads to enhanced transmitter release and the membrane voltage channels play only a secondary role. In both theories, an increase in intracellular calcium is postulated to play a critical role in regulating neurotransmitter secretion, and this postulate is supported by measurements of changes in free calcium during exposure to hypoxia or cyanide (Biscoe 89b, Biscoe 90a). Thus, although it is presently unclear which (if either) theory is correct, it is clear that we are opening a new and exciting window on the internal functioning of the chemoreceptor.

Our own work has focused on the maturational changes which takes place in the electrophysiologic characteristics of glomus cells. We have acutely isolated glomus cells from newborn and adult rabbits and rats and have examined the types of membrane currents expressed at different ages and examined how the membrane currents change during hypoxia. Two differences between newborn and adult are emerging. Virtually all adult glomus cells express voltage-dependent currents (as in Fig. 2), but a high proportion of newborn glomus cells do not evidence voltage dependent currents. This suggests that the expression of these channels may be related to the enhanced chemosensitivity with maturation. Secondly, the magnitude of the decrease in K^+ current which we observe with anoxia is less in the newborn than in the adult (Fig. 2). Although the subcellular mechanisms which alter the K^+ current are unclear, they must necessarily also change with maturation.

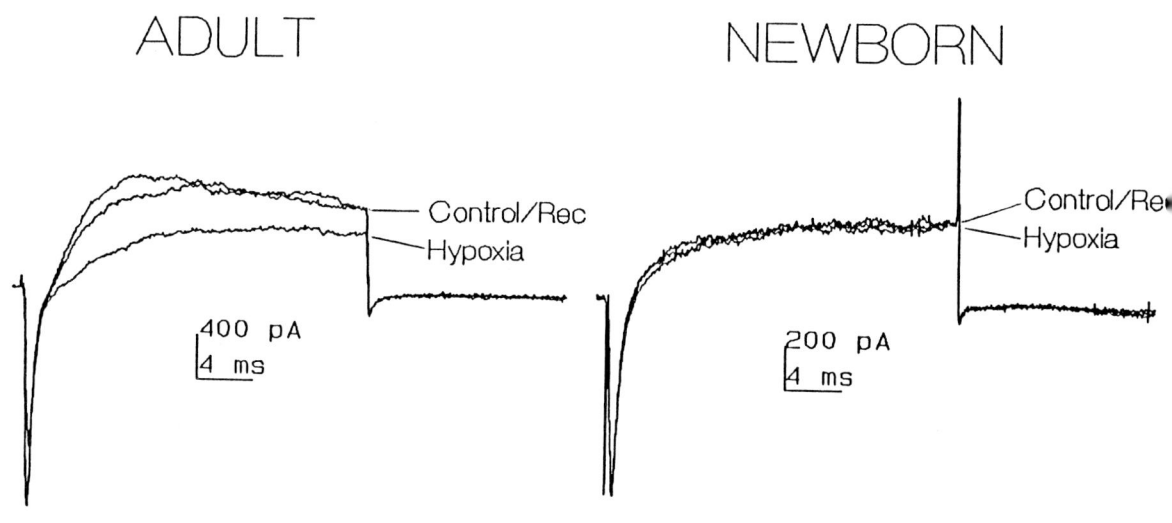

Figure 2. Changes in voltage-dependent currents of glomus cells during hypoxia (left). Whole cell patch clamp recording from an acutely isolated, adult, rabbit glomus cell during step, repetitive (1/sec) depolarizations from -70 mV (holding potential) to -10 mV (command potential). Hypoxia (superfusion with N_2 equilibrated solution) caused a reversible decrease in outward current. (right). Same recording conditions, but the glomus cell was harvested from a 1 day old rabbit. Note minimal change in outward current in newborn cell during hypoxia. Extracellular solution in mM: 140 NaCl, 3 KCl, 1 $CaCl_2$, 1 $MgCl_2$, 25 glucose, 10 HEPES at pH 7.35. Patch electrode: (in mM) 130 KCl, 20 KF, 9 glucose, 1.0 $CaCl_2$, 3 EGTA, 10 HEPES at pH 7.35.

In summary, major developmental changes occur in the post-natal period in the functioning of peripheral chemoreceptors and the dependency of the respiratory system on these receptors. This dependency may take a rather dramatic form in the appearance of spontaneous prolonged apneas and high incidence of death in the post-denervated

period. If apnea and death are the result of loss of chemoreceptive input then, presumably, enhanced survival and more regular breathing may result from enhanced chemosensitivity. However, pharmacologic control of chemosensitivity depends on an improved understanding of the mechanisms of chemotransduction within the carotid body. With the current new experimental techniques using optical and electrophysiologic recordings, the elucidation of these mechanisms should be forthcoming.

REFERENCES

Acker, H, DW Lubbers, MJ Purves and ED Tan. (1980). Measurement of the partial pressure of oxygen in the carotid body of foetal sheep and newborn lambs. *J. Dev. Physiol.* 2: 323-338.

Biscoe, TJ and MJ Purves. (1967). Carotid body chemoreceptor activity in the new-born lamb. *J. Physiol. (London)* 190: 443-454.

Biscoe, TJ and MR Duchen. (1989). Electrophysiological responses of disassociated type I cells of the rabbit carotid body to cyanide. *J. Physiol. (London)* 413: 447-468.

Biscoe, TJ, MR Duchen, DA Eisner, SC O'Neill and M Valdeolmillos. (1989). Measurements of intracellular $Ca2+$ in dissociated type I cells of the rabbit carotid body. *J.Physiol. (London)* 416: 421-434.

Biscoe, TJ and MR Duchen. (1990). Responses of type I cells dissociated from the rabbit carotid body to hypoxia. *J. Physiol. (London)* 428: 39-59.

Biscoe, TJ and MR Duchen. (1990). Cellular basis of transduction in carotid chemoreceptors. *Am. J. Physiol.* 258: L271-L278.

Biscoe, TJ and MR Duchen. (1990). Monitoring PO2 by the carotid chemoreceptor. *NIPS* 5: 229-233.

Blanco, CE, GS Dawes, MA Hanson and HB McCooke. (1984). The response to hypoxia of arterial chemoreceptors in fetal sheep and newborn lambs. *J. Physiol. (London)* 351: 25-37.

Delpiano, MA and J Hescheler. (1989). Evidence for a PO2-sensitive K+ channel in the type-I cell of the rabbit carotid body. *Febs* 249: 195-198.

Donnelly, DF, EJ Smith and RE Dutton. (1981). Neural response of carotid chemoreceptors following dopamine blockade. *J. Appl. Physiol.* 50: 172-177.

Donnelly, DF, EJ Smith and RE Dutton. (1982). Carbon dioxide vs H+ ion as a chemoreceptor stimulus. *Brain Res.* 245: 136-138.

Donnelly, DF and GG Haddad. (1990). Prolonged apnea and impaired survival in piglets following sinus and aortic nerve section. J. Appl. Physiol. 68: 1048-1052, 1990.

Eden, GJ and MA Hanson. (1987). Maturation of the respiratory response to acute hypoxia in the newborn rat. *J. Physiol. (London)* 392: 1-9.

Gonzalez, C and S Fidone. (1977). Increased release of 3H-dopamine during low O2 stimulation of rabbit carotid body in vitro. *Neurosci. Lett.* 6: 95-99.

Haddad, GG, MR Gandhi and RB Mellins. (1982). Maturation of the ventilatory response to hypoxia in puppies during sleep. J. Appl. Physiol. 52: 309-314, 1982.

Haddad, GG and RB Mellins. (1984). Hypoxia and respiratory control in early life. Ann. Rev. Physiol. 46: 629-643, 1984.

Hertzberg, T, S Hellstrom, H Lagercrantz and JM Pequignot. (1990). Development of the arterial chemoreflex and turnover of carotid body catecholamines in the newborn rat. *J. Physiol. (London)* 425: 211-225.

Jansen, AH, MJ Purves and ED Tan. The role of sympathetic nerves in the activation of the carotid chemoreceptors at birth in the sheep. (). J. Dev. Physiol.. 2 305-321: 1980.

Kumar, P and MA Hanson. (1989). Re-setting of the hypoxic sensitivity of aortic chemoreceptors in the new-born lamb. *J. Dev. Physiol.* 11: 199-206.

Lawson, EE and WA Long. (1984). Central neural respiratory response to carotid sinus nerve stimulation in newborns. *J. Appl. Physiol.* 56: 1614-1620.

Leitner, LM, M Roumy and A Verna. (1983). In vitro recording of chemoreceptor activity in catecholamine-depleted rabbit carotid bodies. *Neurosci.* 10: 883-891.

Lopez-Barneo, J, JR Lopez-Lopez, J Urena and C Gonzalez. (1988). Chemotransduction in the carotid body: K current modulated by pO2 in type I chemoreceptor cells. *Science* 241: 580-582.

Peers, C. (1990). Effect of lowered extracellular pH on Ca2+-dependent K+ currents in type I cells from the neonatal rat carotid body. *J. Physiol. (London)* 422: 381-395.

Peers, C and J O'Donnell. (1990). Potassium currents recorded in type I carotid body cells from the neonatal rat and their modulation by chemoexcitatory agents. *Brain Res.* 522: 259-266.

Ponte, J and CL Sadler. (1989). Studies on the regenerated carotid sinus nerve of the rabbit. *J. Physiol. (London)* 410: 411-424.

Stea, A and CA Nurse. (1991). Whole-cell and perforated-patch recordings from O2-sensitive rat carotid body cells grown in short- and long-term culture. *Pflugers Arch.* 418: 93-101.

Verna, A., M Roumy and LM Leitner. (1975). Loss of chemoreceptive properties of the rabbit carotid body after destruction of the glomus cells. *Brain Res.* 100: 13-23.

Résumé

Les corpuscules carotidiens sont les chémorécepteurs primaires chez les mammifères. Ils jouent un rôle important dans le contrôle du système respiratoire mais sont également intégrés à la régulation thermique et cardiovasculaire. Récemment, d'autres auteurs et nous-même avons démontré leur rôle unique et critique au commencement de la vie dans la survie et l'auto-réanimation. Alors que la chémosensibilité carotidienne à l'hypoxie a été décrite depuis plusieurs décennies, les mécanismes responsables de cette sensibilité ont été inconnus jusqu'à une époque récente. Quelques hypothèses de travail et modèles ont été avancés et ont été le résultat d'expériences récentes utilisant les techniques de la neurobiologie moderne incluant les enregistrements à voltage imposé et les méthodes optiques. Bien qu'il y ait encore des controverses, il semble qu'il y ait des modifications majeures des courants membranaires sortants (courants K+) et des variations importantes de calcium intracellulaire lors d'exposition à l'hypoxie. La relation de ces modifications entre elles et avec la transduction et la libération de neuromédiateurs n'est pas claire. Egalement pour la première fois, ont été initiées des recherches sur la compréhension du processus de maturation des cellules du glomus et du développement de leur capacité à "goûter" le niveau de PO_2.

The role of thermometabolism on cardiorespiratory function in postnatal life

P. Johnson and D.C. Andrews

Nuffield Department of Obstetrics, John Radcliffe Hospital, Oxford University, UK

ABSTRACT

Breathing during hypoxia and non-shivering thermogenesis (NST) are both powerfully inhibited during fetal life. These are appropriate responses for fetal survival. Breathing activity is however linked to behavioural thermoregulatory responses, shivering and panting, which are not inhibited.
After birth thyroid function and NST are activated and provide a major "tonic" central stimulus to cardiorespiratory function and arousal state. Body temperature rises above fetal values. A feature of the thermometabolic drive to breathing is periodic breathing (PB), especially prominent in a warm environment and in REM sleep. PB in infancy is not regarded as unstable, vulnerable, or an indication of chemoreceptor abnormality.

Introduction

All newborn mammals, regardless of maturity, have to adapt to an environment where they must, for the first time, meet the demands of regulating body temperature while sustaining a rapid growth rate, mainly during sleep. Thermometabolism, which is actively inhibited in utero, becomes a critical factor in "resetting" central neural thresholds for both arousal state and cardiorespiratory function after birth. It is the nature of this resetting, involving a change in the balance of inhibitory and excitatory states within a well developed central neural network, rather than a definitive respiratory center, that is the focus of this chapter.

Recent studies of cardiorespiratory control and arousal state in late fetal life gives a clear picture of breathing control highly organised to meet the special requirements of fetal life, but also developed for postnatal life. The extent to which the postnatal environment alters, or "distorts", the underlying developmental processes that continue to occur after birth becomes apparent. A concept of cardiorespiratory control emerges which is much more consistent with many of the clinical disorders seen in postnatal life, especially in relation to sleep.

The Fetal Environment

Approaching term, fetal breathing is episodically inhibited (1).Fetal breathing is obstructed, during inspiration, at the level of the larynx and hypopharynx due to a combination of airway dilator incoordination (2) and the dynamics of liquid filled airways (3). This vigorous "obstructed" breathing, which is essential for fetal lung growth (4), would be a potent additional stimulus to breathing and arousal after birth. However it is further inhibited by acute hypoxia in fetal life (1).

Lateral pontine sites are responsible for the hypoxic inhibition of breathing, but this is only demonstrable when the carotid sinus nerves are intact (5), since fetal breathing is not stimulated by hypoxia in their absence. Thus peripheral chemoreceptors are active in fetal life but are initially overridden by central (lateral pontine) inhibition at the onset of hypoxia. Hypercapnia, on the other hand, is a more potent stimulus to fetal breathing (1), but fails to coordinate inspiratory upper airway and diaphragmatic action sufficiently, so that inspiratory obstruction or "obstructive sleep apnea" persists. This contrasts with postnatal air-breathing, where CO_2 inhalation powerfully activates the upper airway dilators (6).

Strikingly, external cooling of the fetus in-utero rapidly coordinated the inspiratory muscles while stimulating breathing and shivering (7). Although appropriate behavioural thermoregulation was activated (ie. shivering), non-shivering thermogenesis, which is actively inhibited in-utero, did not occur (8). External warming of the fetus causes panting, a thermolytic, or heat-losing, behavioural response (9). The fetus, then, normally thrives in a narrow 'clamped' high thermoneutral environment at modest basal levels of metabolic rate (eg 5-8 ml O_2/Kg/min in fetal lambs), cardiac output, and heart rate. Breathing activity is stimulated as part of the thermoregulatory behavioural response above and below a physiologic "apneic window".

Thus in the normal fetal environment, breathing (episodically) and thermoregulation are inhibited. However the infusion of thyrotropin releasing hormone into the lateral ventricle of the fetal lamb caused a dose dependant increase in continuity, amplitude and frequency of breathing during both high and low voltage EEG states, which, significantly, persisted during hypoxia (10). Since after birth, TRH has potent effects on all the mechanisms so far considered; arousal state, temperature control and breathing (11), an executive center of pre-optic anterior hypothalamus-POAH origin seems likely. Although TRH receptors are abundant before birth, TRH secretion is inhibited.

Clearly the thermal environment is a critical factor, and the POAH appears to hold the key to many of the "inhibited" fetal functions including breathing. Inhibition can equally be viewed as an absence of adequate collective stimulation, or a tonic threshold below which even cyclical events such as breathing fail to be initiated.

Onset of breathing and non-shivering thermogenesis at birth

After birth, with the umbilical cord tied and adequate oxygen available, external cooling has immediate and sustained effects on breathing, arousal state organisation, metabolic rate, cardiac output, and heart rate. External cooling causes TSH (and presumably TRH) to increase thus activating non-shivering thermogenesis (12), metabolic rate and ventilation. Some of these effects are "reversible" eg external warming can cause apnea in preterm infants and piglets. Others, such as the large increases in T3 and basal metabolic rate (taking place over hours or days) that accompany the activation of non-shivering thermogenesis (13), become increasingly difficult to "reverse". The onset of effective thermoregulation appears to reset the thresholds for breathing control and arousal state.

The onset of sustained effective breathing after birth can be achieved without peripheral chemoreceptors (14) and usually in the face of hypocapnia and a 'relative' hyperoxia, a so-called physiologic chemodenervation. Carbon dioxide remains a powerful stimulus to breathing after birth whereas hypoxia has very variable effects, greatly influenced by environmental temperature and metabolic rate (MR). Hypoxia (15%) was found to cause an immediate and sustained reduction in minute ventilation in healthy 3 day old infants tested at thermoneutrality (33oC) (15).

It has been assumed that newborns cannot maintain their body temperature at adult levels until maturation of temperature control occurs; 6-7 weeks of age in the cat (42). However litter sizes were abnormally small in those studies, which would compromise the ability of a "critical" litter mass to conserve energy demand and thus body temperature. An adult response to hypoxia (ie a sustained increase in ventilatory response) only occurred after 7 weeks of postnatal age in kittens (43), indicating a direct link between maturation of thermoregulation and the ventilatory response to hypoxia. Our studies in lambs have shown that, even where body temperature rises above fetal values (higher than at any other time in life) in association with elevated T3 levels, hypoxia caused a substantial reduction in MR. A reduction in MR, whether by hypoxia or warming to thermoneutrality, induced PB with a cycle length of 12-15 seconds. The amplitude of the oscillation, and thus the length of the apnea within the cycles, depends on the MR as described above.

Implications for respiratory control theory

PB (appropriately defined), though common in infants, is still considered by many to indicate, unstable respiratory control (22,23), a risk for SIDS (32), and thus the need for monitoring and therapy. While the origin of PB in infancy is closely related to temperature control, in the adult PB, with a longer and more variable cycle length is common during SWS at altitude (hypoxia), during low cardiac output (Cheyne Stokes breathing).

The concept of a tonic neural input being necessary to ensure phasic respiratory activity or breathing is well described. Recently the metabolic influence was demonstrated by the removal of carbon dioxide using an intravenous membrane, which caused prolonged apnea in unanaesthetised spontaneously breathing sheep (44). Since apnea occurred at isocapnia it was difficult to implicate conventional chemoreceptor mechanisms. However this manoeuvre eliminates respiratory metabolism. Why then does PB with such a fixed cycle of 12-15 seconds appear so commonly in infants when warm and asleep (particularly in REM sleep), and in sleeping lambs when other "tonic" inputs have been experimentally removed? Both species exhibit this phenomenon as postnatal thermoregulation develops and metabolic rate is decreasing (2-8 weeks in lamb and 1-6 months in infants). An oscillation, consistant with the thermal vasomotor cycle (45), emerges in both species during this phase of thermal adaptation -in the lamb even after carotid chemodenervation. However the human infant, though less thermally efficient than the lamb, has a much lower basal metabolic rate. It thus could be argued that the basal 'tonic' metabolic drive to breathing in the infant is lower and that when warm, asleep, and aged between 2-5 months, this tonic drive would be minimal.

The mechanism(s) regulating the thermal vasomotor oscillation are poorly understood. One view is that the relaxation time of peripheral vascular smooth muscle is an element in this cycle. If so this cannot simply be considered as a simple feedback loop (46). The potency of this oscillatory rhythm is illustrated by its expression in both sleep states in the warmth. Unlike the adult, in the infant pA CO_2 is lower in REM sleep than in SWS (27). Thus, the tonic CO_2 drive may be less and could explain why PB is more common in REM than SWS in infants (28), whereas PB is uncommon during REM in the adult. However, the constant PB cycle length that occurs while air breathing in infants, with no evidence of hypoxemia or hypercapnia when periodic apnea occurred, does not suggest a vulnerable or unstable pattern of breathing. The fact that PB with a similar cycle length may occur in the newborn during hypoxia is could relate to the same mechanism because hypoxia, like warming to thermoneutrality, rapidly reduces metabolic rate and thus the 'tonic' stimulus to breathing.

The usually close relationship between hypoxia and PB at altitude and in disease tends to endorse the primacy given to chemoreceptor mechanisms in PB. However, there are inconsistancies. The cycle length of PB in normal adults can vary between 19 and 56 (cf Cheyne Stokes breathing) seconds during normoxic sleep at sea level (47).

Also many subjects did not alter their cycle length when made hypoxic, but increased the oscillation amplitude and thus the apnea length. This response is much more akin to the spontaneous and hypoxic induced pattern of PB observed in healthy infants (14,25) where cycle length is comparatively fixed and it is the amplitude that changes. Thus, the pattern of PB, and not simply apnea length, must be considered if scientific and clinical progress is to be made (figure 1).

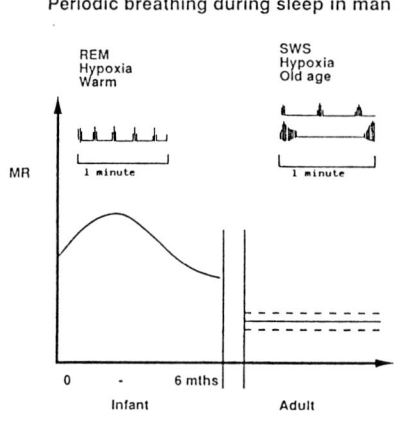

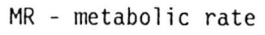

figure 1

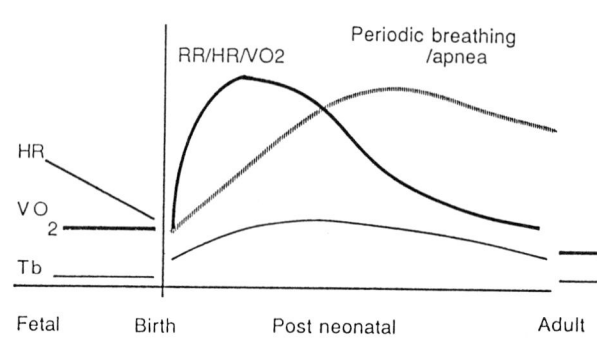

HR - heart rate; RR - respiratory rate
VO2 - Oxygen consumption; Tb - body temperature

figure 2

Defining Periodic Breathing

An increasingly used definition in infants, particularly pertaining to risk for SIDS (32), is inappropriate and misleading. "Three or more apneas of greater than 3 seconds, separated by less than 20 seconds of breathing", is not a description of PB. It will include PB if the amplitude of the oscillation has increased, when intervening apneas occur. However, that definition also includes irregularly occurring apneas, which are rarely seen in healthy infants recorded with sensitive respiratory transducers.

Hypothalamic integration

The concept of an intrinsic central pattern generator, confined to the brainstem, that only requires modulation to alter amplitude and frequency of each breath no longer explains the commonly observed patterns of breathing observed during sleep. Further more, the pre-eminence accorded chemoreception (ie peripheral and central) as the primary modulator of breathing is no longer tenable. The so-called high / low gain state of a feed-back loop mechanism, such as peripheral/central chemoreception (46), may be more usefully viewed as one of many pathways modulating a network (rather than a respiratory center), whose gain is regulated by the POAH, which thus ensures whole-organism thermometabolic control.

Clearly the POAH is one focus that integrates many of the functions observed above. A multitude of mechanisms ranging from, behaviour, neuroendocrine, metabolic, and cardiorespiratory, are regulated from the hypothalamus to achieve effective homeostasis. Their relative priorities change markedly over the course of many weeks or months after birth (figure 2) and greatly influence the expression of periodicities in health and disease.

also described in infants with broncho-pulmonary dysplasia who also have markedly reduced PB (27) despite often being hypoxemic. Warming healthy preterm infants has now also been shown to increase the incidence of PB and apnea (cycle length 12 seconds) in REM sleep, by increasing the amplitude of the oscillation, but its cycle time unchanged (28).

This oscillatory cycle time is the one frequently described in heart rate variability, particularly during "entrainment" tests using cyclical heating (29), and has been demonstrated to exist in infants (30). Our pilot studies have shown that similar entrainment techniques also cause PB in some sleeping infants with a cycle time of 12 -15 seconds. The cycle length of PB during infancy has been reported to decrease from 15 to 12 seconds over the first few months of life (31). Many authors still relate such PB to abnormalities of chemoreceptor function and conclude that such patterns are unstable (22,32) or, if exceeding 5% of sleep time, to be vulnerable and require therapy (32,33). However, we conclude that there is a robust central oscillator, distinct from that usually described as governing inspiratory/expiratory timing (34), with the characteristics of thermal vasomotion that becomes apparent (or exposed) as other combined drives (metabolism, vagal, chemoreceptor) are reduced. Important modulators of this 'tonic' central threshold are BMR, nutrition, growth rate, stage of maturation, arousal state, and ambient temperature (35).

The change in arousal threshold after birth, chiefly a reduction in REM and an increase in wakefullness, more marked in the lamb than the human infant, is greatly influenced by ambient temperature. Both the lamb and human infant increase metabolic rate in response to cooling in both REM or active sleep and slow wave or quiet sleep (13,36). Thus the newborn mammal does not lack active thermoregulation in REM sleep as has been concluded from most experimental studies in adult mammals (37).

The human infant has an higher MR in REM than non-REM sleep, and, in fact, switches preferentially into REM sleep in the neonatal period when confronted by a cool environment. In the lamb over 4 days of age, MR is lower in REM than non-REM sleep, and REM progressively decreased during modest cooling, with a reciprocal increase in SWS. Warming to the upper critical limit, the threshold for thermolysis, on the other hand, increased REM sleep. Warming above this threshold led to panting, sweating and arousal. Species differences in brain size, since brain metabolism is increased in REM, should be taken into account when comparing temperature control in different stages of arousal. Also the studies in infants were relatively acute, whereas in lambs, which have a comparatively short 90 minute interfeed rest-activity cycle, the changes in REM /SWS relating to warm and cool environments persisted during 12 hours of continued exposure (38). Arousal threshold and arousal state is an integral part of behavioural thermoregulation. Thus environmental temperature plays a dominant role in regulating arousal state, metabolism and its related endocrine responses, as well as cardiorespiratory function.

Arousal state modifies the suprapontine influences on cardiovascular and respiratory control (39), notably in REM sleep. This modulation is generally considered to extend to the dissociation of POAH control of temperature regulation (37). However in adult rats, as in lambs, REM sleep is greater at the upper critical limit of the thermoneutral zone (40), indicating that ambient temperature exerts fine control of arousal state organisation. Thus, it may be fair to conclude that temperature "drives" arousal state rather than vice versa.

Ambient temperature, behavioural thermoregulation and ventilatory control

It is well known, of course, that ambient conditions greatly influence postnatal behaviour and development. Neonates, even altricial species, such as rabbits, will behaviourally select, as a first priority, their metabolically thermoneutral environment, reducing this daily as temperature control matures (41). The runts in a litter selected a lower ambient temperature than their normally grown litter mates.

Significantly, a minority of these infants who had a lower minute ventilation while air-breathing, developed periodic breathing (PB) with a cycle time of 12 seconds during hypoxia. Thus, the responses to CO2 and O2 are quite different during postnatal life, initially having similarities with those in fetal life.

Paradoxically it is much later (weeks in the case of the lamb), when basal metabolic rate is falling, that absence of peripheral chemoreceptors (16) or disruption of vagal airway mechanosensory reflexes (upper airway by-pass) (17) may cause breathing dysrhythmia and possible death. It is the large increase in MR, mainly related to thermogenesis, which rapidly becomes a major determinant of cardiorespiratory drive during sleep after birth. There is a sharp increase and then a progressive fall in this 'tonic' stimulus to cardiorespiratory control. Basal body temperature rises from the already high fetal level, directly related to the rise in T3 and BMR before declining with them (13).

As metabolic rate and breathing frequency fall with age, expiratory time lengthens and effective lung volume is threatened, since the chest wall is still relatively compliant. However expiratory phasic activity of the laryngeal constrictors shows a reciprocal increase, generating endogenous expiratory pressure in the process. By-passing the expiratory laryngeal resistance (by opening a tracheal window) leads to increased laryngeal constriction, lengthening of expiratory time, and PB during SWS in older lambs. Since the substitution of positive expiratory pressure abolished expiratory laryngeal braking and PB, and reduced expiratory time, if the vagi are intact, it is clear that vagal mechanosensors provide a tonic "expiratory" stimulus to breathing in the postneonatal period. This is the expiratory stimulus component of the Hering Breuer inflation reflex (18), which is invariably overlooked, since apnea is usually regarded as the sole element of these reflexes. The apparent reemergence of HB reflexes in postneonatal life, elegantly demonstrates the changing postnatal integration of tonic drives to breathing. In the neonatal period the high basal metabolic drive "masks" the presence of these vagal pressor responses, leading to the conventional view that the Hering Breuer inflation (apnea) disappears rapidly after birth (19). The persistance of the HB reflex into postneonatal life in man has also been confirmed (20).

Disturbing vagal mechanosensory control, especially expiratory pressure sensation in the lamb by upper airway by-pass, usually resulted in PB, or periodic apnea, **both** with a remarkably constant cycle time of 10-12 seconds. However, this only occurs if the 'tonic' metabolic stimulus is minimal (ie at thermoneutrality in older lambs after the peak in BMR). Similarly, reducing peripheral chemoreceptor drive with a dopamine infusion caused PB with the same cycle length. Again the amplitude, and thus the length of apnea at the nadir, of the oscillation was similarly influenced by the prevailing metabolic rate. **However**, similar PB persisted after carotid body denervation (21), and, therefore, cannot be primarily dependant on peripheral chemoreceptors as is conventionally thought (22,23). More recent studies in the lamb during pyrexia have again demonstrated similar age-related PB, that not only related to changes in metabolic demand as body temperature changed, but more closely to brain temperature (24).

In the human, where the magnitude and time course of these age-related changes is less and longer, respectively, PB is common in healthy infants (25). Indeed in a detailed study of 67 infants sleeping at home, no obstructive apnea and no central apneas longer than 12 seconds were observed, whereas PB with a cycle length of 10 - 15 seconds was common. Apneas of upto 10 seconds occurred in association with PB, if the amplitude of the oscillation increased. PB, with apnea, occurred predominantly in REM, whereas periodic oscillations in amplitude without apnea were observed in NREM. PB was increased in females, infants in a warm environment, and of a lower weight, but was decreased in those whose mothers smoked during pregnancy. The latter have recently been shown to have decreased pulmonary compliance (26) which would explain the reduction in PB based on increased vagal drive to breathing, a feature

(1) Boddy K., Dawes G.S., Fisher R., Pinter S. & Robinson J.S. Foetal respiratory movements, electrocortical and cardiovascular responses to hypoxaemia and hypercapnia in sheep. J. Physiol. 1974;234: 599-618.
(2) B M Johnston, T R Gunn, P D Gluckman. Genioglossus and alae nasi activity in fetal sheep. J Devel Physiol 1986;8: 323-31.
(3) J E Fewell, P Johnson. Upper airway dynamics during breathing and during apnoea in fetal sheep. J Physiol 1983;339:495-504.
(4) Fewell JE, Hislop AA, Kitterman JA, Johnson P. Effect of tracheostomy on lung development in fetal lambs. J Appl Physiol (1983) 55:1102-1108.
(5) Johnston BM. Brainstem inhibitory mechanisms in the control of fetal breathing movements. in The fetal and neonatal brainstem - developmental and clinical issues. Ed MA Hanson. Cambridge Univ Press (in Press).
(6) England SJ, Bartlett D, Knuth SL. Comparison of human vocal cord movements during isocapnic hypoxia and hypercapnia. J Appl Physiol (1982) 53:81-86.
(7) Johnston BM, Gunn TR, Gluckman PD. Surface cooling rapidly induces coordinated activity in the upper and lower airway muscles of the fetal lamb in utero. Ped Res. 1988. 23.257-261.
(8) Gluckman P.D., Gunn T. & Johnston B.M. The effect of cooling on breathing and shivering in unanaethetized fetal lambs in utero J. Physiol. 1983;343: 495-506.
(9) Johnson P, Rurak D. (unpublished observations)
(10) Bennett L, Gluckman PD, Johnston BM. The central effects of thyrotropin-releasing hormone on the breathing movements and electrocortical activity of the fetal sheep. Ped Res. (1988) 23: 72-75.
(11) Nink M, Krause U, Lehner H, Heuberger, Huber I, Schulz R, Hommel G, Beyer J. Thyrtropin-releasing hormone has stimulatory effects on ventilation in humans. Acta Physiol Scand (1991) 141: 309-318.
(12) Sack J, Beaudry MA, DeLamater PV, Oh W, Fisher DA. Umbilical cord cutting triggers hypertriodothyronemia and non-shivering thermogenesis in the newborn lamb. Pediatr Res (1976) 10:169-175.
(13) Symonds ME, Andrews DA, Johnson P. The control of thermoregulation in the developing lamb during slow wave sleep. J Devel Physiol 1989;11:289-298.
(14) Harned H.S., Herrington R.T., Griffin C.A., Berryhill W.S. & MacKinney. Respiratory effects of the division of the carotid sinus in the lamb soon after the initiation of breathing Ped. Res. 1968;2:264-270.
(15) Andersson D, Sjostrom A, Gennser G, Johnson P. The effect of hypoxia and hyperoxia on breathing and ventilation in newborn infants during sleep: in Physiological Development of the fetus and neonate (ed CT Jones),Perinatology Press, USA.1988:651-56.
(16) Bureau M.A., Lamarsh J., Foulon P. & Dalle D. Postnatal mat-uration of respiration in intact and carotid body-chemodenervated lambs. J.Appl. Physiol. 1985; 59: 869-874.
(17) Johnson P, fewell JE, Fedorko LM, Wollner JC. Vagal mechanisms in respiratory failure in sleeping lambs. in Sudden Infant Death Syndrome. ed Tildon JT, Roeder LM, Steinschneider A. Academic Press (1983) 467-490.
(18) Johnson P. Prolonged expiratory apnea and implications for the control of breathing. Lancet (1985) ii. 877-880.
(19) Cross.KW, Klaus M, Tooley WH, Weisser K. The response of the newborn infant to inflation of the lungs. J Physiol (1960) 151; 798-805.
(20) Rabbette PS, Costeloe K, Stocks J. The persistence of the Hering-Breuer Reflex beyond the neonatal period. J Appl Physiol (1991) in press.
(21) Andrews D.C., Johnson P., & Symond M.E. Metabolic rate and periodic breathing in the developing lamb. J.Physiol 1990;417:137
(22) Fleming P.J., Goncalves A.L., Levine M.R. & Woolard S. The development of stability of respiration in human infants: Changes in ventilatory responses to spontaneous sighs. J. Physiol. 1983; 347:1-16.
(23) Waggener TB, Frantz ID, Stark AR, Kronauer RE. Oscillatory breathing patterns leading to apneic spells in infants. J Appl physiol. (1982) 52;1288-1295.
(24) Andrews D.C. & Johnson P. Breathing pattern and brain sur-face tempera-

ture interactions during pyrogenic responses in the developing lamb. Human Psychopharm. In Press 1990.
(25) Johnson P, Head J, Hughes M, Sands P. Periodic Breathing in healthy infants monitored at home. Am Rev Resp Dis. 1990;141(4)
(26) Hanrahan J P, et al. Lung mechanics in infants whose mothers smoked. Am Rev Resp Dis. 1990;141 (4) : A282.
(27) Carse EA, Wilkinson AR, Whyte PL, Henderson-Smart DS, Johnson P. Oxygen and carbon dioxide tensions, breathing and heart rate in normal infants during the first six months of life. J devel physiol. (1981) 3:85-100.
(28) Berterotteire D., D'Allest AM, Dehan M & Gaultier CL. The Effect of in creasing body temperature on the breathing pattern in premature infants. J. Devl. Physiol. 1990 (In Press)
(29) Kitney R I. An analysis of the thermoregulatory influences on heart rate variability. The study of heart rate variability. Kitney RI, Rompelman O. Oxford Medical Engineering Series. Oxford : Clarendon Press. (1980) 81-106.
(30) Lindqvist A., Oja R., Hellman O. & Valimaki I. Impact of thermal vasomotor control on the heart rate variability of newborn infants. Early Human Dev. 1983;8: 37-47.
(31) Barrington K.J., Finer N.N. & Wilkinson M.H. Progressive shortening of the periodic breathing cycle in normal infants. Pediatr. Res. 1987;21: 247-251.
(32) Kelly DH & Shannon D. Periodic breathing in infants with near-miss sudden infant death syndrome. Pediatrics.1979;63:355-359
(33) Hunt CE, Brouillette RT, Hanson D. Theophylline improves pneumogram abnormalities in infants at risk for sudden infant death syndrome. J Pediatr. 1983;103:969-974.
(34) Clark FJ, von Euler C. On the regulation of depth and rate of breathing. J Physiol (1972) 222; 267-295.
(35) Johnson P, Andrews DC. (1990). Hypoxia, temperature control and periodic breathing in postnatal life. in Hypoxia :the adaptations (eds JR Sutton G Coates JE Remmers). Decker.1990:84-87.
(36) Fleming P J, Levine M R, Azaz Y, Johnson P. The effect of sleep state on the metabolic response to cold stress in newborn infants. Fetal and Neonatal Development (ed CT Jones). Perinatology Press, Ithaca NY.1988:643-647.
(37) Parmegianni PL. Interaction between sleep and thermoregulation: an aspect of the control of behavioural state. Sleep, 1987;10: 426-435.
(38) Andrews D.C., Ball N.J., Symonds M.E., Vojeck L. & Johnson P. The effect of ambient temperature and age on sleep states in developing lambs In: Sleep'90 (ed J. Horne) Pontengel Press, Bochum. (1991)
(39) Frysinger RC, Zhang J, Harper RM. Cardiovascular and respiratory relationships with neuronal discharge in the central nucleus of the amygdala during sleep-waking states. Sleep (1988) 11:317-332.
(40) Szymusiak R, Stainff E. Maximal REM sleeptime defines a narrower thermoneutral zone than does minimal metabolic rate. Physiology and Behaviour. (1981) 26:687-690.
(41) Hull J, Hull D. Behavioural thermoregulation in newborn rabbits. J Comp Physiol Psychol (1982) 96:143-147.
(42) Olunstead CHE, Villiblanca DR, Torbinier M, Rhodes D. Maturation of temperature control in the cat. Physiol and Behav (1979) 23,489-95.
(43) Bonora M, Gautier H. Ventilatory responses to hyoxia in kittens. Resp Physiol (1987) 68,359-70.
(44) Phillipson E.A., Duffin J. & Cooper J.D. Critical dependence of respiratory rhythmicity on metabolic CO2 load. J. Appl. Physiol 1981;50: 45-54
(45) Giddens DP, Kitney RI. Neonatal heart rate variability and its relationship to respiration. J theor Biol (1985) 113;759-780
(46) Khoo MCK, Kronaur RE, Strohl KP, Slutsky AS. Factors inducing periodic breathing in humans: a general model. J Appl Physiol. (1982) 53:644-59.
(47) Carley D, Shannon DC. Relative stability of respiration during progressive hypoxia. J Appl Physiol (1988) 65:1389-99.

Résumé

Pendant la vie foetale, la stimulation de la respiration par l'hypoxie et la thermogénèse sans frisson sont toutes deux puissamment inhibées. Ce sont des réponses appropriées pour la survie foetale. L'activité respiratoire est cependant liée aux réponses thermorégulatrices à l'environnement : frisson et halètement, qui ne sont pas inhibés. Après la naissance, la fonction thyroïdienne et la thermogénèse sans frisson sont activées et constituent un stimulus central "tonique" majeur pour la fonction cardiovasculaire et l'état d'éveil. La température corporelle augmente au dessus des valeurs foetales. Une caractéristique du contrôle thermométabolique de la respiration est la respiration périodique, spécialement importante en ambiance chaude et au cours du sommeil paradoxal. La respiration périodique chez le nourrisson n'est pas considérée comme un état instable ou dangereux ni comme un indice d'anomalie de la fonction chémoréceptrice.

Brain mechanisms underlying cardiorespiratory control during sleep

Ronald M. Harper

Department of Anatomy and Cell Biology and the Brain Research Institute, University of California at Los Angeles, Los Angeles, CA 90024-1763, USA

SUMMARY

Cardiovascular and respiratory patterning control mechanisms are closely integrated; changes in patterning in one system are accompanied by closely-coupled alterations in the other. Thus, sleep state effects on somatic musculature can affect respiratory patterning, which in turn modifies cardiovascular activity. A portion of sleep state effects on cardiac or respiratory patterns appear to be mediated by rostral brain structure influences on brain stem regions; these rostral structures include areas mediating affect. A portion of state-related respiratory and cardiac changes may be modulated by regions within the periaqueductal grey which receive heavy projections from descending rostral sites and has the potential to modulate upper airway and cardiovascular activity.

INTRODUCTION

Any quantification of cardiovascular or respiratory system activity during sleep must consider the interactions between these two systems, and the potential for sleep states, in exerting primary control over one system, to inevitably modify action in the other. This observation appears so obvious and trivial that it barely deserves mention; however, the effects of sleep states on multiple sites within the neuraxis are so profound that the potential for interaction between systems is massive and frequently overlooked. A further consideration is that respiratory patterning (and thus aspects of cardiac activity as well) is one aspect of motor behavior which is tightly coupled with other motor behaviors including locomotion, vocalization, and motoric responses to threatening or affective stimuli. Sleep state influences on respiratory musculature must, therefore, be considered in the context of more widespread influences of state on motor control in general, and on factors which may modify generalized motor control.

RESPIRATORY INFLUENCES ON CARDIOVASCULAR PATTERNING

Of all the state-related interactions between respiratory patterning and cardiovascular activity, the near-synchronous changes in heart rate with the respiratory cycle is perhaps the best known. Negative thoracic pressure, induced by diaphragmatic descent, promotes venous return, with consequent baroreceptor and other sensory sequelae which reflexly modify vagal outflow and result in regular patterns of increases and decreases of cardiac intervals with respiratory cycling; these phenomena have been well described for decades. This "respiratory sinus arrhythmia" is particularly pronounced during quiet sleep, perhaps as a consequence of the prolonged inspiratory timing and relatively slow and unvarying respiratory pattern which is characteristic of that state. The near-synchronous variation of cardiac intervals is so enhanced that assessment of the extent of that source of variability can be used as a primary indicator of sleep state (Harper et al., 1987). The interactions which produce respiratory sinus arrhythmia are powerfully affected by developmental mechanisms, exhibiting an initial decline in amplitude with age followed by a rise (Harper et al., 1978); trends which are partially independent of baseline heart rate effects (Kluge et al., 1988). Assessment of the extent of this measure, of course, requires partitioning of sleep state, since states exert such profound influences on the degree of coupling of cardiac rate with breathing patterns. Moreover, the degree of cardiac variation is markedly dependent on basal heart and respiratory rate; heart rate in particular is markedly affected by state (Harper et al., 1976).

The mechanisms underlying this normal patterning of cardiac variation appear to be exquisitely sensitive to disturbances in central or peripheral nervous system activity which are associated with particular disorders, such as the Sudden Infant Death Syndrome (SIDS). Both the absolute extent of variation with respiratory effort, as well as the degree of coupling on a moment-to-moment basis appear to be altered in infants who later succumb to SIDS (Kluge et al., 1988; Raetz et al., 1991).

Disturbed patterns of breathing during sleep greatly modifies normal physiologic functions including extent of negative thoracic pressure and associated reflexes. Obstructive sleep apnea results in extreme increases in negative thoracic pressure and enhanced venous return. The cardiac response to these actions are dramatic, with extreme rises in arterial pressure and pronounced bradycardic-tachycardic sequences associated with each obstructed breath. The cardiac R-R interval patterns associated with obstructive sleep apnea are so distinctive that they have formed the basis, in some circles, for assistance in clinical detection of the syndrome (Guilleminault et al., 1984). The extent of the variation in heart rate with each obstructed breath depends on the degree of oxygen desaturation and also, of course, the presence of other medical conditions which have the potential to interfere with sympathetic and vagal action, such as long-standing diabetic neuropathy (Trelease et al., 1986). Diabetic neuropathy will greatly diminish extent of respiratory sinus arrhythmia. Other motoric disturbances associated with sleep, including nocturnal myoclonus, i.e., periodic phasic movements of the peripheral musculature, introduce exaggerated tachycardic-bradycardic sequences of cardiac interbeat intervals coincident with the movements (Trelease et al., 1986).

Disordered breathing or disturbed motor functioning during sleep thus leads to dramatic heart rate patterning changes and major alterations in blood pressure; the inverse relationship of cardiovascular influences on respiratory patterning during sleep is equally marked. Transient elevation of blood pressure, by either pharmacologic or mechanical means, induces a suppression of respiratory muscle patterning and amplitude of EMG bursts (Trelease et al., 1985), an effect which is more pronounced on a laryngeal dilator, the posterior cricoarytenoid, than on the diaphragm (Marks & Harper, 1987). Sleep states markedly modify this effect; quiet sleep greatly enhances the suppression. It is not clear how sleep states modify this interaction, but the potential for a blood pressure/respiratory suppression relationship to elicit disruptions of respiratory patterning during sleep is very great. We speculate, for example, that the following scenario might occur: A subject moves during sleep, eliciting a transient blood pressure rise. The blood pressure rise reflexly diminishes diaphragmatic and laryngeal dilator EMG amplitude and patterning, with the upper airway affected more profoundly than the diaphragm. The diaphragm, being less affected, provides negative pressure with increased airflow through a somewhat-constricted upper airway. The upper airway collapses, augmenting negative thoracic pressure, and further increasing arterial pressure, which, in turn enhances the initial suppression of upper airway tone, and potentially leads to an obstructive apnea. That scenario is only speculative, and a number of other factors may override that sequence. However, the scenario does illustrate the potential for considering interactions between somatomotor, respiratory and cardiovascular systems within sleep, when considering disordered breathing during sleep.

CARDIAC INFLUENCES ON RESPIRATORY PATTERNING

One would expect from these experimental manipulations that certain cardiovascular pathologies which modify cardiac output or venous return would also alter respiratory patterning, and that, indeed, appears to be the case. Congestive heart failure, for example, induces dramatic changes in respiratory patterning, and leads to marked changes in moment-to-moment cardiac variability (Woo et al., 1991). Cheyne-Stokes breathing, a state-related respiratory pattern, leads to characteristic patterns observed in plots of successive cardiac R-R intervals (Trelease et al., 1990); these patterns can assist in providing markers for the disease. Periodic breathing, which most likely derives from delays in circulatory time between chemoreceptor structures, appears only during particular sleep states and is also associated with characteristic R-R interval patterns.

The variety of cardiovascular and respiratory changes associated with both normal transitions in state and with pathological conditions within states, suggests that cardiac and respiratory control exerted by a large number of brain structures along the neuraxis may be involved in these changes. The evidence from animal studies suggests that forebrain, midbrain and medullary structures all participate in mediating at least a portion of the cardiac and respiratory changes associated with different states. This evidence is derived from stimulation, lesion, and electrophysiological recording observations.

ROSTRAL BRAIN INFLUENCES ON MIDBRAIN AND BRAIN STEM CARDIORESPIRATORY REGIONS

The available animal evidence suggests that a number of rostral brain structures interact with midbrain and brain stem structures to mediate respiratory and cardiac patterning. These rostral structures have traditionally been associated with "affective" functions of the brain, and include the central nucleus of the amygdala (ACE), anterior frontal cortex, and cingulate regions. The ACE, in particular, has massive projections to the parabrachial pons and to the nucleus of the solitary tract, as well as to the periaqueductal grey (Hopkins & Holstege, 1978). The central nucleus contains neurons which discharge on a breath-by-breath basis as well as an overall rate basis with the respiratory cycle (Zhang et al., 1986a; Frysinger et al., 1988). Moreover, a subset of neurons in the ACE also discharge on an overall rate basis with the cardiac cycle and on a cycle-by-cycle basis with cardiac rate (Frysinger et al., 1988). Bilateral cold blockade of the central nucleus results in loss of an aversive conditioned respiratory and blood pressure response (but not a heart rate response) (Zhang et al., 1986b). The dependencies between discharge of ACE neurons and respiratory and cardiac patterning are extremely state dependent; some dependencies, assessed by cross-correlating neuronal discharge with inspiratory onset or the R wave of the cardiac cycle, only occur in some states, e.g., waking or REM sleep, and disappear in other states, e.g., quiet sleep. Electrical stimulation of the ACE results in a pronounced transient rise in arterial pressure which is slightly reduced in quiet sleep, but virtually abolished in REM sleep (Frysinger et al., 1984). The neuronal relationships are not confined to animal studies. Cycle-by-cycle and rate dependencies between cardiac and respiratory cycling and neural discharge have been found in the human amygdala and hippocampus as well (Frysinger & Harper, 1989). The change in dependencies during different states of sleep, together with the demonstration of a potential to elicit marked state-dependent blood pressure changes, suggest that these rostral brain structures may mediate descending influences which can alter cardiorespiratory patterning during different states.

A principal premotor nucleus to the laryngeal musculature is the nucleus retroambiguus. That nucleus receives substantial projections from portions of the periaqueductal grey (PAG), a large aggregate of cell bodies and axons surrounding the cerebral aqueduct (Holstege, 1989); the PAG can also influence motoneurons projecting to the abdominal musculature. Portions of the periaqueductal grey have been implicated in blood pressure control, and other portions in vocalization behavior through excitatory amino acid stimulation studies and from electrophysiological recording evidence (Bandler, 1988; Larson, 1991). Vocalization, of course, uses abdominal and thoracic respiratory muscles for developing thoracic pressure, and laryngeal "respiratory" muscles for modulating air flow. Thus, one would expect that a parsimonious use of neural control structures might incorporate neurons used in vocalization for roles in respiratory patterning. Indeed, a substantial subset of PAG neurons discharge on a breath-by-breath basis with the respiratory cycle (Ni et al., 1990a) and another set discharge on a cycle-by-cycle basis with the cardiac cycle. Tonic discharge correlations with cardiac and respiratory rate are also found with a large proportion of PAG neurons (Ni et al., 1990b). These correlations are heavily state-dependent; the relationships are present in some states and diminished or absent in others.

The available evidence suggests that a number of rostral brain influences are functionally dissociated from brain stem activity during REM sleep. Electrical stimulation of the ACE, for example, is virtually ineffective in eliciting blood pressure elevations during that state (Frysinger et al., 1984). Temperature-sensitive neurons in the anterior hypothalamus also appear to be dissociated from their functional relationships during that state (Parmeggiani et al., 1983). The functional separation of rostral influences controlling temperature on brain stem stem control during REM sleep could have important implications for respiratory patterning during sleep. Respiratory patterning is extremely dependent on core temperature; even mild elevations in core temperature elicit substantial increases in respiratory rate (Bonora & Gautier, 1989). Thus, state influences on temperature control also could substantially modify respiratory patterning. We speculate that a portion of the temperature effects on respiration may be mediated through the PAG. The anterior hypothalamus massively projects to the PAG (Shipley et al., 1991). Moreover, young rat pups, on cooling, vocalize ultrasonically, a phenomenon that appears to be distinct from distress (J. Alberts, personal communication). Since neurons in the PAG bordering vocalization regions demonstrate respiratory dependencies, we speculate that the mechanisms are in place via an anterior hypothalamic/PAG/laryngeal motoneuron pathway to mediate a portion of temperature-related respiratory effects. Particular attention should be directed toward understanding the state-dependent interactions between rostral temperature control regions and brain stem structures.

CONCLUSIONS

The control of cardiovascular and respiratory patterning during sleep must thus be considered from a perspective of multiple-interacting systems. A most important aspect of this interaction is the dependence of both respiratory patterning and cardiovascular responses on somatomotor control during different states. Clearly, the atonia of postural muscles during REM sleep modifies respiratory musculature to the extent that infants, with already-compliant chest walls, may be placed at special risk with the additional loss of rigidity imposed by REM atonia of the thoracic walls (Henderson-Smart & Read, 1979). There are additional sequelae from this loss of compliance; thoracic pressure is reduced, thus potentially modifying venous return, which subsequently modifies cardiac output. Major questions exist on the responsivity of baroreceptor reflexes to somatomotor changes occurring during different states, and the potential influences on respiratory patterning. The mechanisms by which rostral brain regions affect brain stem cardiorespiratory areas during sleep require exploration. Among these rostral brain influences, temperature, affect and aspects of motion control are particularly important. Answers to those questions will undoubtedly greatly enhance our understanding of breathing and cardiac patterning during sleep.

REFERENCES

Bandler, R. (1988): Brain mechanisms of aggression as revealed by electrical and chemical stimulation: Suggestion of a central role for the midbrain periaqueductal grey region. In *Progress in Psychobiology and Physiological Psychology*, Vol. 13, ed. A. Epstein & A. Morrison, pp. 67-154. New York: Academic Press.

Bonora, M. & Gautier, H (1989): Effects of hypoxia on thermal polypnea in intact and carotid body-denervated conscious cats. *J. Appl. Physiol.* 67(2), 578-583.

Frysinger, R.C. & Harper, R.M. (1989): Cardiac and respiratory correlations with unit discharge in human amygdala and hippocampus. *EEG Clin. Neurophysiol.* 72, 463-470.

Frysinger, R.C., Marks, J.D., Trelease, R.B., Schechtman, V.L. & Harper, R.M. (1984): Sleep states attenuate the pressor response to central amygdala stimulation. *Exp. Neurol.* 83, 604-617.

Frysinger, R.C., Zhang, J. & Harper, R.M. (1988): Cardiovascular and respiratory relationships with neuronal discharge in the central nucleus of the amygdala during sleep-waking states. *Sleep* 11, 317-332.

Guilleminault, C., Connolly, S., Winkle, R., Melvin, K. & Tilkian, A. (1984): Cyclical variation of the heart rate in sleep apnea syndrome: mechanisms and usefulness of 24 h electrocardiography as a screening technique. *Lancet* 1(8369), 126-131.

Harper, R.M., Hoppenbrouwers, T., Sterman, M.B., McGinty, D.J. & Hodgman, J (1976): Polygraphic studies of normal infants during the first six months of life: I. Heart rate and variability as a function of state. *Pediatr. Res.* 10, 945-951.

Harper, R.M., Schechtman, V.L. & Kluge, K.A. (1987): Machine classification of infant sleep state using cardiorespiratory measures. *EEG Clin. Neurophysiol.* 67, 379-387.

Harper, R.M., Walter, D.O., Leake, B., Hoffman, H.J., Sieck, G.C., Sterman, M.B., Hoppenbrouwers, T & Hodgman, J. (1978): Development of sinus arrhythmia during sleeping and waking states in normal infants. *Sleep* 1, 33-48.

Henderson-Smart, D.J. & Read, D.J.C. (1979): Reduced lung volume during behavioral active sleep in the newborn. *J. Appl. Physiol.* 46(6), 1081-1085.

Holstege, G. (1989): Anatomical study of the final common pathway for vocalization in the cat. *J. Comp. Neurol.* 284, 242-252.

Hopkins, D.A. & Holstege, G. (1978): Amygdaloid projections to the mesencephalon, pons and medulla oblongata in the cat. *Exp. Brain Res.* 32, 529-547.

Kluge, K.A., Harper, R.M., Schechtman, V.L., Wilson, A.J., Hoffman, H.J. & Southall, D.P. (1988): Spectral analysis assessment of respiratory sinus arrhythmia in normal infants and infants who subsequently died of sudden infant death syndrome. *Pediatr. Res.* 24(6), 677-682.

Larson, C.R. (1991): On the relation of PAG neurons to laryngeal and respiratory muscles during vocalization in the monkey. *Brain Res.* In press.

Marks, J.D. & Harper, R.M. (1987): Differential inhibition of the diaphragm and posterior cricoarytenoid muscles induced by transient hypertension across sleep states in intact cats. *Exp. Neurol.* 95, 730-742.

Ni, H., Zhang, J. & Harper, R.M. (1990a): Respiratory-related discharge of periaqueductal gray neurons during sleep-waking states. *Brain Res.* 511, 319-325.

Ni, H., Zhang, J. & Harper, R.M. (1990b): Cardiovascular-related discharge of periaqueductal gray neurons during sleep-waking states. *Brain Res.* 532, 242-248.

Parmeggiani, P.L., Azzaroni, A., Cevolani, D. & Ferrari, G. (1983): Responses of anterior hypothalamic-preoptic neurons to direct thermal stimulation during wakefulness and sleep. *Brain Res.* 269, 392-285.

Raetz, S.L., Richard, C.A., Garfinkel, A., & Harper, R.M. (1991): Dynamic characteristics of cardiac R-R intervals during sleep and waking states. *Sleep* In press.

Shipley, M.T., Ennis, M., Rizvi, T.A. & Behbehani, M.M. (1991): Forebrain inputs to the midbrain periaqueductal grey: Evidence for discrete longitudinally organized input columns. In *The midbrain periaqueductal grey matter: Functional anatomical and immunohistochemical organization*, ed. A. Depaulis & R. Bandler, in press. New York: Plenum Publishing Corporation (NATO ASI Series).

Trelease, R.B., Garfinkel, A. & Harper, R.M. (1990): Characteristic dynamics of cardiac R-R interval variation in obstructive apnea, nocturnal myoclonus, and congestive heart failure syndromes during sleep. *Soc. Neurosci. Abstr.* 16, 299.

Trelease, R.B., Harper, R.M., Arand, D.L. & Zimmermann, E.G. (1986): Use of heart rate analysis for differentiation of sleep disorders. *Proc. Eighth Annu. Conf. IEEE Eng. Med. Biol. Soc.* 2, 1203-1206.

Trelease, R.B., Sieck, G.C., Marks, J.D. & Harper, R.M. (1985): Respiratory inhibition induced by transient hypertension during sleep. *Exp. Neurol.* 90, 173-186.

Woo, M.A., Stevenson, W.G., Moser, D.K., Trelease, R.B. & Harper, R.M. (1991): Patterns of beat-to-beat heart rate variability in advanced heart failure. Submitted for publication.

Zhang, J.X., Harper, R.M. & Frysinger, R.C. (1986a): Respiratory modulation of neuronal discharge in the central nucleus of the amygdala during sleep and waking states. *Exp. Neurol.* 91, 193-207.

Zhang, J.X., Harper, R.M., & Ni, H. (1986b): Cryogenic blockade of the central nucleus of the amygdala attenuates aversively conditioned blood pressure and respiratory responses. *Brain Res.* 386, 136-145.

Acknowledgments

This research was supported by HL22418 and HD22695.

Résumé

Les mécanismes des contrôles cardio-vasculaire et respiratoire sont liés de manière intime. Les modifications du schéma d'activité d'un système s'accompagnent de changements précisément couplés de l'autre. De ce fait, les effets du sommeil sur la musculature somatique peuvent modifier le schéma d'activité respiratoire qui à son tour retentit sur l'activité cardio-vasculaire. Une partie des effets du sommeil sur les activités cardiaque et respiratoire semble être liée à l'influence des structures cérébrales supérieures sur le tronc cérébral. Ces structures supérieures incluent les aires du contrôle affectif. Une partie des modifications respiratoires et cardiaques du sommeil peut être modulée par les régions situées dans la substance grise périaqueducale qui reçoit de nombreuses projections descendant des zones supérieures et qui a un potentiel de modulation des voies aériennes supérieures et de l'activité cardio-vasculaire.

II. Pathophysiology of cardiorespiratory control

II. Physiopathologie du contrôle cardio-respiratoire

Gas exchange during apnea : effects on lung and blood oxygen stores

John W. Shepard Jr.

Mayo Sleep Disorders Center, Mayo Clinic and Mayo Foundation, 200 First Street SW, Rochester, MN 55905, USA

During apnea, the metabolic needs of the body for oxygen (O_2) must be provided from the body's endogenous stores of O_2 in the lung, blood and tissues. Seven healthy mongrel dogs were studied to determine how the major O_2 stores in the lung, arterial and venous blood were sequentially utilized during periods of apnea. Each dog was anesthetized, paralyzed, mechanically ventilated and cannulated for sampling of arterial and mixed venous blood. Lung volume was measured at functional residual capacity (FRC) by nitrogen washout, oxygen consumption ($\dot{V}O_2$) by expired gas analysis, and blood volume (BV) by ^{51}Cr radionuclide labeling. Apneas of 30, 60 and 120 seconds duration were performed and the fractional concentration of oxygen in alveolar gas (F_AO_2) measured at apnea termination. Lung O_2 stores were calculated from the equation: $V_LO_2 = (FRC)(F_AO_2)$. Blood O_2 stores were calculated from the following equations which assume that arterial and venous blood volumes represent 25 per cent and 75 per cent of total blood volume, respectively. Arterial blood O_2 stores: $VaO_2 = (0.25)(BV)(CaO_2)$ and venous blood O_2 stores: $VvO_2 = (0.75)(BV)(CvO_2)$. Before apnea, $\dot{V}O_2$ averaged 144 ± 12 ml/min. VvO_2, V_LO_2 and VaO_2 accounted for 46 per cent, 33 per cent and 21 per cent of total O_2 stores (V_TO_2), respectively. VaO_2 decreased linearly and accounted for a consistent 21 per cent of the reduction in V_TO_2 over time. In contrast, the rate of depletion in V_LO_2 was initially rapid and decreased with apnea duration. For VvO_2 the reverse pattern was observed. Minimal reductions in VvO_2 occurred during the initial 30 seconds of apnea, followed by increased utilization of this component of the body's O_2 stores as apnea duration increased. V_TO_2 decreased by 140 ml and 136 ml in the first and second minutes of apnea, respectively. These reductions in V_TO_2 were not significantly different than baseline $\dot{V}O_2$, suggesting that total O_2 stores were adequate to support aerobic metabolism during apneas lasting 120 seconds in duration.

INTRODUCTION

During apnea, the metabolic needs of the body for O_2 must be provided from the body's endogenous stores of O_2 in the lung, blood and tissues. It is widely appreciated that individual patients with obstructive sleep apnea demonstrate widely different rates of arterial oxyhemoglobin desaturation in response to apnea (Bradley et al., 1985; Shepard, 1985). Lung volume, the fractional concentration of O_2 in the lung, oxygen consumption, baseline SaO_2, SvO_2 and cardiac output are all considered to be important variables in determining the rate and extent of oxyhemoglobin desaturation in addition to apnea duration (Bradley et al., 1985; Findley et al., 1983; Shepard, 1989; Strohl & Altose, 1984). Most of the work to date has focused on the role of lung volume and SaO_2 at apnea onset (Series et al., 1989). The present studies were performed to provide an overview of how the body's O_2 stores are sequentially utilized during apnea to meet the body's continuing demands for O_2. Prior to the development of arterial oxyhemoglobin desaturation sufficient to produce tissue hypoxia, it was hypothesized that the rate of oxygen depletion from the O_2 stores within the lung and blood would equal the baseline rate of oxygen consumption.

METHODS

Seven healthy mongrel dogs weighing 18-25 kg were studied. They were anesthetized with sodium pentobarbital, tracheotomized, paralyzed with succinylcholine and mechanically ventilated with a Harvard volume ventilator. Tidal volume was adjusted to 20 ml/kg and frequency set at 10 breaths/min. Blood volume was measured by the radionuclide labeling of red blood cells with ^{51}Cr (Mallinckrodt Diagnostics, St. Louis). Baseline oxygen consumption ($\dot{V}O_2$), carbon dioxide production ($\dot{V}CO_2$) and the respiratory exchange ratio (R) were determined in duplicate by analysis of expired gas (Shepard et al., 1981). Functional residual capacity was then determined in duplicate by the nitrogen washout technique (Minh et al., 1978) After sufficient time (i.e., > 20 minutes) for equilibration on room air, apneas of 30, 60 and 120 seconds duration were performed with sampling of arterial and mixed venous blood at these time intervals. The fractional concentration of oxygen in alveolar gas (F_AO_2) was then measured at apnea termination by compressing the chest wall and monitoring expired gas with a Beckman OM-11 gas analyzer. Four minutes before each procedural measurement, the lung was hyperinflated to 40 cm H_2O pressure to prevent the development of atelectasis. A heating lamp was used throughout the experiment to help maintain body temperature.

Arterial (femoral artery) and mixed venous (pulmonary artery) blood were analyzed for PO_2, PCO_2 and pH using an IL model 813 blood gas analyzer. Oxyhemoglobin saturation was calculated using the following equation for dog blood (Reeves et al., 1982): $S = [(37,900)/(P_s^3 + 205 P_s) + 1]^{-1}$, where S is saturation and P_s is the partial pressure for oxygen under standard conditions of temperature, PCO_2 and pH. Corrections from measured to standard conditions were made according to the following equation (Kelman, 1966):

$$P_sO_2 = [PO_2] [10^{\{0.024(37-temp) + 0.40(pH-7.40) + 0.06(\log 40 - \log PCO2)\}}]$$

Contents were computed from S and hemoglobin concentration (Hgb) by the following equation:
$$C = 1.39(Hgb)(S) + 0.003(P)$$

Total O_2 stores (V_TO_2) were calculated as the sum of lung, arterial and venous blood O_2 stores, where lung O_2 stores: $V_LO_2 = (FRC)(F_AO_2)$, arterial blood O_2 stores: $VaO_2 = (0.25)(BV)(CaO_2)$ and venous blood O_2 stores: $VvO_2 = (0.75)(BV)(CvO_2)$. These equations are based on data indicating that 25 per cent of total blood volume is at arterial O_2 tensions while the remaining 75 per cent is in the venous circulation. The 5 per cent of total blood volume in the systemic capillaries, 9 per cent in the pulmonary vessels, and 7 per cent in the heart were assigned equally between the arterial and venous compartments (Guyton, 1976).

Data are presented as mean ± SEM.

RESULTS

Table 1 presents the baseline data for weight, temperature, hemoglobin concentration, tidal volume, blood volume, FRC and $\dot{V}O_2$ for the seven dogs.

Table 1: Physiologic data for 7 dogs studied during apnea

Weight, kg	22 ± 1
Temperature, °C	39.1 ± 0.1
Hemoglobin, g/dl	16.2 ± 0.7
Tidal Volume, ml	443 ± 22
Blood Volume, ml	1,708 ± 83
FRC, ml	1,313 ± 81
$\dot{V}O_2$, ml/min	144 ± 12

Functional Residual Capacity, FRC; Oxygen Consumption, $\dot{V}O_2$;
Data are mean ± SEM

Figure 1 shows the changes in PCO_2 which occurred during apneas of up to 120 sec duration. Within the initial 30 sec, alveolar, arterial and mixed venous partial pressures for CO_2 have effectively equilibrated with $PaCO_2$ increasing by 9 mmHg from 39 to 48 mmHg while $PvCO_2$ increased minimally from 43 to 45 mmHg. Between 30 and 120 sec, $PaCO_2$ and $PvCO_2$ increased in parallel by 9 and 11 mmHg, respectively. Figure 2 shows the changes in PO_2 which were observed. The decrease in PaO_2 paralleled the decrease in P_AO_2 with both values approaching PvO_2 at 60 sec and effectively reaching equilibrium at 120 sec. In comparison to the rapid 36 mmHg decrease in PaO_2 from 94 to 58 mmHg within the initial 30 sec of apnea, there was only a small reduction of 2 mmHg in PvO_2 from 50 to 48 mmHg. After the initial 30 sec, PaO_2 and PvO_2 decreased by similar amounts of 29 and 21 mmHg, respectively, over the remaining 90 sec of apnea. Despite the fact that PaO_2 decreased to 29 mmHg and V_TO_2 was reduced to only 162 ± 24 ml at the end of 120 sec of apnea, there was no evidence of a significant metabolic acidosis. Over this time period, pH decreased from 7.31 to 7.22 in association with an increase in $PaCO_2$ from 39 to 57 mmHg consistent with an acute respiratory acidosis.

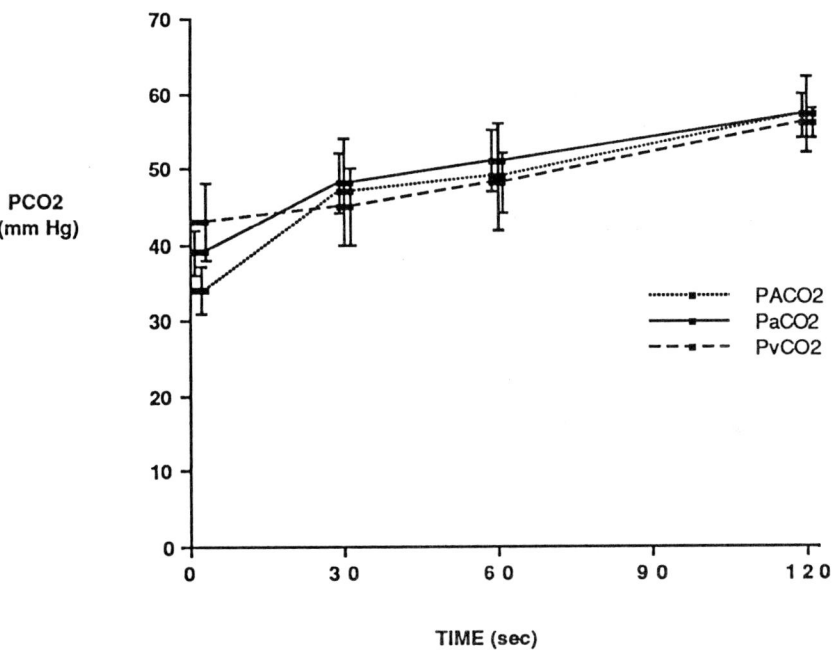

Fig 1. Alveolar, arterial and mixed venous carbon dioxide tensions during apnea in 7 dogs. Data are mean ± SEM.

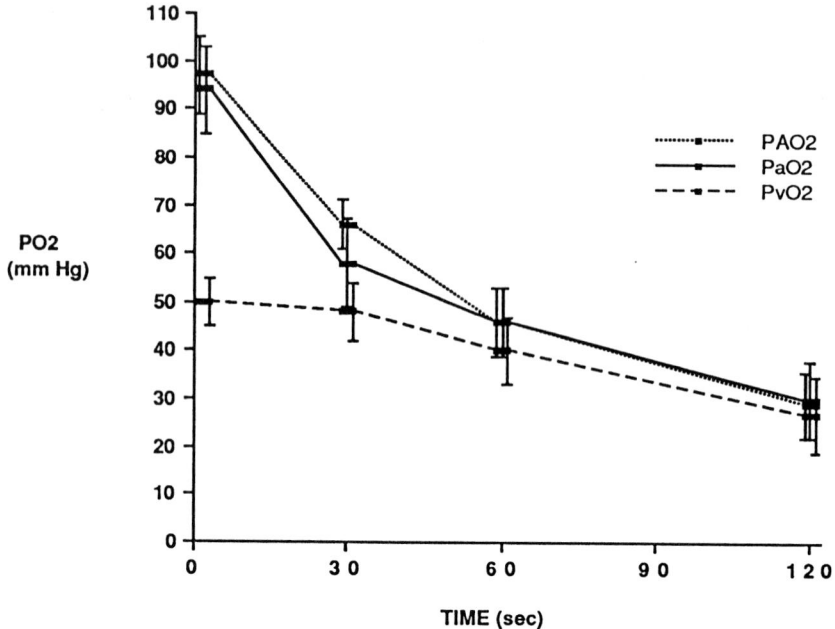

Fig 2. Alveolar, arterial and mixed venous oxygen tensions during apnea in 7 dogs. Data are mean ± SEM.

Figure 3 shows the changes in SaO_2 over time to be essentially linear compared to the prominent curvilinear decrease in PaO_2 that was observed during the initial portion of the apnea. Despite the 17 per cent decline in SaO_2 from 94 per cent to 77 per cent over the initial 30 sec, SvO_2 fell by only 4 per cent indicating relative stability of the O_2 stores in the venous blood. The changes in CaO_2 and CvO_2 directly parallel the changes in SaO_2 and SvO_2.

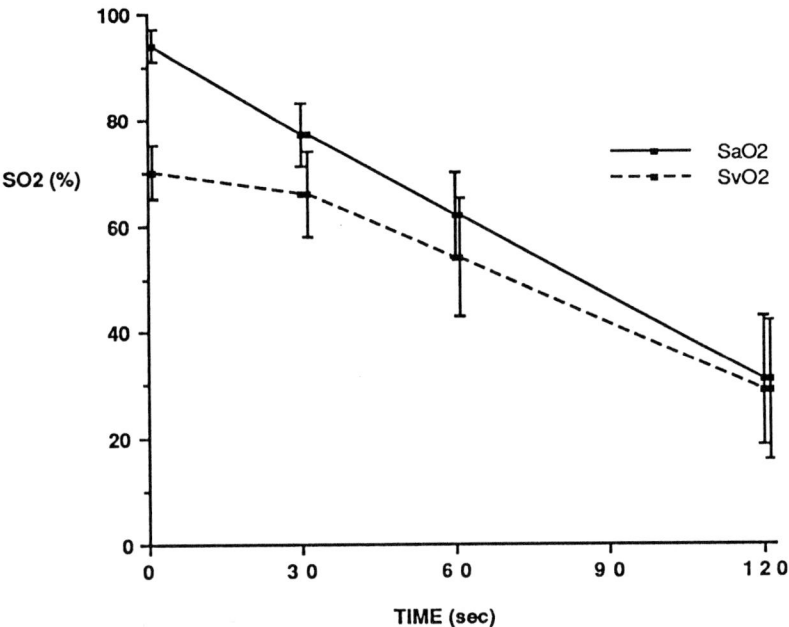

Fig 3. Arterial and mixed venous oxyhemoglobin saturations during apnea in 7 dogs. Data are mean ± SEM.

Figure 4 presents the data for V_TO_2 over time along with the percentages of total O_2 stores that are contributed by each compartment. Calculated V_TO_2 decreased by 140 ml and 136 ml in the first and second minutes of apnea, respectively. These values were slightly less than the measured baseline rate for $\dot{V}O_2$ of 144 ml/min. VvO_2, V_LO_2 and VaO_2 accounted for 46 per cent, 33 per cent and 21 per cent of V_TO_2 prior to apnea. These results indicate that the venous blood contains the greatest reserve of O_2 in the body while the arterial blood contains the least amount of O_2. When combined, the blood compartment contained two-thirds of the dog's O_2 stores compared to one-third in the lung compartment at FRC.

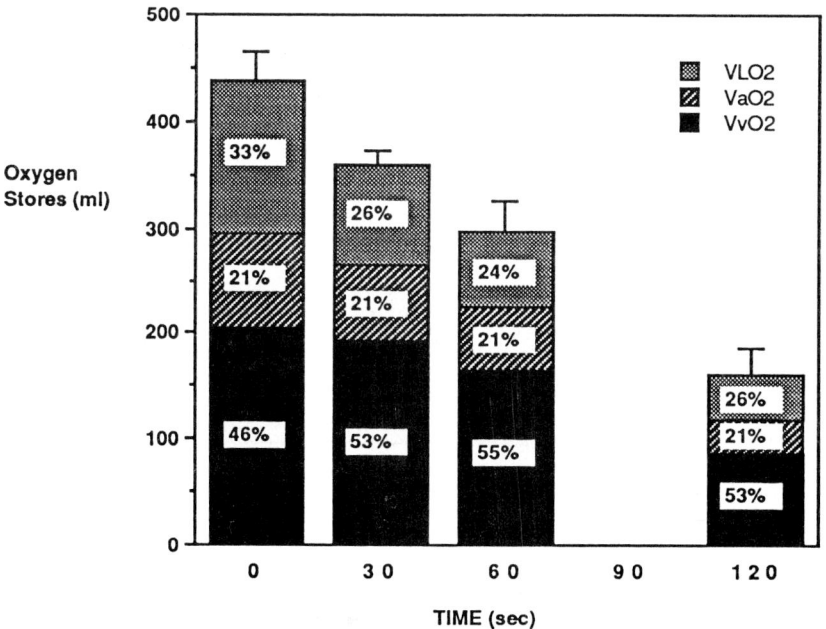

Fig 4. Total (V_TO_2), lung (V_LO_2), arterial blood (VaO_2) and venous blood (VvO_2) oxygen stores during apnea in 7 dogs. Data are mean ± SEM.

Figure 5 shows the relative (per cent) contribution that each of the O_2 storage compartments made to the decrease in total O_2 stores over each specified time interval. During the initial 30 sec, V_LO_2 was preferentially depleted and accounted for 63 per cent of the reduction in V_TO_2. As apnea duration continued, the lung O_2 stores contributed progressive smaller amounts to O_2 consumption. Conversely, the O_2 stores in the venous blood contributed minimally (15 per cent of total) during the initial 30 seconds of apnea compared to providing 57 per cent of the total O_2 requirements of the oxidatively metabolizing tissues during the second minute of apnea. In contrast to the respectively increasing and decreasing roles of the venous blood and lung O_2 stores in meeting total O_2 needs over time, VaO_2 decreased linearly, thereby providing an essentially constant 20-22 per cent of the metabolic needs for O_2 throughout the apneic period.

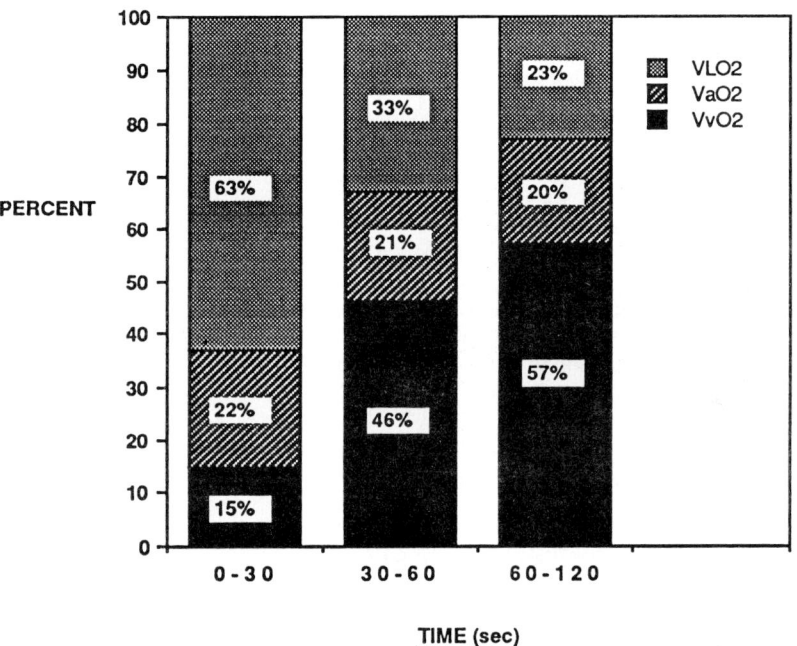

Fig 5. Per cent contributions of the lung (V_LO_2), arterial blood (VaO_2) and venous blood (VvO_2) oxygen stores to total O_2 depletion over initial (0-30 seconds), mid (30-60 seconds) and late (60-120 seconds) phases of apnea in 7 dogs.

DISCUSSION

Direct measurement of the O_2 stores in the lung, arterial and venous blood compartments during apneas of up to 120 seconds duration documented reductions in total O_2 stores which only slightly underestimated baseline oxygen consumption. During the first and second minutes of apnea, V_TO_2 decreased by 140 ml and 136 ml, respectively. These values were not significantly different than the baseline $\dot{V}O_2$ of 144 ml/min. Although PaO_2 reached a nadir of 29 mmHg, there was no evidence for the development of a metabolic acidosis as the decrease in pH of 0.09 was accounted for by the 18 mmHg rise in $PaCO_2$. These results indicate that total O_2 stores in the dog are adequate to meet the tissue demands for oxygen and maintain aerobic metabolism during apneas of up to 120 seconds duration.

The results further indicate that the venous blood compartment is the largest reservoir of O_2 in the dog under the conditions of this study. At FRC, lung O_2 stores were only 33 per cent of total O_2 stores with the arterial and venous blood combined containing 67 per cent of total O_2 stores. Despite the higher content of O_2 in arterial than venous blood, the arterial blood stores of O_2 were only 21 per cent of the total. This is due to the fact that only 25 per cent of total blood volume is considered to be at arterial O_2 tensions.

During the initial 30 seconds of apnea, 63 per cent of the body's needs for O_2 were withdrawn from the O_2 stores in the lung with an additional 22 per cent being provided from the arterial O_2 compartment. Therefore, the O_2 stores in the venous compartment are minimally reduced as reflected by the small decrease in SvO_2 from 70 to 66 per cent. Because the majority of apneas are less than 30 seconds in duration, the O_2 stores of the lung and arterial blood will play the major role in determining the initial rates of O_2 desaturation. During prolonged apneas, the venous O_2 stores become more important with increases in hemoglobin concentration and blood volume playing a greater role.

Although this analysis has neglected tissue O_2 stores, this compartment would represent only a small fraction of total O_2 stores (Cherniak, 1970). Furthermore, since most of the oxygen in tissue is bound to myoglobin, only a small fraction would be utilized as O_2 remains tightly bound to myoglobin until PO_2 falls below 20 mmHg.

In obese patients with obstructive sleep apnea, lung volumes are substantially reduced with many of these individuals essentially breathing at residual volume in the supine position. The reduction in lung O_2 stores that results is considered to play a major role in the rapidity with which these patients desaturate during apnea (Findley et al., 1983). Reductions in F_AO_2 secondary to alveolar hypoventilation will further exacerbate the problem by decreasing O_2 stores within the lung (Strohl & Altose, 1984). Although nasal CPAP works predominantly by maintaining upper airway patency, it has the added benefit of increasing lung volume. This secondary effect of increasing lung O_2 stores would be predicted to have beneficial effects on gas exchange. In fact, it has been demonstrated that increasing lung volume during sleep with continuous negative extrathoracic pressure limits the severity of nocturnal O_2 desaturation in patients with obstructive sleep apnea despite mild prolongations of apnea duration (Series et al., 1989).

REFERENCES

Bradley, T.D., Martinez, D., et al. (1985): Physiological determinants of nocturnal arterial oxygenation in patients with obstructive sleep apnea. *J. Appl. Physiol.* 59, 1364-1368.

Cherniak, N.S. & Longobardo, G.S. (1970): Oxygen and carbon dioxide gas stores of the body. *Physiol. Rev.* 50, 196-243.

Findley, L.J., Ries, A.L., et al. (1983): Hypoxemia during apnea in normal subjects: Mechanisms and impact of lung volume. *J. Appl. Physiol.* 55, 1777-1783.

Guyton, A.C. (1976): The systemic circulation. In *Textbook of Medical Physiology*, ed. A.C. Guyton, pp. 237-249. Philadelphia: W.B. Saunders Company.

Kelman, G.R. (1966): Digital computer subroutine for the conversion of oxygen tension into saturation. *J. Appl. Physiol.* 21, 1375-1376.

Minh, V.-D., Dolan, G.F., et al. (1978): Functional residual capacity and body position in the dog. *J. Appl. Physiol.* 44, 291-296.

Reeves, R.B., Park, J.S., et al. (1982): Oxygen affinity and Bohr coefficients of dog blood. *J. Appl. Physiol.* 53, 87-95.

Series, F., Cormier, Y., et al. (1989): Influence of lung volume in sleep apnea. *Thorax* 44, 52-57.

Shepard, Jr., J.W., Minh, V.-D., et al. (1981): Gas exchange in non-perfused dog lungs. *J Appl Physiol.* 51, 1261-1267.

Shepard, Jr., J.W. (1985): Gas exchange and hemodynamics during sleep. *Med. Clin. North Am.* 69, 1243-1263.

Shepard, Jr., J.W. (1989): Cardiorespiratory changes in obstructive sleep apnea. In *Principles and Practice of Sleep Medicine*, eds. M.H. Kryger, T. Roth, & W.C. Dement, pp. 537-551. Philadelphia: W.B. Saunders Company.

Strohl, K.P. & Altose, M.D. (1984): Oxygen saturation during breath-holding and during apneas in sleep. *Chest* 85, 181-186.

Résumé

Pendant l'apnée, les besoins métaboliques de l'organisme pour l'oxygène doivent être fournis à partir des réserves endogènes d'O_2 dans les poumons, le sang et les tissus. Sept chiens normaux, ont été étudiés pour déterminer comment les principales réserves d'O_2 dans les poumons, le sang artériel et veineux sont utilisées de manière séquentielle pendant l'apnée. Chaque chien était anesthésié, paralysé, ventilé mécaniquement et cannulé pour prélèvements artériel et veineux mêlé. Le volume pulmonaire était mesuré à la capacité résiduelle fonctionnelle (CRF) par élimination d'azote, la consommation d'O_2 (VO_2) par analyse des gaz expirés et le volume sanguin par marquage au ^{51}Cr. Des apnées de 30, 60, 120 secondes ont été réalisées et la fraction alvéolaire (F_AO_2) d'O_2 a été mesurée à la fin des apnées. Les réserves pulmonaires d'O_2 ont été calculées par l'équation : V_LO_2 = FRC x F_AO_2. Les réserves sanguines d'O_2 ont été calculées en supposant que les volumes artériel et veineux représentent respectivement 25 % et 75 % du volume sanguin total. La réserve artérielle d'O_2 est VaO_2 = 0.25 x BV x CaO_2. La réserve veineuse est : V_vO_2 = 0.75 x BV x C_vO_2. Avant l'apnée, la VO_2 était en moyenne de 144 ± 12 ml/min. V_aO_2, V_LO_2, V_vO_2 représentaient respectivement 46 %, 33 % et 21 % des réserves totales en O_2 (V_TO_2). V_aO_2 a diminué linéairement avec le temps d'apnée en représentant dans tous les cas 21 % de la réduction de V_TO_2. A l'inverse, la vitesse de décroissance de V_LO_2 a été initialement rapide puis a diminué avec la prolongation de l'apnée. Pour V_vO_2 l'inverse a été observé. Une diminution minime de V_vO_2 a eu lieu pendant les 30 premières sec d'apnées et a été suivie d'une augmentation de l'utilisation de l'O_2 de ce compartiment avec l'allongement de l'apnée. V_TO_2 a diminué de 140 ml à 136 ml dans la 1ère et la 2ème minute d'apnée. Ces diminutions de V_TO_2 ne sont pas significativement différentes de la VO_2 de base et suggèrent que les réserves totales d'O_2 sont adéquates pour subvenir au métabolisme aérobique pendant des apnées de 120 secondes.

Human sympathetic nerve activity during normal sleep and in sleep apnoea

B. Gunnar Wallin

Department of Clinical Neurophysiology, Sahlgren's Hospital, University of Göteborg, Sweden

INTRODUCTION

During synchronized (non-REM) sleep blood pressure, cardiac output, total peripheral resistance and heart rate have been found to decrease in many species (c.f. Coote, 1982). A further (tonic) fall of blood pressure may occur during desynchronized (REM) sleep but this lower level is often interrupted by irregular shortlasting increases of blood pressure and heart rate. In the cat renal sympathetic nerve traffic was found to decrease during synchronized sleep (Baust et al., 1968). In decerebrated cats exhibiting desynchronized sleep-like (REM) periods mean activity decreased in renal and splanchnic sympathetic fibres but increased in muscle sympathetic fibers (c.f. Coote 1982). During this sleep stage the variability of sympathetic activity in all nerves was much higher because of short-lasting marked increases of sympathetic traffic.

In awake humans the microneurograhpic technique has been used extensively for measurements of sympathetic outflow to skin and muscle (Wallin and Fagius, 1988). Such recordings have shown that sympathetic outflow is differentiated: skin sympathetic activity (SSA) consists of a mixture of impulses (sudomotor, vasoconstrictor and possibly also vasodilator and piloerector impulses) involved in thermoregulation and highly sensitive to emotional reactions. Muscle sympathetic activity (MSA) is dominated by vasoconstrictor impulses contributing to homeostatic blood pressure control. The present report summarizes 1) findings from recent studies of sympathetic nerve traffic in humans during normal sleep (Hornyak et al, 1991) and 2) MSA-data from a group of patients with sleep apnoea (Hedner et al, 1988).

METHODS

Multi-unit nerve recordings were made in the peroneal nerve at the fibular head with tungsten microelectrodes with tip diameters of a few micrometers. A reference electrode was placed subcutaneously 1-2 cm away. The recording electrode was inserted manually into a muscle or in some cases a skin branch and small adjustments were made until a site with good signal to noise ratio for sympathetic impulses was found. In some experiments, blood pressure was recorded in the brachial artery, in others finger blood pressure was monitored continuously with a non-invasive device (Finapres). For sleep staging the following parameters were recorded: 13 bipolar EEG derivations from the fronto-temporal, temporo-central, temporo-temporal, temporo-occipital, centro-parietal, parieto-occipital and the Fz-Cz regions; a submental electromyogram; an electro-oculogram by electrodes at the outer canthi; electrocardiogram by precordial surface electrodes; respiratory movements by a strain gauge attached around the chest with a rubber strap; in some cases nasal and oral air flow was monitored by thermistors. In apnoea patients oxygen saturation was measured continously with a finger oximeter (Biox 3700).

The strength of MSA was analyzed with a computer program which measured the number of sympathetic bursts/min and mean burst area in the integrated neurogram. Total MSA is given as number of bursts x burst mean burst area. For methodological details see Sundlöf and Wallin (1977) and Hornyak et al (1991).

RESULTS

MSA during spontaneous sleep i normal subjects

The normal temporal pattern of MSA did not change during sleep. Thus, in all sleep stages there were irregular sequences of sympathetic bursts which occurred predominantly during temporary blood pressure reductions (see Wallin and Fagius 1988). With increasing depth of synchronized sleep MSA decreased successively and in stage 2 the number of bursts/min was 90 ± 8 % and total MSA was 89 ± 5 % of the value in the awake state (n=14, $P < 0.05$ for both). In deep sleep (stage 3-4) total MSA was 71 % of the awake control value (n=5), which corresponded to a further decrease in four and unchanged level in one subject. Quantitative data from all sleep stages are summarized in fig. 1.

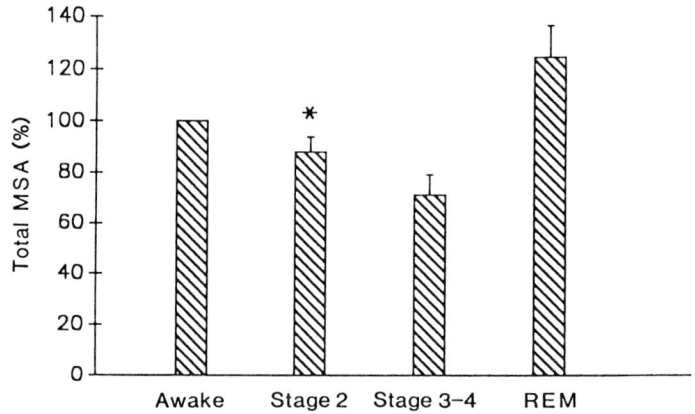

Fig. 1. Total muscle sympathetic activity (MSA) in 5-min periods of sleep stage 2, stage 3-4 and during the whole period of desynchronized (REM) sleep (mean duration: 7.4 min). Total MSA is expressed in percent of the awake value. * indicates significant difference from awake ($p < 0.05$). n=14 in the awake state and stage 2; n=5 in stage 3-4 and in desynchronized (REM) sleep. Reproduced with permission from Hornyak et al (1991).

During desynchronized (REM) sleep total MSA increased to a mean of 124 ± 12 % of the awake value. The increases occurred mainly in short (10-30 s), irregular periods of high amplitude bursts. These periods of high sympathetic activity during desynchronized sleep were often but not always related to rapid eye movements. The increase of total MSA was inversely correlated to the duration of the desynchronized (REM) sleep which may be related to the finding that the longer the period of desynchronized sleep the shorter the relative duration of rapid eye movements.

These findings agree well with data from neural (Baust et al 1968, Coote 1982) and haemodynamic (Mancia et al 1971) recordings in cats and it seems likely that the changes of MSA partly explain the changes of blood pressure during sleep which have been reported previously in humans (e.g. Snyder et al 1964, Kathri and Freis 1967).

The relationship between MSA and K-complexes. In sleep stage 2, high amplitude K-complexes were accompanied by short lasting increases of MSA which had a maximum during the second heart beat following the K-complex (fig. 2). After the peak MSA fell successively to values below the control level and at the sixth heart beat after the K-complex MSA was significantly less than the control, i.e. the value during the cardiac cycle immediately preceding the K-complex. Instantaneous heart rate and blood pressure also increased but reached their peaks at the third and the sixth heart beat after the K-complex, respectively.

Since blood pressure did not fall before or during the MSA-peak our interpretation is that a K-complex is associated with a non-baroreflex mediated increase of vasoconstrictor drive to skeletal muscle vessels which contributes to a succeeding blood pressure increase. In contrast, the MSA reduction following the primary increase coincided with the blood pressure peak (fig. 2) and therefore probably was a baroreflex response. The increase of MSA occurred approximately one second after the first sharp-wave of the K-complex. Since there is a conduction delay for MSA from the brain to the peroneal nerve at the knee of slightly more than one second (Wallin and Fagius 1988) it is likely that activation of sympathetic centres occurs at the same time as cortical activation, i.e. in terms of time relationship both phenomena may have the same origin.

K-complexes are considered to be signs of abortive arousal (Roth et al 1956, Johnson and Karpan, 1968). This interpretation is supported by the finding that K-complexes often are associated with signs of cutaneous vasoconstriction and sweating. In recent microneurographic recordings we have also found that around one second after a K-complex there is a strong discharge of SSA in the peroneal nerve (Noll, Kunimoto, Elam and Wallin, unpublished data). Although MSA is insensitive to arousal in the awake state we hypothetize that conditions are different during sleep and that the K-complex related increase of MSA also is an arousal phenomenon (Hornyak et al 1991).

The functional importance of a K-complex is unknown. However, if the K-complex related increase of sympathetic activity is an indicator of an (internally evoked?) generalized arousal, one may speculate that it has survival value. During deep sleep the low responsiveness to external stimuli makes the individual vulnerable to external threats. Perhaps, therefore, stage 2 sleep is a preparation for deep sleep during which the K-complex related partial awakenings allow the individual a long enough appraisal of the "danger situation" before and between periods of deep sleep.

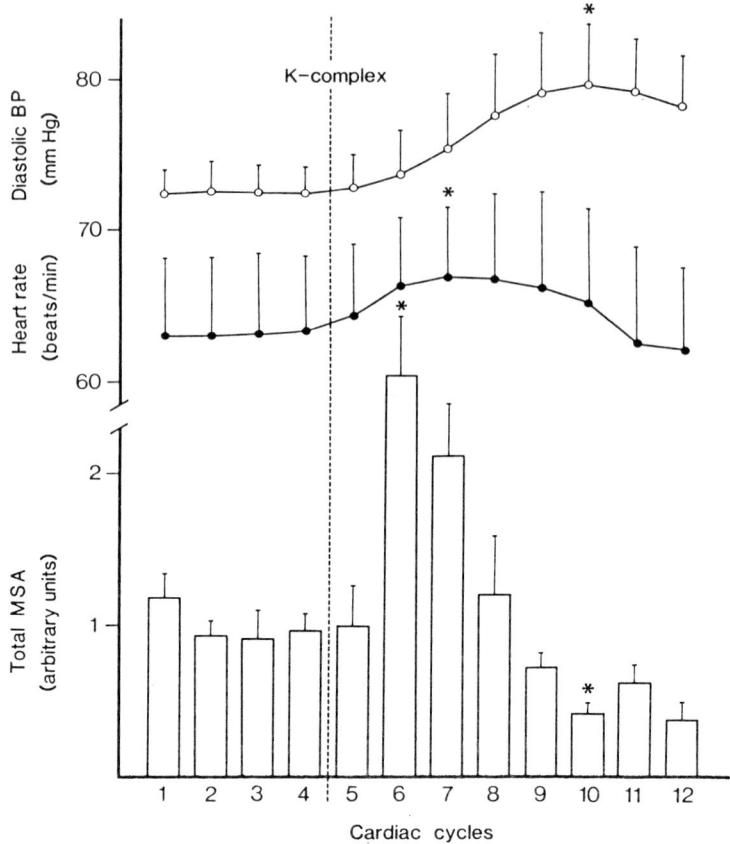

Fig. 2. Changes of total MSA, heart rate and diastolic blood pressure (BP) during 4 cardiac cycles preceding and during 8 cardiac cycles following the first sharp-wave peak of K-complexes (indicated by dashed line) in 6 subjects. MSA values are normalized the mean of the values obtained in 4 heart cycles preceding to a K-complex. * indicates significant difference from the control level (the cardiac cycle immediately preceding the K-complex). Reproduced with permission from Hornyak et al (1991).

MSA in sleep apnoea

A small group of male patients with the sleep apnoea syndrome (n=6, age 47, range 40-52 years, 4 hypertensive and 2 normotensive) have been studied with respect to the level of MSA at rest in the awake state and the change of activity occurring with apnoeic periods during sleep (Hedner et al 1988). The resting level of activity was compared with an age and sex-matched normotensive control group selected blindly from a large material of previous MSA-recordings. In the patients the level of activity was 75 ± 13 bursts/min and in the control group 36 ± 4, (mean ± SE), a difference which was statistically significant ($p < 0.05$, Wilcoxons signed rank test). In an ongoing prospective study results are similar (Karlsson, Hedner, Elam, Cejnar, Ejnell, Wallin, unpublished data).

When the patients were sleeping and had repeated apnoeas there was a typical pattern of sympathetic activity characterized by continously increasing activity during the apnoea, followed by a sudden reduction or cessation of MSA upon onset of ventilation (fig. 3). The pattern was similar during central and obstructive apnoic events. Blood pressure was highly variable and in most patients a clear association with the apnoic breathing pattern was seen. Thus, during the periods when oxygen saturation fell, systolic and diastolic blood pressures were significantly increased.

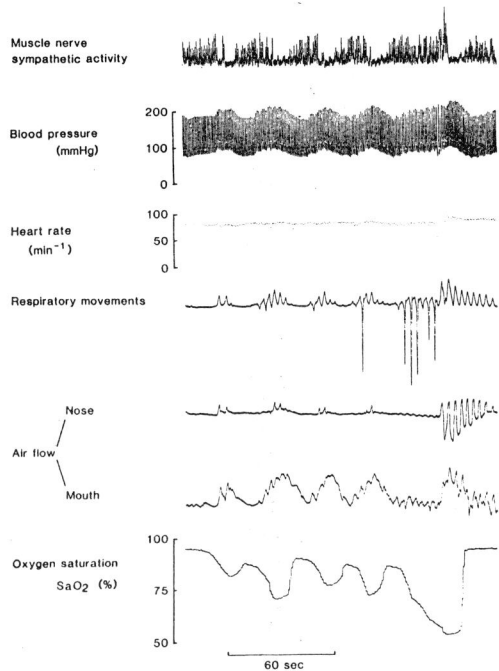

Fig. 3. A representative recording of apnoic events during sleep in a patient with sleep apnoea syndrome. Note that central as well as obstructive apnoic events appear during the recording. The integrated muscle sympathetic activity, arterial blood pressure, heart rate, thoracic movements, nose and mouth air flow, and oxygen saturation curve are shown. The time-scale is indicated at the bottom of the figure. Reproduced with permission from Hedner et al (1988).

Our data suggest that the cyclic changes of blood pressure during repeated apnoeas are due, at least in part, to the periodic variations of MSA which in turn may be caused by a combination of arterial baroreceptor, chemoreceptor and lung receptor reflexes. The mechanisms underlying the increased level of MSA at rest in patients with sleep apnoea is unclear but chemoreceptor mechanisms may be involved since hypoxia and hypercapnea are known to increase MSA in healthy subjects (Somers et al 1989 a,b). If the high MSA-level is a primary phenomenon it may contribute to the development of hypertension in some patients with sleep apnoea.

Acknowledgement: Supported by Swedish Medical Research Council Grant No B91-04X-03546-21A.

REFERENCES

Baust, W., Weidinger, H., Kirchner, F., (1968). Sympathetic activity during natural sleep and arousal. Arch. Ital. Biol., 106, 379-389.

Coote, J.H. (1982). Respiratory and circulatory control during sleep. J. Exp. Biol., 100, 223-244.

Hedner, J., Ejnell, H., Sellgren, J., Hedner, T., Wallin, G. (1988). Is high and fluctuating muscle nerve sympathetic activity in the sleep apnoea syndrome of pathogenetic importance for the development of hypertension? In J. Hypertension, 6 (suppl. 4), 529-531.

Hornyak, M., Cejnar, M., Elam, M, Matousek, M. and Wallin B.G. (1991). Sympathetic muscle nerve activity during sleep in humans. Brain: In press.

Johnson, L.C., Karpan, W.,E. (1968). Autonomic correlates of the spontaneous K-complex. Psychophysiol., 4, 444-452.

Khatri, I.M., Freis, E.D. (1967). Hemodynamic changes during sleep. J. Appl. Physiol. 22, 867-873.

Mancia, G., Baccelli, G., Adams, D.B., Zanchetti, A. (1971). Vasomotor regulation during sleep in the cat. Am. J. Physiol 220, 1086-1093.

Roth, M., Shaw, J., Green, J. (1956). The form, voltage distribution and physiological significance of the K-complex. Electroenc. Clin. Neurophysiol., 8, 385-402.

Snyder, F., Hobson, J.A., Morrison, D.F., Goldfrank, F. (1964). Changes in respiration, heart rate and systolic blood pressure in human sleep. J. Appl. Physiol., 19, 417-422.

Somers, V.K., Mark, A.L., Zavala, D.C. and Abboud, F.M. (1989a). Influence of ventilation and hypocapnia on sympathetic nerve responses to hypoxia in normal humans. J. Appl. Physiol, 67, 2095-2100.

Somers, V.K., Mark, A.L., Zavala, D.C. and Abboud, F.M. (1989b). Contrasting effects of hypoxia and hypercapnia on ventilation and sympathetic activity in humans. J. Appl. Physiol, 67, 2101-2106.

Sundlöf, G., Wallin, B.G. (1977). The variability of muscle nerve sympathetic activity in resting recumbent man. J. Physiol (Lond), 272, 383-397.

Wallin, B.G., Fagius, J. (1988). Peripheral sympathetic neural activity in conscious humans. Ann. Rev. Physiol, 50, 565-576.

Spectral analysis of heart rate and blood pressure in sleep apnea syndrome

T. Penzel, J.H. Peter and P. von Wichert

Medizinische Poliklinik of Philipps, Universitat of Marburg, Baldingerstrasse 1, D-3550 Marburg, Germany

Sleep related breathing disorders have important implications on the cardiovascular system (Podszus 1990). They cause severe sequela and present a major health risk (Peter 1990). One major finding of the cardiovascular implications in sleep related breathing disorders are excessive variations of blood pressure which do exceed changes as they occur in normal sleep. Variations are found to be most prominent in arterial blood pressure and heart rate. The variations accompany the changes of disturbed nocturnal respiration and are tightly connected to the breathing disorder. They are so pronounced that they can be used to detect and to diagnose sleep related breathing disorders. A spectral analysis approach was selected and the application on blood pressure and heart rate was compared in patients with obstructive sleep apnea.

INTRODUCTION

In the past many studies investigated the variation of heart rate and blood pressure. Some studies were based on longterm recordings and thus could analyse sleep related changes (Bond et al. 1973, Zemaityte et al. 1986). Usually heart rate was the subject of this type of investigation (Sayers 1980). Arterial blood pressure was recorded in fewer studies because exact quantitative values were obtained only by invasive techniques (Sleight et al. 1979). Several different rhythms were distinguished in heart rate (Akselrod et al. 1981) which could be found in blood pressure too.
  a) low-frequency: < 0.1 Hz (i.e. > 10 seconds)
  b) mid-frequency: 0.1-0.3 Hz (i.e. 3-10 seconds)
  c) high-frequency: 0.3-0.5 Hz (i.e. 2-3 seconds)
The variations were investigated for many different reasons. Some studies wanted to determine autonomic function (Köpchen 1962, Akselrod et al. 1981, Loula 1991). Under parasympathetic blockade all rhythms were diminished, but low-frequency components could still be found. They also disappeared in the case of total autonomic blockade. Other studies investigated the circadian variation of heart rate. Beside the circadian pattern (i.e. heart rate during sleep is lower than during the day) changes of the ultradian rhythms were analysed. It was found that heart rate variability did rise during sleep (Malpas & Purdie 1990). Some studies recorded blood pressure in normals and in hypertensive patients to look for differences in the corresponding circadian patterns. Differences in the circadian pattern often are very pronounced and then intermittent non-invasive blood pressure recording is perfectly sufficient to recognize these differences. Some studies slightly changed frequency bands for their rhythm analysis or they even adapted the frequency bands according to the individual frequency pattern of every patient (Zemaityte et al 1986). Respiratory sinus

arrhythmia was found in almost all heart rate studies and was subject for intensive investigations (Melcher 1976). Few studies especially looked for 10-second rhythms but interpretation of this particular rhythm still is not clarified.

Only few studies did set variations of heart rate in relation to sleep related breathing disorders (Guilleminault et al. 1984, Penzel 1987a, Ichimaru & Yanaga 1989). The typical cyclical variation of heart rate (CVHR) as accompanies sleep apnea was used as a screening methodology for obstructive sleep apnea. The recurrent temporal pattern of CVHR characterized by relative bradicardia and relative tachycardia has a duration of 30 to 60 seconds which corresponds directly to the duration of an "apnea cycle". This is defined as the sum of apnea duration and the duration of compensating hyperventilation. It was described that cyclical variation of blood pressure (CVBP) does acompany obstructive sleep apnea in the same way as CVHR (Mayer et al. 1988, Peter 1990). As continuous invasive blood pressure recordings only were performed under clinical supervision, this technique never was used as a screening technique. Technical innovation allows non-invasive continous blood pressure recording using finger photo-plethysmography (Wesseling et al. 1986). Today this technique was improved and becomes portable. Thus it is possible to use CVBP instead of CVHR as a screening technique for sleep apnea. To show the use of CVBP we performed spectral analysis in both signals (i.e. heart rate and arterial blood pressure) in patients with sleep apnea. The goal was to compare the recognition of the apnea associated 30 to 60 second rhythms as detected in the two different signals.

METHODOLOGIC APPROACH

52 patients with hypertension and sleep apnea underwent polysomnography in a sleep laboratory with parallel invasive arterial blood pressure recording. All signals were recorded on an eight-channel FM tape recorder for the duration of the entire night. Blood pressure and ECG were digitized by computer (Intertechnique IN 1200) at 32 times realtime with a sampling rate corresponding to 60 Hz. The ECG was evaluated to calculate heart rate beat to beat. With each R-wave detected in the ECG a search started in the sampled blood pressure signal to find the next minimum. This is diastolic blood pressure. The next maximum was taken as systolic pressure. This ECG triggered method of blood pressure analysis has the advantage that only a short undisturbed segment of the blood pressure signal is required (Kalli 1987, Penzel et al. 1987b). For data compression the values of heart rate, systolic and diastolic pressure are stored at a low sampling rate of 1 Hz. Mean blood pressure does not need ECG and is calculated once per second as the mean of all 120 signal samples within two seconds. All together four values are stored once per second in a compressed data file. Thus the data file contains values which are equidistant in time. This is a prerequisite for spectral analysis.

Compressed systolic blood pressure and heart rate underwent spectral analysis by means of Fast Fourier Transform (FFT). Signals were divided in consecutive segments of five minutes (300 seconds) and FFT was performed on windows of 1024 samples after removal of the mean value of the data segment. Thereby a frequency resolution of 0.00195 Hz was reached. Compressed spectral arrays (Cerutti et al. 1989) were plotted for each parameter and each recording.

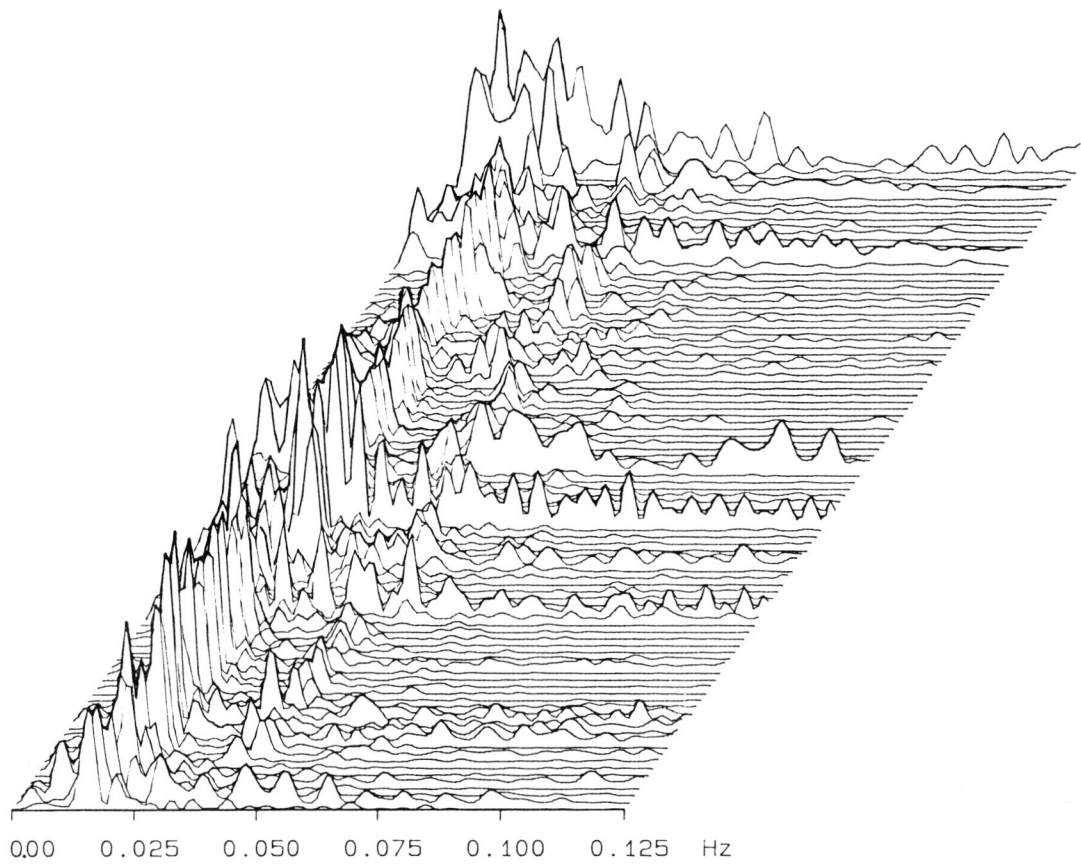

Fig. 1. A compressed spectral array of heart rate. Each single line was calculated out of 5 minutes of data. The entire plot covers eight hours. This subject shows pronounced heart rate variations and an apnea index of 70 phases/hour. The regularly recurring apneas are reflected in a clear periodicity at about 0.015 Hz (this corresponds to a periodicity of 66 seconds). Two major disturbances can be recognized: one in the middle of the plot and the other one at the end of the plot. Both correspond to episodes of REM sleep. The very end of the plot was disturbed due to awaking of the patient.

APPLICATON OF SPECTRAL ANALYSIS: RESULTS AND DISCUSSION

The application of spectral analysis could reveal the occurance of the cyclical pattern of apnea associated heart rate, CVHR (fig. 1) and blood pressure (fig. 2) changes, CVBP. The absence of this particular rhythm can be proved by this method also (fig. 3). The limitations of spectral analysis must be mentioned here. Spectral analysis is not the appropriate method if the temporal pattern of signals is disturbed in a way that no consistent rhythm is preserved. This happens typically during REM sleep but occurs also in patients with other cardiovascular diseases beside sleep apnea. These difficulties are present in patients with autonomic dysfunction, persistent arrhythmias

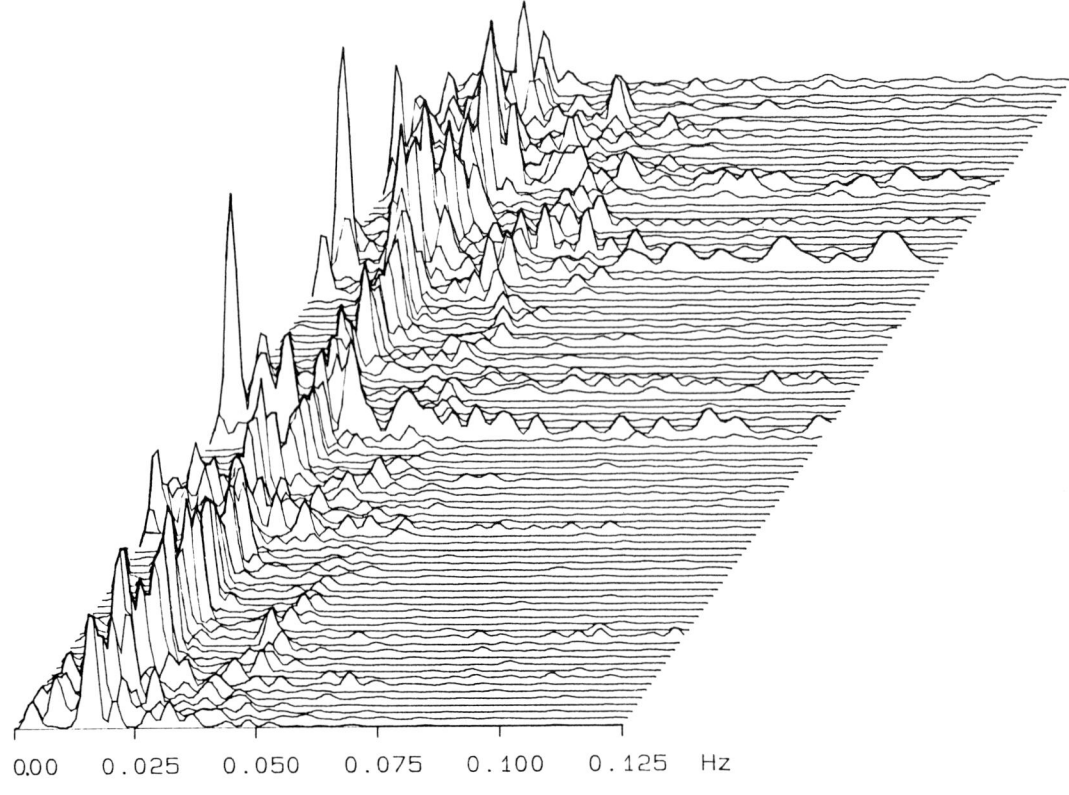

Fig. 2. A compressed spectral array of systolic blood pressure of the same subject as fig. 1. The same method as in fig. 1. was applied to the same recording. Comparing the two spectral arrays the same disurbances can be recognized. Over all this spectral array of systolic blood pressure is less disturbed than the corresponding one calculated from heart rate.

and hypoventilation syndromes. This means the absence of apnea related rhythms CVHR or CVBP in a spectral analysis does not exclude sleep related breathing disorders. But the presence of these rhythms gives clear indications for further investigations.
Comparing the spectral analysis of heart rate and blood pressure it became evident, that systolic blood pressure variation is less likely to be disturbed. The influence of some ectopic beats is less remarkable than in the analysis of heart rate. In addition it becomes clear that blood pressure variation CVBP is more sensitive to obstructive apnea and hypopnea than heart rate variation CVHR and can be used more effective to preselect patients with sleep related breathing disorders.

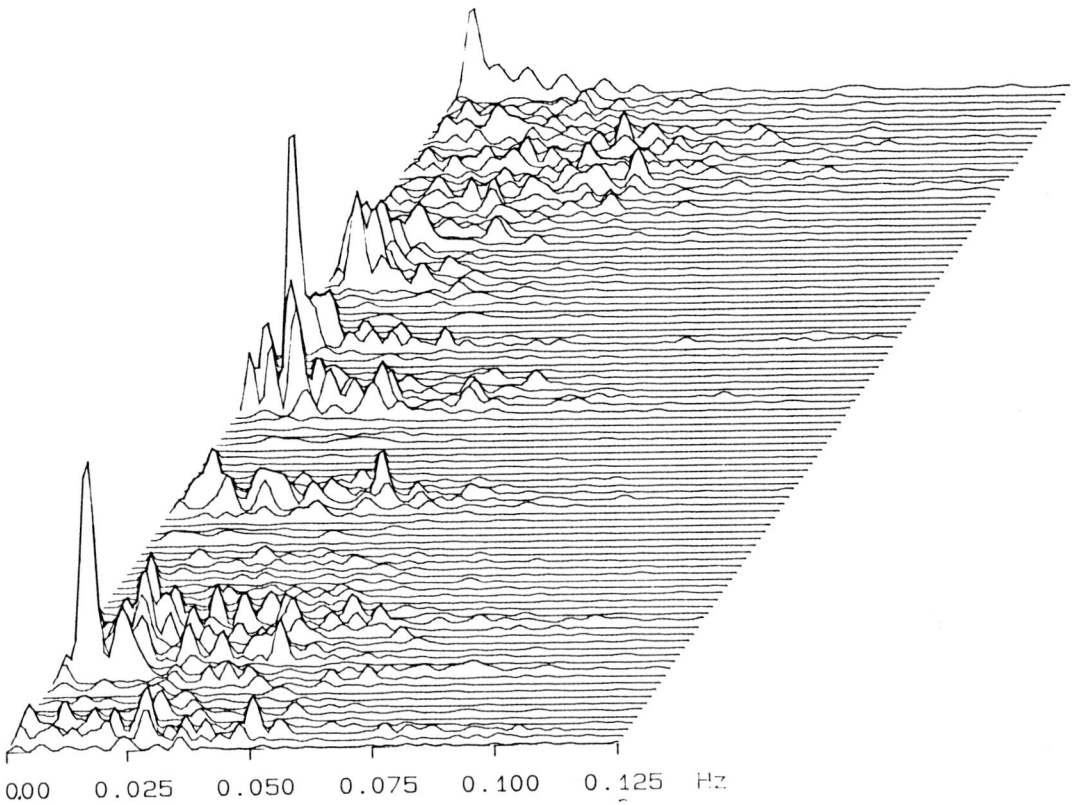

Fig. 3. A compressed spectral array of heart rate. The same method as described in fig. 1 was applied. This patient had only few apneas during this night of recording. The apnea index was 3 phases/hour. Compared to fig. 1. and fig. 2. the absence of typical apnea associated rhythms is obvious. The occurance of the disturbance may be caused by some irregular apneas and hypopneas as well as by heart rate fluctuations during REM sleep.

CONCLUSION

The application of spectral analysis on heart rate and systolic blood pressure can give indications for sleep related breathing disorders, if they appear in a clear periodicity. Some types of sleep related breathing disorders (i.e. hypoventilation syndromes) do no longer have a periodic occurance. As a consequence the variation of heart rate CVHR and blood pressure CVBP do not occur periodically. Than the spectral analyis approach fails. The analysis of blood pressure is less disturbed than heart rate. The non-invasive continuous recording of blood pressure thus allows easier recognition of sleep related breathing disorders than using heart rate. As for this type of analysis absolute blood pressure values are not important, an absolute accuracy of non-invasive blood pressure values are not required this approach. Only relative changes in pressure must be recorded in acceptable accuracy which can be done by finger photo-plethysmography. Future screening devices for sleep apnea may then replace their heart rate recording by systolic blood pressure recording by means of non-invasive techniques to gain sensitivity on sleep apnea recognition and periodic hypoventilation diagnosis.

REFERENCES

Akselrod, S., Gordon, D., Ubel, F.A., Shannon, D.C., Barger, A.C., Cohen, R.J. (1981): Power spectrum analysis of heart rate fluctuations: a quantitative prove of beat-to-beat cardiovascular control. Science 213:220-222.

Bond, W.C., Bohs, C., Ebey, J. and Wolf, S. (1973): Rhythmic heart rate variability (sinus arrhythmia) related to stages of sleep. Condit. reflex 8:98-107.

Cerutti, S., Bianchi, A., Baselli, G., Civardi, S., Guzzetti, S., Malliani, A., Pagani, A., Pagani, M. (1989): Compressed spectral arrays for the analysis of 24-hr heart rate variability signal: enhancement of parameters and data reduction. Comp. and biomed. res. 22:424-441.

de Boer, R.W., Karemaker, J.M., Strackee, J. (1985): Relationships between short-term blood-pressure fluctuations and heart-rate variability in resting subjects I: a spectral analysis approach. Med. & Biol. Eng. & Comput. 23:352-358.

Findley, L.J., Farkas, G.A. and Rochester, D.F. (1985): Changes in heart rate during breathing interrupted by recurrent apneas in humans. J. Appl. Physiol. 59: 536-542.

Guilleminault, C., Connolly, S., Winkle, R., Melvin, K. and Tilkian, A. (1984): Cyclical variation of the heart rate in sleep apnoea syndrome. Mechanisms, and usefulness of 24h electrocardiography as a screening technique. Lancet I: 126-131.

Ichimaru, Y. and Yanaga, T. (1989): Frequency characteristics of the heart rate variability produced by Cheyne-Stokes respiration during 24-hr ambulatory electrocardiographic monitoring. Comput. Biomed. Res. 22:225-233.

Kalli, S. (1987): Computerized analysis and modelling of blood pressure. Espoo, Technical research center of Finland, publ. 35.

Köpchen, H.P. (1962): Die Blutdruckrhythmik. Darmstadt, Steinkopff Verlag pp:1-139.

Loula, P. (1991): Analysis of EEG and heart rate signals during anaesthesia and autonomic function tests. Thesis, Tampere (Finland) pp 1-89.

Malpas, S.C. and Purdie, G.L. (1990): Circadian variation of heart rate variability. Cardiovasc. res. 24:210-213.

Mayer, J., Becker, H., Brandenburg, U., Penzel, T., Peter, J.H., Podszus, T., Weiner, T. and von Wichert P. (1988): Blood pressure variability and nocturnal blood pressure profile in sleep apnea under nasal continuous positive airway pressure (nCPAP) therapy. In: Duron, B. and Lévi-Valensi, P. (eds.) Sleep Disorders and Respiration. Colloque INSERM/John Libbey Eurotext Ltd. vol. 168 pp 241-243.

Melcher, A. (1976): Respiratory sinus arrhythmia in man. Acta physiol. scand. suppl. 435:1-31.

Penzel, T. (1987a): Monitoring cyclical variation of heart rate in patients with nocturnal disturbances in respiratory regulation. In: Hildebrandt, G., Moog, R. and Raschke, F. (eds.) Chronobiology & Chronomedicine. Basic Research and Applications. Frankfurt, Bern, New York, Peter Lang Verlag pp 155-159.

Penzel, T., Peter, J.H. and von Wichert, P. (1987b): Konzepte für die rationelle Erfassung und Auswertung polysomnographischer Daten bei Pateinten mit schlafbezogenen Atemregulationsstörungen. Prax. Klin. Pneumol. 41:411-416.

Peter, J.H. (1990) Sleep apnea and cardiovascular diseases. In: Guilleminault, C. and Partinen, M. (eds.) Obstructive sleep apnea syndrome: clinical research and treatment. New York, Raven press pp 81-98.

Podszus, T. (1990) Hemodynamics in sleep apnea. In: Issa, F.G., Suratt, P.M. and Remmers, J.E. (eds.) Sleep and Respiration. New York, Wiley-Liss Inc. pp 353-361.

Sayers, B.McA. (1980): Signal analysis of heart-rate variability. In: Kitney, R.I. and Rompelman, O. (eds.) The study of heart-rate variability. Oxford, Clarendon press pp 27-58.

Sleight, P, Floras, J., Jones, J.V. (1979): Automatic analysis of continuous intra-arterial blood pressure recordings. In:Clement, D.L. (ed.) Blood pressure variability. Proc. of the Int. Workshop on blood pressure variability Ghent 1978. MTP press pp 61-88.

Wesseling, K.H., Settels, J.J. and de Wit, B. (1986): The measurement of continuous finger arterial pressure noninvasively in stationary subjects. In: Schmidt, T.H., Dembroski, T.M. and Blümchen, G. (eds.) <u>Biological and psychological factors in cardiovascular disease.</u> Berlin, Heidelberg, Springer Verlag pp 355-375.

Zemaityte, D., Varoneckas, G., Plauska, K., Kaukenas, J. (1986): Components of the heart rhythm power spectrum in wakefulness and individual sleep stages. <u>Intl. J. of Psychophysiol.</u> 4:129-141.

Résumé

Les anomalies respiratoires du sommeil ont des conséquences importantes sur le système cardio-vasculaire (Podszus 1990) ; elles sont responsables de séquelles sévères et sont un risque majeur de santé publique (Peter 1990). Une des principales modifications cardio-vasculaires des anomalies respiratoires du sommeil est la variabilité excessive de pression artérielle qui dépasse celle qui est normalement constatée au cours du sommeil normal. Les variations les plus importantes concernent la pression artérielle et la fréquence cardiaque. Ces variations accompagnent les modifications des anomalies respiratoires nocturnes et sont intimement liées à la maladie respiratoire. Elles sont si importantes qu'elles peuvent être utilisées pour dépister et diagnostiquer les anomalies respiratoires du sommeil. Une approche par analyse spectrale appliquée à la pression artérielle et à la fréquence cardiaque a été comparée chez des patients porteurs de syndrome d'apnées du sommeil.

Cardiorespiratory autonomic reflex behaviour during sleep

Michael D. Goldman, Kenneth R. Casey* and Christopher R. Jones**

*Sleep Disorders Center, Medical College of PA, Phila, PA, *Virginia Mason Clinic, Seattle, WA, and **University of Utah, Salt Lake City, UT, USA*

ABSTRACT: Digital (finger) plethysmography is a well established technique to assess skin sympathetic vasoconstrictor tone. Vasoconstriction is transiently observed during wakefulness and sleep after a deep breath, and is accompanied by increased discharge in skin sympathetic nerves. Vasodilation during nonREM sleep has been reported in young normal subjects at sea level. In the present study at 1400 M altitude, middle aged normal subjects show vasodilation during nonREM sleep and variable changes in REM sleep. Middle aged patients with sleep apnea (OSA) show vasoconstriction during regular respiration during both nonREM and REM sleep; and hypertensive OSA patients show greater vasoconstriction during nonREM sleep than normotensive OSA patients. Skin vasoconstriction for 20-30 seconds immediately after the onset of hyperpnea following obstructive apnea is prominent in the present study in OSA patients at sea level as well as 1400 M altitude. At both altitudes, blood pressure increases markedly during this hyperpnea. In contrast, middle aged patients at sea level with OSA have been reported to show decreased muscle sympathetic nerve discharge during the hyperpnea following obstructive apnea. This raises the question of the significance of the association between skin sympathetic vasoconstrictor activity and the hypertensive response during episodic hyperventilation during sleep in patients with OSA.

This paper considers some recent findings relating to simple noninvasive cardiorespiratory measurements in humans. These findings are modest extensions of previous work, and make use of old and well established measurement techniques, as well as newer technology. Measurements presented in this paper concern digital (finger) plethysmography, finger arterial pressure, and respirtory movements of the thorax and abdomen. It is appropriate that this paper follows closely after that of Dr. Wallin, since it was his studies that stimulated our analysis of these results.

Digital plethymsography was shown more than 50 years ago (Burton, 1939) to be useful in characterizing autonomic reflex behaviour of the peripheral (skin) circulation. The size of the volume pulsation with each cardiac cycle is closely correlated with blood flow to the finger. Marked decreases in volume pulsation were seen with a deep breath, and in response to the stimulation of pain or startle. Skin vasoconstriction was more sensitive to these latter influences than changes in heart rate or blood pressure.

Changes in skin blood flow show bilateral symmetry, and are simultaneous over large portions of the peripheral vascular bed. Simultaneous changes in cardiac rate and blood pressure are consistent with sympathetic and vagal modulation, such that blood pressure rises during skin vasoconstriction. Heart rate shows a biphasic response with an initial increase during vasoconstriction, followed by a decrease in response to the rise in blood pressure. Corresponding changes in electrical activity in sympathetic nerves have been known for decades. In contrast, changes in skin blood flow are in phase with those of systemic blood pressure in sympathectomized limbs, consistent with passive increases in flow in response to blood pressure changes.

Subsequent studies (Khatri and Freis, 1967a,b) of finger pulse volume have shown that pulse volume increases in normal subjects during sleep compared with wakefulness and pilot data suggested that hypertensive patients showed similar vasodilation during sleep. However, a more recent study (Zweifler et al, 1982) in normals and patients with borderline hypertension showed decreased finger volume pulsation in hypertensive patients.

Changes in skin circulation differ from those occurring simultaneously in muscles, and this is reflected in corresponding differences in muscle and skin sympathetic nerve activity (Delius et al, 1972, Wallin and Fagius, 1986). Skin sympathetic nerve activity shows changes relative to respiratory events which are closely comparable to those of skin vasoconstriction.

Recently, a noninvasive automated method has been developed for continuously recording arterial pressure in the finger and a device for measuring finger arterial pressure is now commercially available which yields measurements which correlate closely with invasive intraarterial pressures (FINAPRES).

The present studies have focused on noninvasive measurements of digital arterial pulsation volume and pressure in relation to respiratory events during wakefulness compared with sleep. Respiratory movements of the thorax and abdomen have been measured with the respiratory inductive plethysmograph.

An initial pilot study at 1400 M altitude evaluated digital (finger) plethysmographic volume changes as an index of changes in skin sympathetic vasoconstrictor tone during wakefulness and sleep. We monitored 28 middle aged patients referred for evaluation of clinically suspected sleep apnea syndrome. We measured pulse volume amplitude during the first half of the night during epochs of stage 2 NREM and REM sleep, avoiding periods of large changes in tidal volume. Patients were monitored with the usual polysomnographic parameters, and in addition, brachial artery blood pressure was measured automatically at 5-10 min intervals during one hour of wakefulness prior to sleep onset and throughout the night.

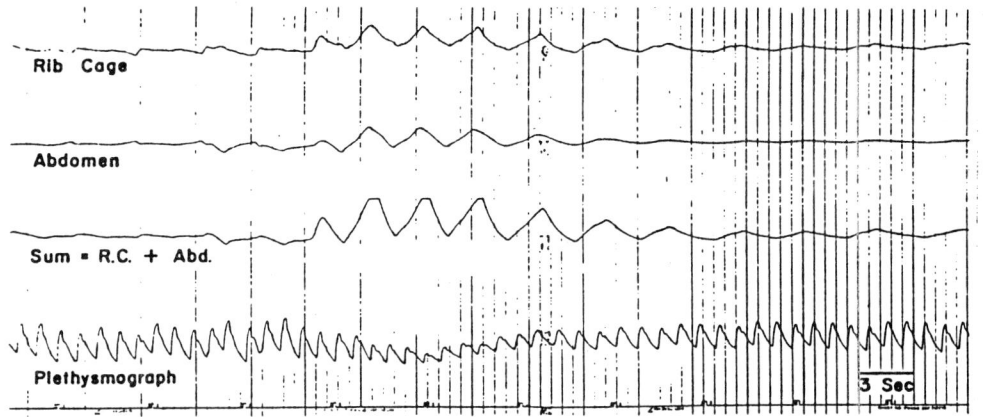

Figure 1. Polygraphic tracings of thoracic and abdominal movements and finger plethysmograph in a patient with OSA during stage 2 sleep. Note paradoxical movements of rib cage and abdomen typical of obstructive apnea, followed by hyperpnea. Finger plethysmograph tracing shows vasoconstriction after the deep inspirations begin.

Figure 1 shows recordings of finger pulse volume and respiratory movements in a patient with obstructive sleep apnea (OSA) during transitional (stage 2) sleep. Note the decrease in finger arterial pulsations following the deep inspirations. Such periods of intermittent apnea were avoided for the purpose of measuring baseline wakeful and sleeping finger pulse volume amplitudes in the present investigation.

We found that finger pulse volume decreased significantly during early NREM sleep in 19 patients with OSA to 70 ± 22 % of waking baseline (WB), in contrast to an increase to 130 ± 42 % WB in 9 patients without apnea. These changes could not be attributed to passive responses to changes in mean arterial or pulse pressures which were comparable in the two groups. During REM sleep, pulse amplitude in patients with OSA was 62 ± 22 % WB, while in patients without apnea it was 123 ± 98 % WB. These differences also could not be attributed to passive responses to changes in arterial pressures.

Among patients with OSA, 11 patients with daytime hypertension had significantly smaller finger pulse amplitudes during NREM sleep (60 ± 16 % WB) than 8 normotensive patients (83 ± 22 % WB). During REM sleep, hypertensive patients had no further change in pulse amplitude (59 ± 19 % WB), while normotensive patients showed a trend toward decreased (relative to NREM) finger pulse amplitudes (67 ± 26 % WB).

These preliminary results suggest that middle aged patients with OSA manifest peripheral skin vasoconstriction during both NREM and REM sleep at 1400 M altitude. This is in contrast to similar patients without sleep apnea, whose finger pulsation amplitude changes are consistent with vasodilation during NREM, and for the most part, during REM sleep as well. The patients without sleep apnea manifested similar results to those reported in young healthy normal subjects at sea level (Khatri and Freis, 1967a) during NREM sleep, while there was substantial variability during NREM sleep.

Patients with daytime hypertension and sleep apnea manifest more severe vasoconstriction during NREM sleep than normotensive sleep apnea patients. This apparent difference in skin sympathetic reactivity occurred in spite of no difference in severity of apnea, as measured by cumulative arterial oxygen desaturation. The significance of differences in skin sympathetic vasoconstrictor activity is not clear from these studies. However, Hedner and coworkers (Hedner et al, 1988) have recently shown greater muscle sympathetic nerve activity in OSA patients than in controls during wakefulness and sleep. Further observations of blood pressure changes and skin and muscle sympathetic activity may shed more light on this issue.

We have further evaluated autonomic reflex behaviour from continuous noninvasive measurements of arterial pressure (FINAPRES, OHMEDA). We report here representative results from among 21 nocturnal studies in young subjects with asthma, middle aged males with occasional snoring, and middle aged patients with OSA.

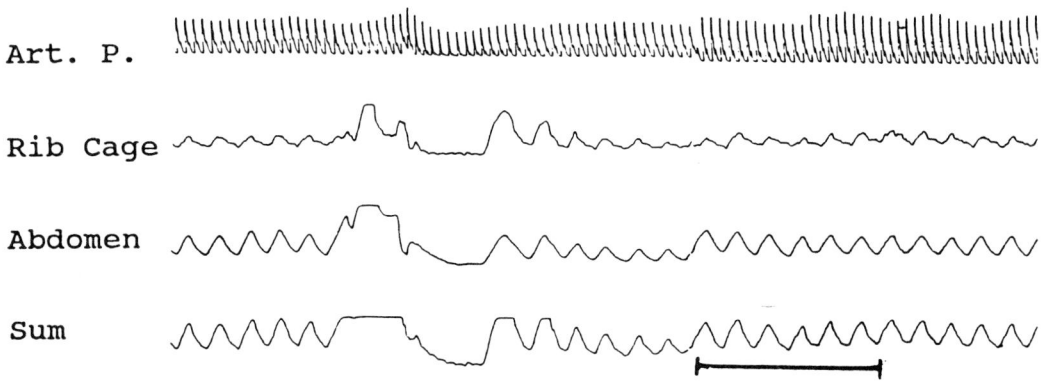

Figure 2. Polygraphic tracings of arterial pressure (FINAPRES) and thoracic and abdominal movements in a normal middle aged male during wakefulness. Note the spontaneous deep breath (sigh) after the fifth breath, followed by an increase in arterial pressure. After several subsequent breaths, arterial pressure shows oscillations with a period of approximately 20 seconds. Time marker = 30 seconds.

Figure 2 shows a recording of finger arterial pressure and respiratory movements during wakefulness in a middle aged male with occasional snoring. Slow oscillations of pressure are seen which have a period of approximately 20 seconds. These oscillations may correspond to the so-called Traube-Hering-Mayer waves, although we have no direct evidence of their mechanism in normal humans. The effect of a spontaneous sigh during wakefulness is also illustrated. The rise in arterial pressure is greater after the deep inspiration, and is followed by cardiac slowing.

Figure 3 shows a recording of finger arterial pressure (FINAPRES) and respiratory movements during wakefulness in a normal subject. Records are obtained by computer assisted data acquisition. The effect of high inspiratory airflow resistance is illustrated: with each inspiration, arterial pressure falls and rises during expiration ("pulsus paradoxus").

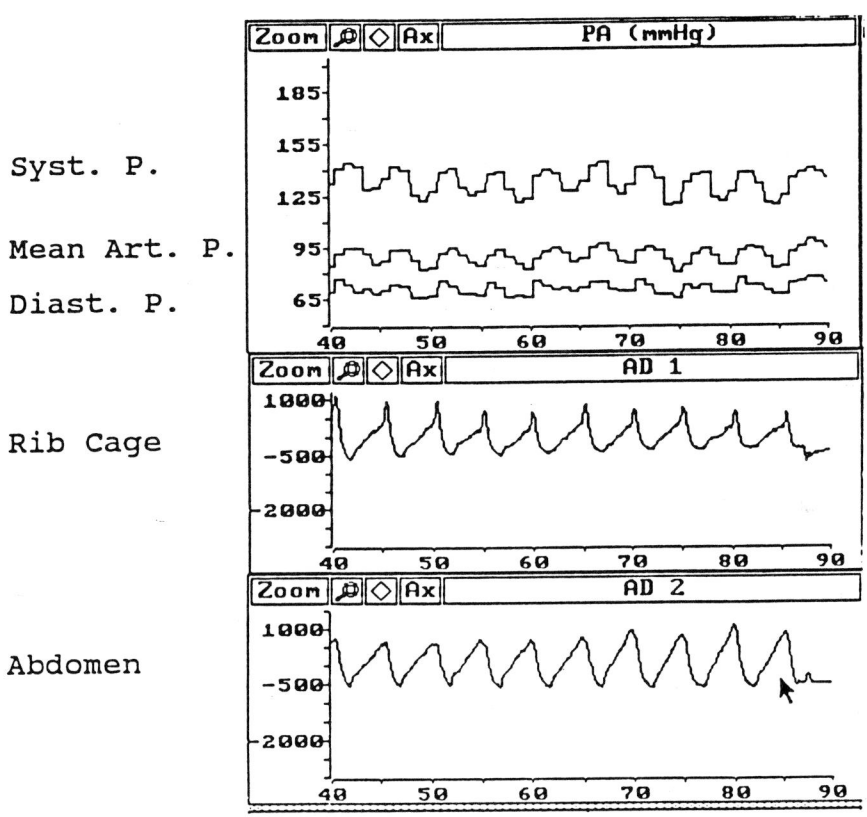

Figure 3. Computer assisted data acquisition of finger arterial pressure (FINAPRES) and thoracic and abdominal movements in a normal subject during wakefulness, breathing through an inspiratory resistance. The individual values of systolic, mean, and diastolic pressure are plotted for each cardiac cycle, and the computer draws a line connecting each value. Note the fall in arterial pressures during each inspiration ("pulsus paradoxus") and abrupt increase in ribcage movements at the end of inspiration, associated with release of "negative" intrathoracic pressure. Time axis labeled in seconds.

Figure 4 shows similar computer assisted data acquisition in a normal human subject and a patient with OSA during sleep. The upper panel shows a normal subject, illustrating small (5-10 mm Hg) oscillations in systolic pressure with a period of about 15 seconds occurring one to four times per minute. These oscillations appear similar to those during wakefulness illustrated in figure 2. In addition, very small (1-2 mm Hg) changes in systolic and diastolic pressure occurring with a respiratory rhythm (16-18 times per minute) are seen (pulsus paradoxus).

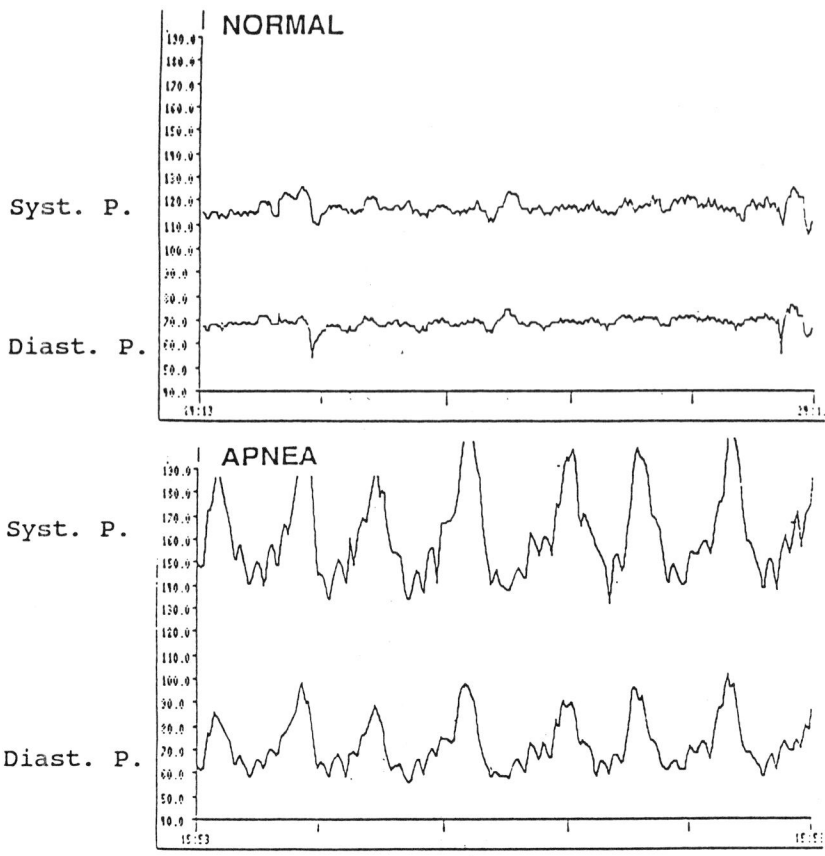

Figure 4. Computer assisted data acquisition from FINAPRES. Individual values of systolic and diastolic pressure are plotted for each cardiac cycle, and the computer draws a line connecting these values. Each tic on time axis indicates one minute.

The lower panel of figure 4 shows similar recordings in a patient with OSA. Cyclic rises in arterial pressures are seen approximately every 40 seconds, in phase with the hyperpnea following each apneic cycle. During each apnea a marked pulsus paradoxus is seen (10-15 mm Hg), which occurs with each obstructed inspiratory effort. These cyclic rises in arterial pressure during the hyperpnea following apnea have been described previously (Shephard, 1985). They are identical in character to those seen in anesthetized animals, mediated via chemoreceptor pathways (Andersson et al 1950). There is also an important chemoreceptor influence on arterial pressure in normally sleeping animals (Guazzi et al, 1966).

Hedner observed (Hedner et al, 1988) that muscle synpathetic nerve activity progressively increases during apnea and suddenly decreases markedly at the onset of ventilation (hyperpnea) following apnea. This finding is in contrast to our findings of marked finger vasoconstriction and hypertension during the hyperpnea following apnea. It raises the possibility that skin sympathetic vasoconstrictor activity, in contrast to muscle sympathetic nerve activity is closely associated with the hypertensive response during episodes of hyperventilation in patients with OSA. Whether this association is fortuitous, or whether it reflects a relatively greater influence of the skin circulation during sleep when muscle activity is normally reduced and skin circulation normally increased remains to be investigated.

It may be argued that, in view of the simultaneous EEG arousal which commonly occurs during the hyperpnea following apnea, some degree of increase in arterial pressure would be expected. On the other hand, it is of interest that patients with OSA do not show the expected progressive fall in arterial pressure during sleep, as occurs in normal subjects and even patients with essential hypertension (Tilkian et al, 1976). It is possible that the increase in sympathetic autonomic tone associated with hypoxia (Sylvester et al, 1979) is associated with both the increased arterial pressure and increased skin sympathetic vasoconstrictor tone in patients with OSA. This is consistent with a finding of increased skin vasoconstrictor tone in our patients with OSA.

REFERENCES

ANDERSSON, B., R.KENNEY and E.NEIL (1950). The role of the chemoceptors of the carotid and aortic regions in the production of the Mayer waves. Acta. Physiol. Scand. 20:203-220.

BURTON, A. (1939). The range and variability of the blood flow in the human fingers and the vasomotor regulation of body temperature. Am. J. Physiol. 127:437-453.

DELIUS, W., K.HAGBARTH, A.HONGELL and B.WALLIN (1972). Manoeuvres affecting sympathetic outflow in human skin nerves. Acta Physiol. Scand. 84: 177-186.

ECKBERG, D., M.DRABINSKY and E.BRAUNWALD (1971). Defective cardiac parasympathetic control in patients with heart disease. N. Engl. J. Med. 285:877-883.

HEDNER, J., H. EJNELL, J. SELLGREN, T. HEDNER, G. WALLIN (1988). Is high and fluctuating muscle nerve sumpathetic activity in the sleep apnoea syndrome of pathogenetic importance for the development of hypertension? J. Hyperten. 6 (suppl 4):S529-S531.

KHATRI, I. and E.FREIS (1967a). Hemodynamic changes during sleep. J. App. Physiol 22:867-873.

KHATRI, I. and E.FREIS (1967b). Hemodynamics of sleep in hypertensive patients. Clin. Res. 15:451.

SHEPARD J.(1985). Gas exchange and hemodynamics during sleep. Med. Clinics of North Amer. 69:1243-1263.

SYLVESTER, J., S. SCHARF, R. GILBERT, R. FITZGERALD, R. TRAYSTMAN (1979). Hypoxic and CO hypoxia in dogs: hemodynamics, carotid reflexes and catecholamines. Am. J. Physiol. 236:422-428.

TILKIAN, A., C. GUILLEMINAULT, J. SCHROEDER, K. LEHRMAN, F. SIMMONS, W. DEMENT (1976). Hemodynamics in sleep-induced apnea. Ann Intern Med. 85:714-719.

WALLIN, B., J.FAGIUS (1986). The sympathetic nervous system in man-aspects derived from microelectrode recordings. Trends in Neuroscience 9:63-64.

WALLIN, B., and C.NERHED (1982). Relationship between spontaneous variations of muscle sympathetic activity and succeeding changes of blood pressure in man. J. Autonomic Nerv. System 6:293-302.

ZWEIFLER, A., and M. NICHOLLS (1982). Dimished finger volume pulse in borderline hypertension: Evidence for early structural vascular abnormality. Am. Heart. J. 104:812-815.

Résumé

La pléthysmographie digitale est une technique bien établie pour évaluer l'activité tonique du sympathique cutané. Une vasoconstriction est observée transitoirement pendant l'éveil et le sommeil après une inspiration profonde ; elle s'accompagne d'une augmentation de la décharge de nerfs sympathiques cutanés. Une vasodilatation pendant le sommeil lent a été rapportée chez des sujets jeunes normaux au niveau de la mer. Dans l'étude actuelle à 1400 m d'altitude, chez des sujets normaux d'âge moyen, une vasodilatation est mise en évidence pendant le sommeil lent et des modifications variables du tonus apparaissent au cours du sommeil paradoxal. Les malades porteurs de syndrome d'apnées obstructives du sommeil ont une vasoconstriction pendant la respiration régulière à la fois en sommeil lent et en sommeil paradoxal ; les patients SAS hypertendus ont une vasoconstriction plus importante pendant le sommeil lent que les patients normotendus. Une vasoconstriction cutanée durant 20 à 30 secondes apparaît immédiatement après le début de l'hyperpnée suivant l'apnée obstructive enregistrée au niveau de la mer et à 1400 m d'altitude. Aux deux altitudes la pression artérielle augmente fortement pendant l'hyperpnée. Au contraire, il a été montré que les sujets d'âge moyen apnéïques au niveau de la mer ont une diminution des décharges sympathiques musculaires pendant l'hyperpnée de la reprise ventilatoire. Ces faits posent la question de la signification de l'association entre l'activité vasoconstrictrice du sympathique cutané et de la réponse hypertensive pendant l'hyperventilation épisodique du sommeil chez les patients apnéïques.

Echocardiographic studies in adults and children presenting with obstructive sleep apnea or heavy snoring

Christian Guilleminault, Toshiaki Shiomi, Riccardo Stoohs and Ingela Schnittger*

*Sleep Research Center and *Department of Cardiovascular Medicine, Stanford University School of Medicine, Stanford, California 94305, USA*

To better understand the hemodynamic changes observed during sleep in association with obstructive sleep apnea syndrome (OSAS), we performed an echocardiographic study during sleep of children and middle-aged adults presenting with OSAS or simply with heavy snoring. Heavy snorers who do not present obstructive sleep apnea or hypopnea as classically described may present a pathology we call "upper airway resistance syndrome" (Guilleminault & Stoohs, 1991).

POPULATION

A. <u>Adults</u>: Ten patients (9 men, 1 woman) previously diagnosed with OSAS participated in our study after signing an informed consent. They had a mean age of 43.3 ± 3.8 years and a mean respiratory disturbance index (RDI) of 69.1 ± 56.6 (range: 11-189). [RDI = number of apneas (complete airway occlusions) or hypopneas (partial airway occlusions) per hour of sleep]. Most of the subjects were overweight; the mean body mass index (BMI) was 33.5 ± 8.4 kg/m^2 (up to 27.8 kg/m^2 is considered normal for the US population). None of the subjects presented any lung disease or hypoxia while awake and seated, as determined by pulmonary function tests performed no more than six months prior to the study. Most of them had restrictive chest-bellow problems when supine which were related to obesity. However, none of them had oxygen saturation (SaO_2) below 93% when kept awake and on their backs for 15 minutes. The only woman in the group had clear retrognathia. When the subjects performed Valsalva maneuvers (Bannister, 1983; Levin, 1966) while awake and seated, all had normal Valsalva ratios, eliminating the possibility of any significant autonomic nervous system dysfunction.

B. <u>Children</u>: Six boys whose mean age was 7.9 ± 5.3 years (range 3-14 years) were referred for heavy snoring at night and daytime fatigue or somnolence. Parents reported restless sleep and nocturnal sweat in all cases. Other symptoms included morning headaches (2 cases), behavioral problems at home and in school (2 cases), intermittent nocturnal enuresis (1 case) and nocturnal bruxism (1 case). One child (#5) presented with very significant obesity; the others were of normal weight. None had hypertension or clinical signs of acute cardiovascular complications.

METHODS

All subjects had been polygraphically monitored during sleep prior to the echocardiographic study. For the purpose of this study, patients were monitored during nocturnal sleep for one baseline night and again for a night with nasal CPAP administration, once nasal CPAP had been set at an appropriate level which completely relieved the obstruction. The measurements were performed during NREM and REM sleep (if patients presented REM sleep).

The following variables were systematically monitored: EEG (C3/A2 - C4/A1 of the 10-20 international placement system); EOG (electro-oculogram); EMG (chin and leg electromyogram); ECG (modified V-2 lead); and cardiotachograph. Respiration was monitored by measurement of airflow with oro-naso thermistors; thoracic and abdominal efforts with inductiv respiratory plethysmography; and esophageal pressure (Pes) through an esophageal balloon. The technique described by Baydur et al (1982) was used for balloon placement and calibration. Oxygen saturation was monitored with pulse oximetry (Biox-Ohmeda^{TM}). In adults, blood pressure was continuously monitored after cannulation of the non-dominant limb radial artery. In two children, a non-invasive continuous blood pressure measurement was performed using Finapres^{TM} (Ohmeda - Colorado) equipment. These two children had fingers wide enough to wear the finger cuff of the equipment, and their sleep was not disturbed by this procedure.

All variables were monitored on a Grass polygraph in combination with a time code. Simultaneous echocardiograms were taken, with the subjects awake and supine and also during nocturnal sleep. We used a Hewlett-Packard 77020-A echocardiograph with a 2.5 MHz transducer. The echocardiographs were recorded continuously on videotape and intermittently on heat-sensitive paper for a hard copy. The M-mode and two-dimensional echocardiograms in the parasternal long-axis view were monitored during nocturnal sleep. The echocardiographic probe was attached to the subject's chest through the use of a table designed and previously used in Japan, which prevented significant sleep disturbances during the monitoring.

Pes, ECG, and time code were simultaneously monitored on videotape and on the polygraph. Pes was calibrated on both sets of equipment during supine wakefulness.

ANALYSIS

Sleep, sleep stages, and apneas and hypopneas were scored following the international criteria (Rechtschaffen & Kales, 1968). Lowest oxygen saturation and most negative Pes (Pes nadir) during all-night recordings were determined, and a train of apneic events associated with these extreme values were analyzed. In addition to these most severe events, we also randomly selected groups of apneic events throughout nocturnal sleep for analysis. Each group consisted of three apneic events; thirty groups were chosen from recordings of stage 2 NREM sleep and 12 groups from REM sleep. Apneic episodes with atrial or ventricular premature beats were excluded. Measurements were performed on the hard copies of the echocardiograms, which were taken during at least one hour of quiet wakefulness with the subject supine, and then during sleep.

M-mode echocardiographic measurements were made according to the recommendations of the American Society for Echocardiography (Sahn et al, 1978), with the leading-edge-to-leading-edge convention. End-diastole was defined by the onset of the QRS complex, and end-systole was defined by the smallest ventricular dimension between the septum and the posterior wall. The M-mode echocardiographic measurements were made during both inspiration and expiration (or attempts at inspiration and expiration, with obstruction), and they were performed both during unobstructed breathing and during complete obstruction during sleep. Our measurements of apneas were taken as follows: from the first heartbeat occurring at the onset of the first obstructed breath through the last beat before the first non-obstructed breath. As noted before, a train of three successive apneas were always analyzed. Heart rate, right and left ventricular internal end-diastolic dimensions (RVIDd and LVIDd), left ventricular end-systolic dimensions (LVIDs), and Pes were measured. The 2-D images were obtained systematically just prior to and just after hard-copy M-mode image recordings, and regularly throughout the monitoring, to ensure appropriate placement of the movable cursor. The Pes values reached at end diastole (determined by analysis of the QRS complex) during each apnea were determined, and the interventricular septal motion ("septal motion") was qualitatively analyzed using the formula of Pearlman et al (1976): $100 [(RV - S)d - (RV - S)s] / TCDd$. The variables (RV - S)d and (RV - S)s are the end-diastolic and end-systolic dimensions, measured from the right ventricular epicardium to the right ventricular side of the interventricular septum, at mid-septum. Total cardiac diameter (TCDd) is the measurement at end-diastole from the right ventricular epicardium to the left ventricular epicardium. A negative sign (-) indicates normal motion of the interventricular septum, while a positive sign indicates a leftward shift of the interventricular septum (LSIVS), i.e. a paradoxical septal motion. Pes values during obstructed breathing were measured both at the nadir of the esophageal pressure curve and when end-diastole occurred. As end-diastole occurred both during inspiratory-type motion (performed against a closed glottis) and during expiratory-type motion (with absence of air exchange), the two kinds of end-diastolic measurements were called "inspiration-type" and "expiration-type" measurements. The percentage of fractional shortening (%FS) was calculated with the following equation: $\%FS = (LVIDs - LVIDd) / LVIDd$ (see Table 1).

During nasal CPAP administration, similar measurements were taken, but normal inspiration and expiration were now occurring. We compared the measurements taken during obstructed breathing and during non-obstructed, CPAP breathing. Comparison of results obtained with and without nasal CPAP were always made with measurements taken from the same sleep stages and from the same time of night.

Finally, in adults, left ventricular mass, expressed in grams, was calculated from echocardiographic measurements performed during quiet wakefulness, using the Troy et al (1972) formula. Criteria for left ventricular hypertrophy (LVH) were derived from the Framingham heart study (Levy et al, 1987). The values for LVH corresponding to two standard deviations above the mean for calculated left ventricular mass/ body surface area (LVM/BSA) are 150 g/m^2 for men and 120 g/m^2 for women.

STATISTICAL ANALYSIS

One-way analysis of variance was used for statistical analysis.

RESULTS

All patients presented with symptoms of obstructive sleep apnea, but RDI and lowest SaO_2 values during sleep varied, as indicated in Tables 1 and 2. The greatest difference was in maximum Pes nadir during sleep, which oscillated between -4 cm H_2O and -80 cm H_2O.

A. <u>Adults</u>:

Table I: Clinical Characteristics of Obstructive Sleep Apnea Syndrome With and Without a Leftward Shift of the Interventricular Septum (LSIVS)

Legend

Septal motion (%) calculations have been found using the formula of Pearlman et al (1976). BMI = body mass index; RDI = respiratory disturbance index;

SaO$_2$ = arterial oxygen saturation; Pes nadir = the nadir of esophageal pressure; LVM/BSA = left ventricular mass / body surface area.
C (Control), N-CPAP = variations in stage 2 non-REM sleep before and during nasal continuous positive airway pressure (CPAP) administration.
@@ p < 0.01 : LSIVS+ vs. LSIVS-
*** p < 0.001; ** p < 0.01; * p < 0.05 : C (apneic period) vs. CPAP

Patient	Septal Motion (%)	Gender	Age (yrs.)	BMI (kg/m^2)	RDI (A+H)I	Lowest SaO$_2$ (%) Control	N-CPAP	Maximum Pes Nadir (cmH$_2$O) Control	N-CPAP	Blood Pressure (mmHg) office (seated)	X values during apnea	Pulsus Paradoxus	LVM/BSA (g/m^2)	Final N-CPAP Value (cmH$_2$O)
1	+3	M	31	32	82	64	96	-80	-4	140/102	171/94	+	78	12
2	+5	M	35	33	11	91	95	-40	-3	140/100	137/98	+	129	8
3	+8	M	32	42	86	64	95	-66	0	122/80	140/97	+	201	17
4	+3	M	41	28	38	86	95	-72	-3	130/80	....		90	7.5
5	+2	M	30	42	96	65	93	-52	-4	110/70	....		136	12
Mean SD	+4.2@@ 2.6	LVIVS (+)	33.8@@ 4.4	35.4 6.2	62.6 36.5	74.0 13.4	94.8** 1.1	-62.0@@ 16.0	-2.8*** 1.6	129/86 14/14	149/96 19/2		126.8 48.3	11.3 3.8
6	-4	M	56	28	14	88	96	-4	-3	104/70	105/66	-	122	7.5
7	-5	M	57	25	19	89	99	-14	-2	120/78	129/80	-	168	15
8	-8	F	64	26	38	84	94	-24	-2	136/70	113/62	-	273	11
9	-3	M	46	49	189	74	93	-46	-12	140/80	....		146	15
10	-3	M	41	50	118	61	94	-22	0	170/110	....		219	12.5
Mean SD	-4.6 2.0	LSIVS (-)	52.8 9.2	35.6 12.9	75.6 76.1	79.2 11.8	95.2* 2.4	-22.0 15.6	-3.8* 4.7	134/82 25/17	116/69 12/10		185.6 60.6	12.2 3.1
Mean SD	n=10 Total Group		43.3 12.1	35.5 8.4	69.1 56.6	76.6 12.2	95.0*** 1.8	-42.0 25.8	-3.3*** 3.4	133/83 23/16	133/83 23/16		156.2 60.2	11.8 3.4

When qualitative analysis was performed, five patients (#1-5) presented with marked LSIVS, while five (#6-10) had normal motion. We called the first group LSIVS+ and the second group LSIVS-. The two groups of subjects were analyzed separately. As can be seen in Table 1, the LSIVS+ patients were significantly younger (mean age: 33.8 ± 4.4 versus 52.8 ± 9.2) and presented much more negative maximum Pes nadirs (mean Pes: -62.0 ± 16.0 versus -22.0 ± 15.6 cm H$_2$O). There were no significant differences between the two subgroups in BMI, RDI, or lowest SaO$_2$. The ratio LVM/BSA was not significantly different in the two groups (126.8 ± 48.3 versus 185.6 ± 60.6 g/m), but in individual analysis, echocardiographic criteria for LVH were fulfilled in only 1/5 of the LSIVS+ patients, while 3/5 of the LSIVS- patients fulfilled the criteria. In LSIVS+ patients, LVIDd and LVIDs decreased with increasingly negative Pes nadir. The progressively more negative Pes at end-diastole correlated significantly with the increase in RVIDd (r = .72, p < 0.001) and the decrease in LVIDd (r = .79, p < 0.001). There was also a correlation between Pes and LVIDs (r = 0.40, p < 0.01). Arterial blood pressure measurements were collected with valid results during sleep in only 6 out of the 10 patients. The LSIVS+ patients with continuous arterial blood pressure measurements presented pulsus paradoxus, while none of the LSIVS- patients with continuous sleep-related blood pressure monitoring presented this pattern. Pulsus paradoxus was defined as an inspiratory (or inspiratory effort against a closed upper airway) decrease in systolic blood pressure of 10 mm Hg or more (Shabetai et al, 1970). Pulsus paradoxus was noted with simultaneous significantly negative Pes nadir and associated LSIVS during obstructed breathing. The most important falls in systolic blood pressure during obstructed breathing were in subjects #1, 2 and 3; their values were 28, 25 and 30 mm Hg, respectively. None of the patients had clinical evidence suggesting pericardial restriction or echocardiographic evidence of pericardial effusion.

In examining Pes at baseline with obstructed inspiration, we looked at the Pes values corresponding to points of end-diastole, as end-diastole is the point at which a collapse due to LSIVS is likely to occur. We observed an increase in RVIDd and a decrease in LVIDd at these points as Pes increased. Although all our subjects had significant negative esophageal pressure at baseline, as we have mentioned the LSIVS+ patients had much more marked Pes negativity. LVIDd during baseline attempted inspiratory effort was significantly smaller in the LSIVS+ than in the LSIVS- patients (35.2 ± 4.9 versus 45.2 ± 6.9 mm, p < 0.05) (see Fig. 1).

*Diastolic Left Ventricular Collapse during Obstructed Inspiration

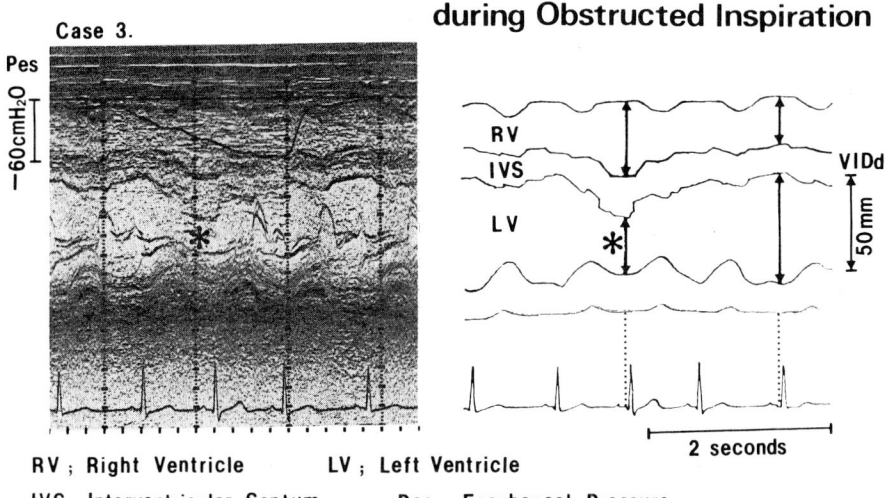

RV ; Right Ventricle   LV ; Left Ventricle
IVS ; Interventricular Septum   Pes ; Esophageal Pressure
VIDd ; Ventricular Internal Diastolic Dimension

B. Children:
Table II: Polygraphic Results of Children's Population
Legend
BMI = Body mass index; RDI = Respiratory disturbance index; Baseline = Measurements obtained while untreated; Nasal CPAP = Measurements obtained during treatment with nasal continuous positive airway pressure

Patient		1	2	3	4	5	6	Mean	SD
Gender		M	M	M	M	M	M		
Age (yrs.)		5	4	14	3	11	8	7.5	4.3
BMI (kg/m^2)		15.4	16.3	21.9	14.7	34.2	17	19.9	7.4
RDI [(A+H)I]		67.5	14.5	82.3	12.0	14.5	3.5	32.4	33.5
Lowest SaO$_2$ (%)	Baseline	64	92	64	70	60	93	73.8	14.8
	N-CPAP	95	96	95	96	95	96	95.5	0.5
Maximum Pes nadir (cm H$_2$O)	Baseline	-80	-5	-35	-17	-30	-12	-29.8	27.0
	N-CPAP	-3	-3	-6	-3	-9	-5	-4.8	2.4
Nasal CPAP (cm H$_2$O) pressure		7.5	5.0	12.0	12.0	12.5	4	8.8	3.8
Septal motion (%)		+3.5	-10.0	0	-3.9	-7.8	-3.0	-3.5	5.0

Current clinical wisdom would have classified subject #6 as not having obstructive sleep apnea syndrome and subject #2 as being a mild to moderate case, considering respiratory disturbance index (RDI) and lowest SaO_2 findings. Cases #4 and #5 also had moderately elevated RDI, but a few apneic events were very long and resulted in very low saturation readings (70% and 60%, respectively). However, these two subjects spent cumulative times of, respectively, 4 and 7 minutes out of total sleep times of 409 and 427 minutes with SaO_2 below 85%. Cases #1 and #3 presented more partial than complete obstruction of the upper airway. Subject #1's hypopnea index was 39 and subject #3's was 61. Their RDI (including apnea and hypopnea) were 67 and 85 events per hour of sleep. The partial obstructions were frequently, but not always, associated with SaO_2 drops to between 93% and 85%.

Mechanical changes induced by inspiratory efforts were greatest in case #1, as indicated by maximum Pes nadir (see Table 1). However, mean Pes nadirs in the segments submitted to analysis were smaller overall: when the mean right ventricular internal dimension at diastole (RVIDd), left ventricular internal dimension at diastole (LVIDd), and left ventricular internal dimension at systole (LVIDs) measurements during obstructed breathing were calculated from those segments, the mean changes in internal right and left ventricular dimensions were for the most part non-significant when mean values before and after nasal CPAP were compared.

Subjects in this children's group, despite the clinical complaint of EDS, had different echocardiographic findings. Case #1 was the most abnormal and presented changes similar to those seen in the LSIVS+ adult group. Interestingly, this subject presented a leftward shift of the interventricular septum even during partial obstruction and continuous heavy snoring, with Pes nadir oscillating between -30 and -40 cm H_2O and with SaO_2 often maintained at 94%. He had a paradoxical motion with a positive percentage of septal motion. One child (#3) had an intermittent leftward shift, and calculation of his percentage of septal motion was nul. All the other children had negative percentages of septal motion, as is normally seen. Case #5 did present intermittent leftward shift of the interventricular septum but to a much smaller degree than case #3. There was a direct relationship between these findings and the peak Pes nadir noted during the night: subject #1 had a Pes nadir of -80 cm H_2O, subject #3 of -35 cm H_2O, and subject #5 of -30 cm H_2O, while the others had values no lower than -20 cm H_2O. We had no measurements of arterial pressure in subjects #1 and #3, but case #5 presented pulsus paradoxus while #6 did not.

In our children the most negative Pes nadirs were seen during stage 2 NREM sleep. Leftward shift of the interventricular septum and pulsus paradoxus were seen at that time, even in children who only snored and had partial obstruction. The longest apneas were seen during REM sleep, and lowest SaO_2 was also noted during this state. There was thus a dissociation between the most important interventricular shift and lowest SaO_2 measurements. The echocardiographic findings were related to the mechanical changes associated with the complete or partial obstruction, as was pulsus paradoxus. All interventricular shifts and pulsus paradoxus were eliminated by nasal CPAP.

LIMITATIONS OF THE INVESTIGATION

Undoubtedly, the more equipment is fitted to a subject, the more disturbed his or her sleep may be, and certain sleep states may not occur. The sleep disturbance led two adult subjects to request discontinuation of the arterial blood pressure line. We did obtain good measurements in all individuals during NREM sleep. Echocardiographic signals were obtained during apneic events, even in cases of significant obesity, as subjects presented very low lung volumes and very limited movement. This absence of air exchange allowed great reduction in artefacts related to cardiac movements. However, signal distortions existed during the post-apneic hyperventilation period, due to hyperventilation and movements.

COMMENTS

Echocardiographic studies allow the investigation of some of the cardiovascular changes which occur in obstructive sleep apnea patients and heavy snorers.

Two types of abnormal septal motion were described by Popp et al (1969). In Type A, the left ventricular posterior wall echo and the septal echo move simultaneously in the same direction: anteriorly during systole and posteriorly during diastole (a paradoxical motion). In Type B, the septal echoes become flattened during systole. Almost all the abnormal septal motions detected during our study were Type B rather than Type A, and the greatest abnormal septal motion was seen when the most negative Pes nadir coincided with end diastole.

Left ventricular end-diastolic volume, or pre-load, is thought to be reduced through ventricular interdepenence mechanisms. Changes in left ventricular configuration induced by increased right ventricular volume during obstructed inspiration (Bromberger-Barnea, 1981) have been postulated to reduce left ventricular compliance (Robotham et al, 1979; Santamore et al, 1976), limit left ventricular filling and reduce LV stroke volume (Robotham et al, 1979; Santamore et al, 1976; Scharf et al, 1979). Leftward shift of the interventricular septum during obstructed inspiration has been demonstrated by Brinker et al with two-dimensional echocardiography in normal subjects (1981) and by Santamore et al with cineradiography in dogs (1976).

Right ventricular volume has been shown to increase during obstructed inspiration and a significant increase in Pes nadir (Brinker et al, 1981). LSIVS may thus result from a transient right ventricular volume overload temporally related to the strong inspiratory effort performed with a partially or completely obstructed airway.

During obstructed inspiration, LSIVS+ patients had a significantly smaller LVIDd than LSIVS- patients. This suggests a decrease in left ventricular end diastolic volume (LVEDV) during obstructed inspiration, even though the true LVEDV could not be measured. These data point in the same direction as previous reports (Robotham et al, 1979; Santamore et al, 1976; Brinker et al, 1981) which indicate that obstructed inspiration or a Muller maneuver may limit left ventricular filling through ventricular interdependence mechanisms. They may also be related to the data obtained from animals and humans which show that, during the Muller maneuver, hemodynamic alterations are induced by markedly negative pleural pressure (Scharf et al, 1979; Winer et al, 1977).

The ventricular dimension changes with abnormal septal motion are similar to those reported in adults with cardiac tamponade (Appleton et al, 1988), constrictive pericarditis (Gibson, 1976), acute pulmonary embolism (Winer et al, 1977), severe bronchial asthma (Jardin et al, 1982), and COPD (Settle et al, 1980). The latter observed in COPD patients that the inspiratory effort apparently causes overdistension of the right ventricle, which in turn displaces the interventricular septum posteriorly into the left ventricle, possibly impairing the filling of the left ventricle. A similar phenomenon may occur here.

The pulsus paradoxus in OSA may result from an interplay of several mechanisms similar to those noted in chronic airway disease:

1) The increased variations of intrathoracic pressures (indicated by Pes) are transmitted to the left ventricle and to the intrathoracic arterial vessels, causing a decrease in blood pressure during inspiration and an increase during expiration.

2) There is an increased filling of the right ventricle during the

inspiratory effort against a closed upper airway, with displacement of the interventricular septum. As shown in our study, this will limit the filling of the left ventricle by reducing its compliance (Robotham et al, 1978), thus lowering left ventricular stroke volume and decreasing the arterial blood pressure during inspiration. It is also possible that the abnormal systolic motion of the interventriclular septum during inspiration may have the same action without compliance changes.

In the investigation of breathing during sleep, much attention is given to SaO_2 values and complete obstruction of the upper airway, while little attention is given to the impact of the mechanical changes associated not only with apnea but also with snoring. These mechanical changes are commonly seen in children. The importance of these mechanical changes can be appreciated indirectly by measurement of Pes. The more negative Pes is, the more mechanical changes can be expected. LSIVS with significant changes is seen when Pes is profoundly negative at end diastole. Pulsus paradoxus is noted at that time. These significant negative Pes values during laborious inspiration are seen in children and in middle-aged adults. In follow-up work (unpublished data) we have found that out of 30 successively seen adult OSAS patients, 20 presented pulsus paradoxus (PP), 8 with systolic blood pressure (BP) drops > 20 mm Hg, and 12 with BP drops > 10 and < 20 mm Hg. The only differences between groups were age and Pes nadir. Pes nadir dissociated PP+ and PP- groups, but age statistically dissociated all 3 groups: the older the subject, the smaller the likelihood of very negative Pes and PP. The age at which children develop enough muscular strength to create very negative intrathoracic pressure has not been determined. However, the continuous changes in ejection suggested by our results must in some cases have an impact on tissue vascularization and normal functioning of the heart, brain, and other organs, and this effect must be exacerbated by any concurrent acute problems.

ACKNOWLEDGEMENTS

This work was supported by National Institute of Aging grant #AG-07772 and Clinical Research Center Grant #RR-00070.

REFERENCES

Appleton, C.P., Hatle, L.K., Popp, R.L. (1988). Cardiac tamponade and pericardial effusion: respiratory variation in transvalvular flow velocities studied by Doppler echocardiography. J Am Coll Cardiol 11: 1020-1030.

Bannister, R. (1983): Testing autonomic reflexes. In Autonomic Failure: A Textbook of Clinical Disorders of the Autonomic Nervous System (1st edition), ed. R. Bannister, pp. 52-63. Oxford: Oxford University Press.

Baydur, A., Behrens, P.K., Zin W.A., Jaeger, M., Milic-Emili, J. (1982). A simple method for assessing the validity of the esophageal balloon technique. Am Rev Resp Dis 126: 788-791.

Brinker, J.A., Weiss, J.L., Lappe, D.L., Rabson, J.L., Summer, W.R., Permutt, S., Wiesfeldt, M.L. (1981). Leftward septal displacement during right ventricular loading in man. Circulation 61: 626-633.

Bromberger-Barnea B. (1981). Mechanical effects of inspiration on heart functions: a review. Federation Proc 40: 2172-2177.

Gibson, T.C., Grossman, W., McLaurin, L.P., Moos, S., Craige, E. (1976). An echocardiographic study of the interventricular septum in constrictive pericarditis. Br Heart J 38: 738-743.

Guilleminault, C. and Stoohs, R. (1991): Upper airway resistance syndrome (UARS). Sleep Res: 20:250.

Jardin, F., Farcot, J.C., Boisante, L., Prost, J.F., Gueret, P., Bourdarias, J.P. (1982). Mechanism of paradoxic pulse in bronchial asthma. Circulation 66: 887-894.

Levin, A.B. (1966): A simple test of cardiac function based upon heart rate changes induced by the Valsalva maneuver. Am J Cardiol 18: 90-99.

Levy, D., Savage, D.D., Garrison, R.J., Anderson, K.M., Kannel, W.B., Castelli, W.P. (1987). Echocardiographic criteria for left ventricular hypertrophy: the Framingham heart study. Am J Cardiol 59: 956-960.

Pearlman, A.S., Clark, C.E., Henry, W.L., Morganroth, J., Itscoitz, S.B., Epstein, S.E. (1976). Determinants of ventricular septal motion: influence of relative right and left ventricular size. Circulation 54: 83-91.

Popp, R.L., Wolf, S.B., Hirata, T., Feigenbaum, H. (1969). Estimation of right and left ventricular size by ultrasound: a study of the echoes from the interventricular septum. Am J Cardiol 24: 523-530.

Rechtschaffen, A., Kales, A. (1968). A manual for standardized terminology, techniques, and scoring system for sleep stages of human subjects. Washington, D.C.: Public Health Service, U.S. Government Printing Office.

Robotham, J.L., Rabson, J., Permutt, S., Bromberger-Barnea, B. (1979). Left ventricular hemodynamics during respiration. J Appl Physiol 47: 1295-1303.

Sahn, D.J., DeMaria, A., Kisslo, J., Weyman, A. (Committee on M-mode standardization of the Americal Society of Echocardiography) (1978). Recommendations regarding quantitation in M-mode echocardiography: results of a survey of echocardiographic measurements. Circulation 58: 1072-1083.

Santamore, W.P., Lynch, P.R., Meier, G., Heckman, J., Bore, A.A. (1976). Myocardial interaction between the ventricles. J Appl Physiol 41:362-368.

Scharf, S.M., Brown, R. Saunders, N., Green, L.H. (1979). Effects of normal and loaded spontaneous inspiration on cardiovascular function. J Appl Physiol 47: 582-590.

Settle, H.P., Engel, P.J., Fowler, N.O., Allen, J.M., Vasallo, C.L., Hackworth, J.N., Adolph, R.J., Eppert, D.C. (1980). Echocardiographic study of the paradoxical arterial pulse in chronic obstructive lung disease. Circulation 62: 1297-1307.

Shabetai, R., Fowler, N.O., Guntheroth, W.G. (1970). The hemodynamics of cardiac tamponade and constrictive pericarditis. Am J Cardiol 26: 480-489.

Troy, B.L., Pombo, J., Rackley, C.E. (1972). Measurement of left ventricular wall thickness and mass by echocardiography. Circulation 45: 602-611.

Winer, H., Kronzon, I., Grassman, E. (1977). Echocardiographic findings in severe paradoxical pulse due to pulmonary embolization. Am J Cardiol 40: 808-810.

Extraction of cardiorespiratory parameters

François Kauffmann[1] and Bruno Cauchemez[2]

[1] Université de Caen, Département de Mathématiques, 14032 Caen Cedex, France;
[2] Hôpital Lariboisière, Service de Cardiologie, 75010 Paris, France

ABSTRACT

Digital processing is now widely used for studying physiological signals. We have focused our interest on quantification of heart rate and respirarory rate variability. In this paper we describe some processings to extract some of these parameters. We have split these processings in four categories : acquisition of digital recordings (named Analogic to Digital processing; A/D processings), treatment of electrocardiogram and respiratory recordings (named ECG and RES processings), and those which describe heart and respiratory rate variability (named HRV processings).

Pre-treatments such as A/D and ECG processings are crucial to measure HRV. We show two specific problems that influence HRV : the stability of the playback recorder's speed and the detection algorithm.

HRV processings are of great importance. Here we describe two algorithms which are able to quantify the power spectrum of HRV in a specific frequency band (FB). The reference algorithm for power spectrum analysis is the discrete Fourier transform with a well known algorithm : the Fast Fourier Transform (FFT). This algorithm gives an estimation of the power spectrum over a rather long period of time and works in stationary conditions. Other algorithms are able to give instantaneous power spectrum evaluation over very short periods of time with weaker assumptions. This dynamic evaluation of HRV in a FB is particularly suitable for studying sudden changes of amplitude or periods of periodic oscillatory patterns (OP). They are providing some new information that cannot be obtained by classical spectrum analysis. They evaluate the duration where the amplitude of OP is greater than a threshold. The first algorithm is the oscillation wave detection (OW) method developed in the Lariboisière hospital, the second one is a short Fourier transform magnitude (SF). Both algorithms are described and tested over clinical recordings.

We have chosen RES processings which are able to give instantaneous informations about respiratory rates. In order to compare heart rate and respiratory variability with any averaging.

We have written a modular system which is able to treat polygraphic recordings. It is actually implemented in Fortran, and is running on Sun4 machine. With this system Clairambault (1989) studied heart rate variability of a databank of 12 healthy premature infants. Medigue (1991) tries to study maturation of autonomous nervous system from a databank of 100 Doepler heart rate recordings. All algorithms have been tested on several databases. In this paper, we use a database of 10 24-hour Holter recordings to test HRV processings. A/D, ECG and RES processings are tested with thirty-five cardio-respiratory Holter recordings of newborn infants which are extracted from the analog database on Sudden Infant Death Syndrome of Monod (1986).

ANALOG TO DIGITAL PROCESSING

This is of course the first step of any digital processing and is often a difficult one. As we are concerned with heart rate variablity, speed's stability of the playback deck is of great importance. We are obliged to use a sampling rate which depends on tape's clock channel. Theses algorithms are called Phase lock loop (PLL). Figure 1 shows two spectra of a short series of RR intervals which are calculated from a simulated analog recordings with two different A/D processings. Left Figure is obtained without any PLL algorithms, whereas on the right the PLL is ON. In this example the square root of the total artefactual power (due to variations of the speed) is less than one ms. But some stable periodic components appear with PLL OFF. These components can be misinterpreted. Specially for premature newborn infants where respiratory arrhythmias can have a periodic variabilty whose amplitude can be low.

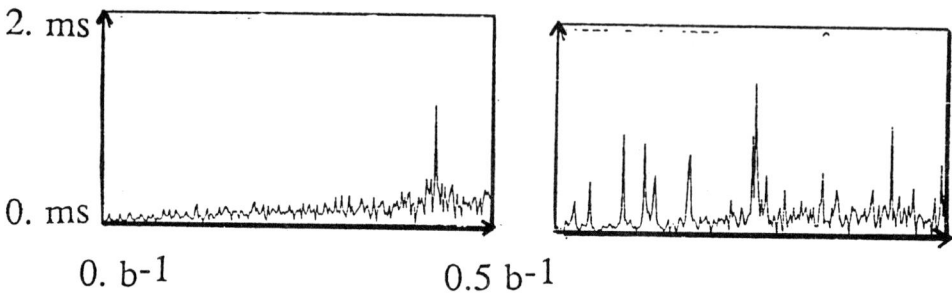

Fig. 1: Spectrogram of a tachogram from a test tape, on the left PLL if OFF, on the right PLL is ON.

E.C.G PROCESSINGS

Detection

This is the main processing. Here we describe a method based on classical estimation of signal to noise ratio. We have implemented an algorithm which is able to follow rapid variations of noise. It is unaffected by variations of QRS wave's amplitude. And it requires a minimum a-priori knowledge of QRS wave. We note $Var(Y)_t$ and $Var(E)_t$ estimations of variances of the ECG and noise signal at time t. The parameters of this module are :

- frequency bandwidth for the ECG signal
- window length to calculate $Var(Y)_t$
- time constant (A) for the estimation of $Var(E)_t$
- maximum relative variation (B) between two sampled data for the estimation of $Var(e)_t$
- minimum and maximum duration of QRS wave (QRSmin and QRSmax)
- minimum and maximum duration for a RR interval (RRmin and RRmax)
- trigger's values for the signal to noise ratio. Three values are required : for the beginning, the validation and the end of the QRS wave: (SNRbegin, SNRvalid, SNRend)
- refractory period. This is he period after a QRS wave during which it is not possible to detect another one.

We can describe the algorithm with the following formula. Let X_t be the original ECG signal at time t , and Y_t the filtered bandpass signal, with the specifications given earlier. The power of the signals Y_t and E_t are evaluated with :

$$Var(Y)_t = y_t^2 + y_{t-1}^2 + \ldots + y_{t-L+1}^2.$$
$$Var(E)Min = (1-A) * Var(E)_{t-1}$$
$$Var(E)Max = (1+A) * Var(E)_{t-1}$$
$$Var(E)_t = \max(Var(E)Min, \min(Var(E)max, a*Var(E)_{t-1} + (1-a)*Var(y)_t))$$

The signal to noise ratio at time t, SNR(t) is simply :

SNR(t) = Var(y)$_t$ /Var(E)$_t$.

The decision step is described by the following automata which can take the following value (INIT, SEARCH, VALIDATE_BEGIN, VALIDATE_EVENT, SEARCH_END, REFACTORY). In the INITIALIZING STEP, Var(E)$_t$ is set to the middle sample of the current series var(Y)$_t$. A VALIDATED BEGINNING TIME is an interval of time (T0,T1) which lasts for at least QRSMin samples, and during which SNR(t) is always greater than SNRbegin. A VALIDATED EVENT at time T1 is constituted of a validated beginning time T0 and time T1 in the interval (T0,T0+QRSmax), such that SNR(T1) is greater than SNRvalid. The END OF A VALIDATED EVENT is the first time T2 greater or equal to T1 such that the signal to noise ratio at time T2 is less than SNRend or if T2 is greater than T0+QRSmax.

These tests allow us to follow rapid variations of the noise power. Is is also robust to aberrant values, for the detection test oblige the signal to noise ratio to be greater than SNRbegin, during an interval of time. Prefiltering step allows us to eliminate slow frequency variations of baseline and high frequency noise.

Fiducial point algorithm

Localization of fiducial points for each QRS complexes can introduce some disturbances in HRV. Sharp R waves, large T waves can also be misinterpreted. In this system we can localize fiducial points such as minimum, maximum, longuest monotone subsequence, averaging of time (the leads are proportional to positive signal), on a window defined around an already calculated event.

Results

First trace in Figure 2 presents the original ECG signal. Second trace presents the bandpath filtered signal. On third trace, continuous line shows the estimate of the power of the signal Var(Y)t, whereas dashed line is the estimation of the power of noise. Vertical dashed lines show the fiducial points in each detected QRS wave.

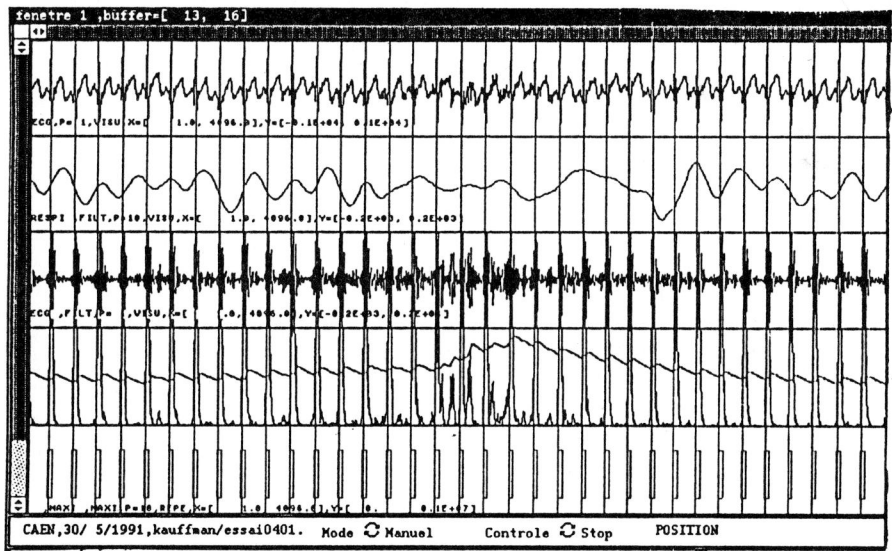

Fig. 2: Results of ECG processings

HRV PROCESSING

Data

Ten 24-hour analog ECG recordings are digitized and processed with a MARKET system. The RR annotated list (beat label and RR values) are transferred towards a PC and then to a Sun4. These series are stored in successive buffers of 512 beats.

Artefact correction module

A simple algorithm is used to detect and correct aberrant RR values. This module evaluates a mean RR series and compares the current value to the estimated mean. If this difference is greater than a threshold or if the current value is outside a normal interval, the RR label is set to false and corrected with the previous RR correct value.

Linear Filter Bank module

We define three non-overlapping frequency bands of interest : the rapid one or high frequency band (HF); the slow one or middle frequency band (MF); the very slow one or low frequency band (LF). As we are using a time scale expressed in a number of beats with no resampling methods, each period is expressed in a number of beats. The HF band has periods ofbetween 3 and 8 beats, the MF band has periods ofbetween 10 and 25 beats, the LF band has periods ofbetween 30 and 100 beats. We use linear filtering to extract from the corrected RR series, three signals corresponding to the HF,MF and LF bands. Each filter is an infinite impulse response band-pass filter of elliptic type (order 4 with a precision of -40dB in the stop and pass-band).

Decimation

We also use decimation to minimize post-treatment computation time. The high frequency series (HF) is decimated with a factor one (all RR are used), but the middle frequency band is decimated with a factor four (one RR over four is used), and the slow frequency series is decimated with a factor twelve (one RR over twelve is used). This method can be applied because of the limited frequency bandwidth of each filtered series.

Oscillation wave detection module

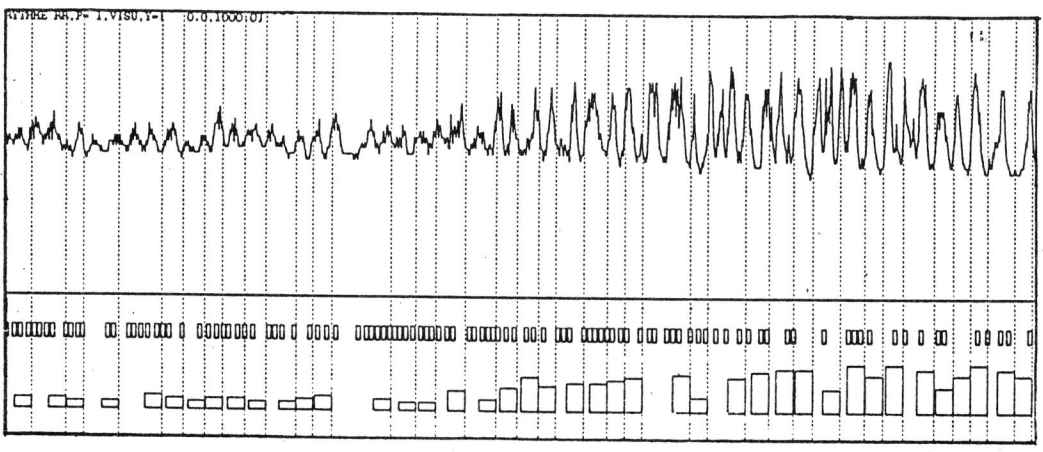

Fig. 3: Results of the OW method for the high and mid frequency band. The first trace is the raw tachogram, the second trace corresponds to the OW method's output for the HF and MF band.

The aim of this algorithm is to detect, measure and count simple patterns (Coumel (1985), Kauffmann (1988)). An oscillatory pattern (OP) is composed of a decelerating slope surrounded by two slopes of inverse tendencies. Each slope is defined by its length and its amplitude. A slope is decelerating if the number of consecutive decreasing pairs of RR intervals in this subsequence is above a fixed percentage (ER) of the slope's length. This oscillation wave detection algorithm detects OP whose periods are inside a prescribed interval : HF,MF,LF bands and whose amplitude is greater than a fixed threshold. The error percentage in this study is set to 20%. The minimum amplitude threshold is set to 20 ms, but it is set to 10 ms when we want to evaluate mean power in a FB since all OP must be detected. The inputs of the OW module are the decimated outputs of the linear filter bank. The outputs of the OW module are firstly graphical. Figure 3 shows the results of OW module for HF and MF band, the width and height of squares are proportional to period and amplitude respectively of the detected OP. Secondly we evaluate for each buffer the percentage of time (%OW) during the current buffer where there are OP, and the mean power (AOW) which is simply the product of the mean amplitude of the detected OP with %OW.

Short time Fourier transform magnitude

Short time Fourier transform (SF) is particularly suitable to study time-varying spectral characteristics of HRV. Whereas discrete Fourier transform supposes a stationary signal, SF can work with small windows and give dynamic evaluation of power in a specific frequency band (Dalton (1986), Shin (1989)). Amplitude at time n for the frequency f $|X(n,f)|$ of signal x is given by the formula (Lim (1988)) :

$$|X(n,f)| = |\sum x(j)w(n-j)\exp(-2\pi i f)|$$

where w is a series for the window coefficients. Here we have chosen for the low pass-filter, w, an infinite impulse response low-pass filter with a width equal to half the studied frequency bandwidth (elliptic filters with a dynamic of -40db in stop and pass-band). Then the module $|x(n,f)|$ can be interpreted as an estimation of the instantaneous power in HF,MF and LF bands. The inputs of the SF module are the decimated outputs of the linear filter bank, but this method can be applied to the corrected RR series. We calculate for each buffer the mean of instantaneous power (ASF) and the percentage of time (%SF) where this amplitude series is greater than a fixed threshold which is set as for the OW method to 20 ms. Figure 4 shows the results of this algorithm for a short period of a tachogram which is recorded on a patient with sleep apnea syndrome. On the right panel, the first trace is the tachogram (x scale 2048 RR, y scale 1000ms), the second and third traces are the outputs for the HF and the LF respectively (y scale 400ms). Dashed lines represent the outputs of the linear filter banks. Continuous lines in traces 2 and 3 correspond to the outputs of the SF module. The left panel shows histograms corresponding to traces on the right (x scale from 0 to 100ms, y scale 0 to 25%). The two peaks in this histogram show that the amplitude in the MF band has changed, whereas the HF and LF histograms show that there is no activity in these bands.

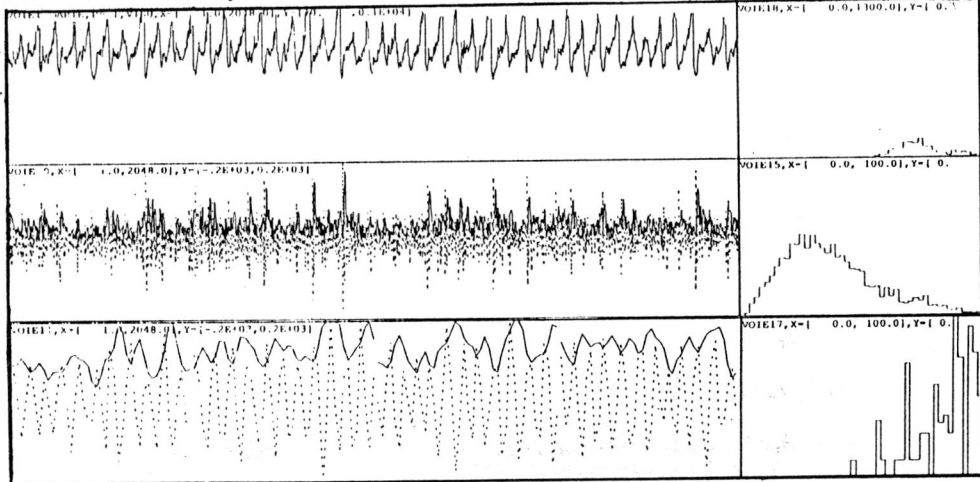

Fig. 4 Results of the linear filter bank and SF algorithm.

Results

We have studied FFT, OW and SF methods with a database of ten patients with 100 buffers per record. We correlate mean power estimated by FFT, OW and SF methods, and the mean duration time where the amplitudes of OP were greater than a threshold estimated with OW and SF methods which can evaluate instantaneous power. The results are quite significant. The estimation of the power spectrum and percentage of time (Table 1) where there are OP, give comparable quantitative and qualitative results in all FB.

POWER	FFT,AOW	FFT,ASF	%AW,%SF
HF	0.76±0.23	0.89±0.10	0.83±0.21
MF	0.87±0.29	0.90±0.08	0.94±0.03
LF	0.87±0.06	0.85±0.07	0.84±0.10

Table 1: Correlations between estimated power spectrum

Patients with lower correlation between FFT, OW and SF power spectrum have the lowest activity in the studied band. This assumption can be verified in Table 2 (patients 5,8 and 10 for HF band). If this activity is greater (patients 6 and 9 Table 3) then correlations are better. Firstly we can say that the OW method depends on the detection algorithm. As the minimum amplitude threshold is set to 10 ms (in the case of power estimation), it is normal that if the mean power spectrum is lower than 10 ms, the OW method cannot detect all OP. Secondly as the results with SF methods are lower, it can be supposed that this phenomenon can be attributed to precision of the RR measurements. The same discussion may apply to the estimation of percentage of time %OW, %SF.

PATIENT	FFT	AOW	ASF	cor(FFT,OW)	cor(FFT,SF)
5	7.8	4.6	6.25	0.41	0.73
8	10.6	8.0	8.9	0.68	0.81
10	8.6	9.6	7.1	0.49	0.87
6	30.0	33.7	25.4	0.97	0.99
9	33.2	30.5	30.0	0.98	0.99

Table 2: Individual correlations for power spectrum evaluation. All results for power are expressed in ms (square root of the power)

Table 3 shows results of the OW method on the raw RR series without any preprocessing in the HF and MF on the same database. The results here are lower for the MF band : 0.61 ±0.32. With preprocessing correlations are 0.87 ±9. But results are comparable for the high frequency band. The oscillation wave method can work with the highest frequency band on raw data.

BAND	cor(OW,FFT)
HF	0.79±0.10
MF	0.61±0.32

Table 3: Correlations between FFT and OW without any preprocessing.

RESPIRATORY PROCESSING

Respiratory signal is a signal whose frequency components are few and in the low frequency band. It can be modelized by :

$$y_t = a_t * \cos(2*\pi*(F0 + F_t + Phi_t))$$

where a_t is the amplitude, $F0+F_t$ is the frequency signal (slowly varying), and Phi_t is a phase. Numerous algorithms give estimations of these parameters (complex demodulation , ARMA modelization, ...) In this paragraph, we describe a method which is able to describe instantaneous interactions between heart rate and respiratory rate.

Examination of cross-spectrum between resamples RR series or interval RR series defined by ROEL (1984) and respiratory signal has shown an exact synchronisation between these two signals during some periods of quiet sleep in polygraphic infant's recording. Witte (1988) shows that complex interferences such as aliasing phenomenon can be seen between heart rate variability (on the interval RR series) and respiratory signal.

All these methods are working on the interval series and are methods which are FFT-like. The first assumption is that the real clock of cardiac events is a clock expressed in seconds. The second assumption supposes the signal is stationary of the signal. Because FFT-like methods give a correct estimation in mean. For example FFT gives a mean power over periods of 512 points.

Our objective is to correlate instantaneous variability of cardiac rate and respiratory rate. Thus we have chosen the simplest clock : the cardiac one. If Ti is the ith occurence of a QRS wave, the index i is taken as the time, which is referred as cardiac clock. Then sampling of others physiological signals is made of a frequency which depends on the heart variability. Whereas previous methods uses equispaced times to sample their informations.

In this way, all HRV processings use time which is indexed by the number of QRS wave. Consequently each frequency must be expressed in a unit proportionnal to the inverse of a number of beats.

In order to minimize effect of averaging, we use a least-mean square algorithm to identify unknown parameters. Figure 5 shows both results ECG processing and RES processing. First trace is the ECG processing, second trace is the respiratory signal, third trace is the estimated amplitude one, the fourth one is the phase.

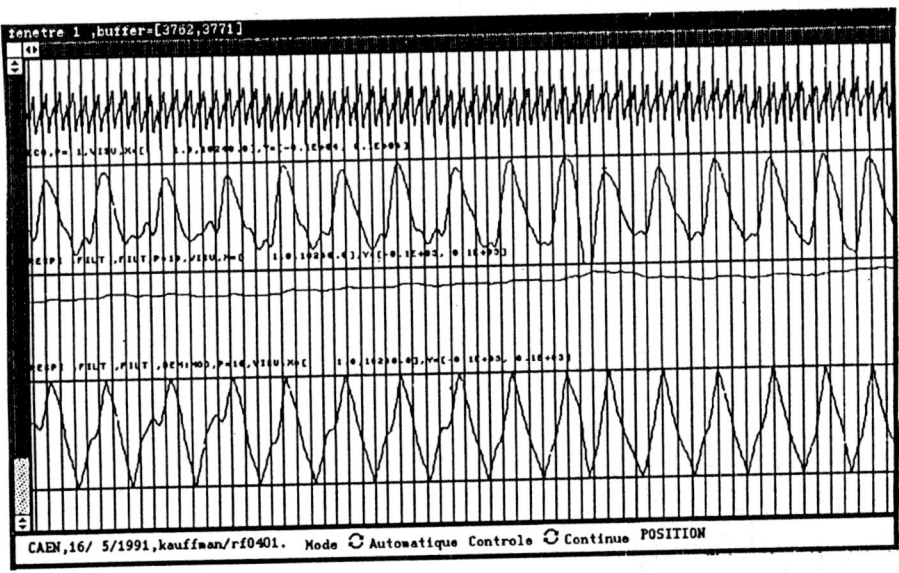

Fig. 5 : Results of ECG and RES processings

CONCLUSION

The playback unit can induce low amplitude periodic activity in HRV. PLL techniques for sampling frequency can reduce these false components. The detection algorithm can induce HRV in the high frequency band. Removing aberrant cardiac cycles is necessary for classical spectrum analysis(FFT). Linear filter banks techniques can separate frequency bands. Decimation drastically reduces computation time. The FFT method is a rapid method to evaluate the power spectrum over a period of time. The OW method works quite well on separate frequency band. It gives the location in time of each oscillation, but is limited by the minimum amplitude threshold. The SF methods give instantaneous value of power in each frequency band. A simple histogram module can evaluate ASF and %SF. But this module can work with the corrected RR series. This algorithm is able to zoom in on the frequency axis and the time axis. It can work on narrow bands and gives results over a very short period of time.

To study the interactions between heart rate and respiratory signal, we have used a variable sampling time. All results are then instantaneous, so we are able to quantify exact heart rate variability induced by the respiratory rate. All these methods are employed to study the SIDS databank. We are working during periods of strong strong arrhythmias, during periods which preceeds cardiac pose, and of course during all the recordings.

REFERENCES

Appel M.L., Cohen R.J.(1988) : Use of Phase-locked loop to correct heart rate variability. In Computers in Cardiology.307-310.
Clairambault J. : (1989) :Thèse de Doctorat en médecine, Univesité de Paris 6.
Coumel P., Leclercq JF et al : (1985) : Computerized analysis of dynamic electrocardiograms : a tool for comprehensive electrophysiology. A description of the Atrec II system.Clinical Progress,3,181-201.
Dalton K.J, Denham D.W, Dawson A.J., Hoffman H.J. (1986) : Ultradian rhythms in human fetal heart : a computerized time series analysis.Int. J. Biom. Comp. 18:45-60.
KauffmannF., Maison-BlancheP., CauchemezB., Coumel P.(1988). A study of non stationary phenomena of HRV during 24-hour ECG ambulatory monitoring.In Computers in Cardiology,303-306.
Lim J.S., Oppenheim A.V.(1988) : Advanced topics in signal Processing.eds Printice Hall.
Medigue C., Kauffmann F., Clairambault J.,Rapport Inria to appear.
Monod N., Plouin P., Sternberg B. (1986): Are polygraphic and cardiopneumographic respiratory patterns useful for predicting the risk of sudden death Infant Syndrome ? Biol. Neonate 50 :147-153 .
Roel W. Be Boer, & (1984) : Comparing spectra of series of points events particulary for heart rate variability data. IEEE Trans. Biom. Comp. BME 31,384-387.
Shin S.J., Tapp W.N., Reisman S.S., Natelson B.H.(1989) : Assessment of Autonomic regulation of heart rate variability by the method of complex demodulation. IEEE Trans. Biom. Eng.:36,274-283.
Witte H., Zwiener U., Rother M., Glasers (1988) : Evidence of a previously undescribed form of respiratory sinus arrhytmia: the physiological manifestation of cardiac aliasing. Pflugers Arch.,412,442-444.

Résumé

Nous présentons plusieurs algorithmes permettant d'évaluer la variabilité du rythme cardiaque ainsi que celle du rythme respiratoire. Premièrement nous décrivons brièvement un des problèmes de l'acquisition du signal : la stabilité de la vitesse de déroulement de l'enregistreur magnétique. Deuxièmement ,un algorithme de détection des ondes QRS est présenté. Enfin nous présentons les algorithmes relatifs à la variabilité du rythme cardiaque, ainsi qu'un algorithme de démodulation pour l'étude du signal respiratoire.

Tous ces algorithmes ont été testés sur de nombreuses banques de données. Ici nous utilisons 35 enregistrements cardio-respiratoires extraits de la banque de donnée sur la mort inexpliquée du nourisson du Dr Monod (1986).

III. Pathophysiology of cardiorespiratory control. Clinical and diagnostic aspects

III. Physiopathologie du contrôle cardio-respiratoire. Aspects cliniques et diagnostiques

Systemic hypertension and sleep apnoea

John Stradling

Osler Chest Unit, Churchill Hospital, Oxford, OX3 7LJ, UK

There is some evidence that obstructive sleep apnoea (OSA) leads to an increased rate of cardiovascular deaths [Partinen & Guilleminault, 1990; Thorpy & Ledereich, 1988; He et al, 1988; Gonzalez-Rothi et al, 1988; Partinen et al, 1988]. Although no proper controlled prospective study exists to prove this, retrospective and uncontrolled studies have shown an excess of cardiovascular deaths in untreated or poorly treated groups. For example, Partinen [Partinen & Guilleminault, 1990; Partinen et al, 1988] traced 198 patients with OSA up to 11 years post diagnosis. In 71 patients who had received a tracheostomy the 11 year survival rate was 95%, but in the 127 who received only conservative therapy the 11 year survival was significantly lower at 87% (1 death versus 14 deaths). Although the two groups were not matched, the treated patients were in fact more severe (heavier, older, higher apnoea rate) although the presence of cardiovascular disease at presentation was similar. Thorpy et al [Thorpy & Ledereich, 1988] found a poorer survival of only 85% in a group of patients with OSA, followed on average for 6.5 years. There was no significant difference in the overall survival between treated and untreated groups, although cardiovascular deaths were significantly less in those treated. He et al [He et al, 1988] contacted about half of a group of 706 OSA patients. Eight year survival was 63% in the >20 apnoeas/hr group compared to 96% in the <20/hr group. Survival was greatly improved by treatment (no deaths in the tracheostomy and nasal CPAP group) except that UPPP did not improve survival when compared to no treatment.

Although these studies strongly suggest that OSA is bad for the cardiovascular system, it must be admitted that full control for confounding variables such as upper body obesity, insulin resistance, lipidaemia and smoking has not been achieved. In view of the availability and success of nasal CPAP as a treatment for OSA it is unlikely that fully satisfactory data on these points will ever be collected.

If we assume that there is an excess of cardiovascular deaths in patients with OSA then there has to be a pathogenetic mechanism linked to the recurrent obstruction, asphyxia and arousal. Various hypotheses have been suggested that operate through known factors such as sustained hypertension [Guilleminault et al, 1980], increased catecholamines [Fletcher et al, 1987; Goldstein, 1983; Clark et al, 1980], increased lipids [Freidman et al, 1958], hypoxaemia and cardiac arrhythmias [Guilleminault et al, 1983]. In addition an increased cardiac workload due to excessive blood pressure swings and the negative intrathoracic pressure swings during the obstruction, have been postulated to add in some way to myocardial damage [Tolle et al, 1983].

This short review examines the possible contribution of a link through hypertension to OSA-induced cardiovascular morbidity and mortality.

SLEEP APNOEA AND SUSTAINED HYPERTENSION.

Depending on definition, the prevalence of systemic hypertension in patients with OSA varies enormously. Different authors have usually reported figures based on casual, one-off, readings done in outpatients or on the admission night for sleep studies. Careful, matched control, studies using ambulatory monitoring have not been reported. Usually the prevalence of hypertension in most series has been in the range of 30-50% [Guilleminault et al, 1976]. This hypertension was at first assumed to be due to the sleep apnoea, essentially for two reasons. Firstly that OSA was a "stressful" condition leading to catecholamine release. Studies had shown an increased release of catecholamines during sleep in OSA patients [Fletcher et al, 1987; Clark et al, 1980] as well as an increase in resting sympathetic tone [Hedner et al, 1988; Hedner et al, 1990]. In other disorders, that also raise catecholamines, sustained hypertension may be found [Goldstein, 1983; Oparil, 1986]. The stimulus for this catecholamine release might be hypoxaemia [Somers et al, 1988; Balter et al, 1990] or just the effect of recurrent arousals. Secondly, because there were repeated rises in blood pressure during sleep perhaps baro-receptor mechanisms were down-regulated.

Recently, however, several studies have seriously questioned whether OSA, in its own right usually provokes significant hypertension. Because most OSA patients are obese (in most clinics they are on average 30% overweight, $W/Ht^2=30$) there will be the problem of this confounding variable when analysing the cause of blood pressure elevation. In addition upper body obesity, the fat distribution pattern most associated with hypertension and cardiovascular mortality [Blair et al, 1984; Weinsier et al, 1985; Welin et al, 1987; Larsson et al, 1984; Knight, 1984], may also be particularly related to OSA through the greater propensity for neck obesity to provoke OSA [Davies & Stradling, 1990; Katz et al, 1990]. Hoffstein et al [1988] used multiple linear regression to show that in a group of 372 patients who snored (194 with OSA), 8% of the variance in diastolic blood pressure was "explained" by obesity, 4% by age and only 1.7% by the number of apnoeic episodes/hr of sleep. An epidemiological survey that identified 15 individuals with OSA found the prevalence of hypertension in these 15 subjects to be no higher than in 46 controls without OSA [Gislason et al, 1988]. More recently Escourrou et al [1990] studied 50 patients with a diagnosis of sleep apnoea syndrome (AH index >10) and found no relationship between apnoea severity and the presence of hypertension.

Although treatment of obstructive sleep apnoea has been reported to lead to falls in blood pressure there have been no trials with untreated controls. The blood pressure falls found have been no bigger than might have been expected from remeasuring a hypertensive population some months later (regression to the mean).

Because persistent snoring in population surveys is likely to be an epidemiological marker for OSA it is perhaps permissible to look at unselected populations and ask whether there is a link between hypertension and snoring. For example Lugaresi et al [1980] collected data on 5713 men and women. Hypertension correlated with older age, obesity and snoring. Allowance for obesity removed any significant effect of snoring in the >15% overweight group, but in the thinner group snoring was still correlated with hypertension, although allowance for weight differences within this group was not made. In a sample of 4064 men aged 30-69, surveyed by questionnaire, snoring prevalence was higher in the 9.3% who reported a history of hypertension [Gislason et al, 1987]. However this was significant only in the 40-49 year old group once obesity (but not upper body obesity) was allowed for. Because snoring correlates not only with obesity [Stradling et al, 1991] but also with cigarette smoking, alcohol or hypnotic use [Bloom et al, 1988] and some other diseases [Norton & Dunn, 1985] it is difficult to be convinced that an association with snoring is not through another variable.

Two more recent epidemiological surveys have found that the apparent association between snoring and hypertension is entirely explained by obesity. Schmidt-Nowara et al [1990] surveyed 1222 adults and found snoring to be initially correlated with measured blood pressure but after correction for obesity this was no longer the case. Stradling and Crosby [1990] found in 748 men aged 35-65 that obesity, age and alcohol consumption accounted for 9% of the variance of measured diastolic blood pressures, with no significant contribution from a history of snoring.

Another approach to assessing if sleep apnoea and hypertension are related is to look at patients with a primary diagnosis of hypertension to see if they have a higher prevalence of sleep apnoea. This has been done by several authors [Kales et al, 1984; Lavie et al, 1984; Williams et al, 1985; Fletcher et al, 1985] who claimed that up to 40% of hypertensives had sleep apnoea. However, all the studies can be questioned on various accounts. The studies of Lavie et al [1984] and Kales et al [1984] had no suitable weight-matched control groups for the heavier hypertensive population and in addition many were studied whilst on drugs. Some hypertensive drugs (eg diuretics, beta blockers and alpha methyl dopa) may potentially provoke sleep apnoea [Sullivan et al, 1985; Lahive et al, 1988; Boudoulas et al, 1983; Fletcher et al, 1985]. Other studies have had different problems which were extensively discussed elsewhere [Stradling, 1989]. Heart failure has also been shown recently to cause respiratory oscillations which could be mistaken for primary sleep apnoea [Hanly et al, 1989] and some patients treated for hypertension will be at risk of left ventricular failure. Warley et al [1988] studied 30 untreated hypertensive men with 30 control subjects matched for age, weight, height, smoking habit and alcohol consumption. Despite a clear difference in blood pressures there was no difference in the amount of nocturnal hypoxaemic dipping. Although overnight oximetry may not diagnose all patients with OSA this study clearly showed that overnight hypoxaemia (one of the possible promoting causes of hypertension in OSA) could not be a common aetiological factor in "essential" hypertension as previously hypothesised. This was confirmed in a study by Hirshkowitz et al [1989] who studied 175 hypertensive men and 110 normotensives. In the untreated hypertensives (113) the apnoea index was no different from the normotensives, but the treated hypertensives had higher apnoea rates. This suggested that some of the earlier results described above might well have been due to the anti-hypertensive medications.

It may be that the apparent high rates of apnoea in hypertensives found in some studies (which included central apnoea as well as obstructive) could be because both abnormalities are being provoked by a third factor. There is a clear association between hypertension and increased carotid body sensitivity to hypoxaemia [Vlachogianni et al, 1989; Prybylski et al, 1980]. This increased activity of the carotid body could well provoke apnoeas and irregular respiration during sleep, as occurs at altitude [Reite et al, 1975]. This might explain why the apnoeas that have been found in hypertensives are more often central and less frequent than seen in classical obstructive sleep apnoea.

If the evidence is poor that OSA produces sustained diurnal hypertension, could a hypertensive link between OSA and cardiovascular morbidity and mortality be through nocturnal hypertension, but with relatively normal daytime values? It has been shown recently, for example, that left ventricular hypertrophy in hypertensive disease correlates better with nighttime pressures than with daytime figures [Verdecchia, 1990].

SLEEP APNOEA AND NOCTURNAL HYPERTENSION

One of the most striking cardiovascular findings in OSA are the violent swings in blood pressure that occur both during an apnoea and upon arousal. We have seen patients whose systolic blood pressure swings from a nadir of 90mmHg to a maximum of 200mmHg with every apnoea, ie 300-400 times a night, Fig. 1. The usual swings we find with each arousal, though, are in the region of 30mmHg [Ali et al ,1991b].

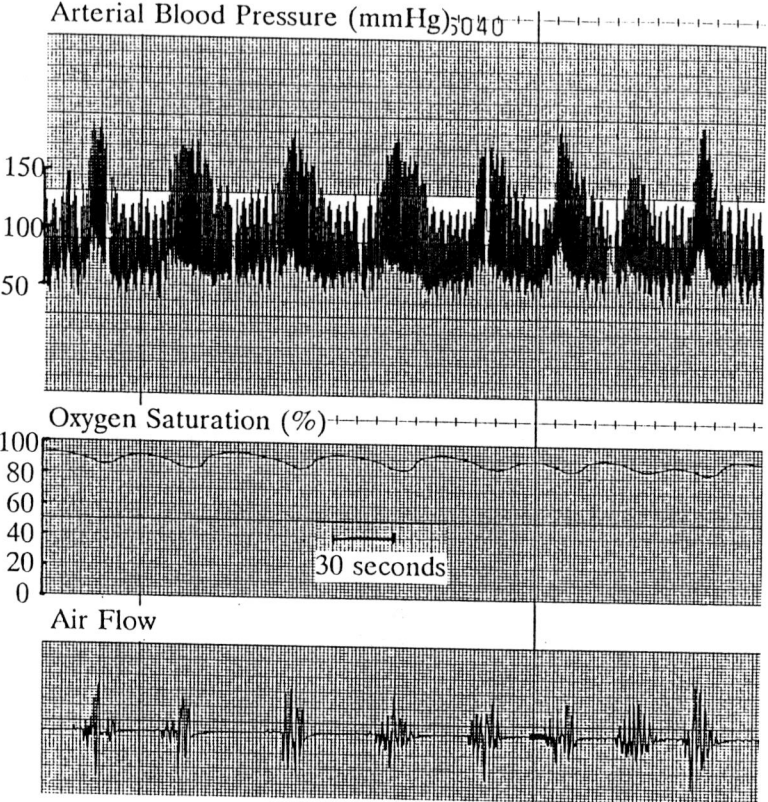

Fig 1. Continuous tracing of arterial BP in a patient with obstructive sleep apnoea. Note the rises with each resumption of airflow (on arousal), and the faster swings during the apnoea due to the obstructed inspiratory efforts (pulsus paradoxus).

The causes of these swings in BP are not entirely clear. As the apnoea progresses the mean BP actually falls, but this is mainly due to increasing transient falls with each frustrated inspiratory effort (pulsus paradoxus). Because the heart is in the chest the blood pressure, in the arteries emerging from the thorax, swings in concert with the pleural pressure [Lea et al, 1990]. This is because during these short Mueller manoeuvres there is very little in the way of adaptatory increases in left ventricular transmyocardial pressure to maintain peripheral pressures.

During the apnoea there is also a bradycardia thought to be part of the diving reflex [Zwillich et al, 1982], ie apnoea and hypoxaemia provoking peripheral arterial vasoconstriction and bradycardia (reducing cardiac output) which reduces oxygen consumption, thus preserving oxygen deliveries to the brain without big rises in arterial blood pressure [Angell-James et al, 1969]. This is clearly useful to the diving mammal [Andersen, 1964]. Superficial nerve studies have shown an increasing sympathetic activity to arterioles during apnoeas that disappears upon arousal [Hedner et al, 1988].

At, or just before, cortical arousal the blood pressure rises over about 20 seconds before settling again, although by then a new apnoea has usually started. Originally, because the post apnoea blood pressure rise correlated with the nadir of the hypoxaemia, it was felt that the hypoxaemia itself had caused the BP rise [Shepard, 1985]. However a recent study has shown that this is not the case since added O_2, to abolish the hypoxaemia during the apnoeas, hardly alters the post-apnoeic blood pressure rise [Ali, 1991b]. It is the apnoea length that most closely correlates with post-apnoeic BP rise. The apparent correlation with hypoxaemia was because longer apnoeas cause greater hypoxaemia. In this study 25% of the variation in post-apnoeic BP rise was "explained" by apnoea length, 15% by the rise in heart rate and none by the degree of hypoxaemia [Ali et al, 1991b]. Since transient rises in blood pressure occur following arousals of any kind [Ali et al, 1991a; Shimizu et al, 1990], it may simply be the extent or "violence" of the arousal which determines the size of the post-apnoeic BP rise. Although the peripheral sympathetic nerve studies suggest a fall-off of activity on arousal [Hedner et al, 1988], there presumably exists continuing vasoconstriction for a few seconds after. A unifying hypothesis might be that the length of the apnoea determines the degree of recruitment of the diving reflex (and thus degree of peripheral vasoconstriction) and that the post-apnoeic BP rise consists of two components - a rise in heart rate and cardiac output (following release of the diving reflex) in the face of transiently persisting peripheral vasoconstriction; and an arousal-related phenomenon perhaps acting on visceral sympathetic tone rather than peripheral. It is clear from the above that the mechanism of the post-apnoeic rise in BP is not fully understood!

During the Mueller manoeuvres of an obstructive apnoea the intra-thoracic pressure falls and systolic BP falls as well, Fig. 1, [Lea et al, 1990]. If the intra-pleural and arterial falls are similar then no increase in left ventricular transmyocardial wall pressure occurs. But if there is any defence of peripheral arterial pressure then this must be at the expense of increased left ventricular transmyocardial wall pressures. Thus an increased afterload on the heart will exist. Whether this does occur is not clear [Podzus, 1990] but there is some evidence that patients with OSA have left ventricles more hypertrophied than can be accounted for by their daytime hypertension or obesity alone [Hedner et al, 1990].

Despite an incomplete understanding of the cause of these post-apnoeic BP rises we can still postulate what consequences they might have. In our experience the patients with the worst sleep apnoea (longest apnoeas and worst hypoxaemia) have the biggest BP swings. So that the patients who probably have the worst prognosis are the ones with the greatest BP swings. Normal people have falls in nocturnal BP [Khatri & Freis, 1967] but these patients do not [Ali et al, 1991b], and thus mean 24 hr blood pressure will be elevated even if the daytime values are not. If a group of cardiologists were told that there was a patient whose average 24hr BP was raised, and that in addition it rose further by 30mmHg or more over 300 times a night, then they would surely be happy to accept that this was bad for the heart and peripheral vasculature. Pulsatile blood pressure rises may be more important than average pressures in the pathogenesis of haemorrhagic strokes, aortic dissections and atheroma generation.

Thus in summary, there is some evidence that OSA provokes increased cardiovascular morbidity and mortality. This does not seem to be explained by higher levels of daytime arterial BP which, when raised in patients with sleep apnoea, are probably due mainly to their obesity. However, cardiovascular damage may result from increased average 24hr BP levels due to lack of the normal overnight fall, and also from the recurrent upward surges that occur hundreds of times a night following each apnoea.

REFERENCES

Ali, N.J., Davies, R.J.O., Fleetham, J.A. and Stradling, J.R. (1991a): Periodic movements of the legs during sleep associated with rises in systemic blood pressure. Sleep. in press.

Ali, N.J., Davies, R.J.O., Fleetham, J.A. and Stradling, J.R. (1991b): The effects of oxygen and CPAP on systemic blood pressure during obstructive sleep apnoea. Thorax. in press.

Andersen, H.T. (1964): Physiological adaptations in diving vertebrates. J. Appl. Physiol. 19, 417-422.

Angell-James, J.E., and DeBurgh-Daly, M. (1969): Cardiovascular responses in apnoeic asphyxia: role of arterial chemoreceptors and the modification of their effects by a pulmonary inflation reflex. J. Physiol. 201, 87-104.

Balter, M.S., Chapman, K.R., Maleki-Yazdi, M.R., Leenen, F.H.H. and Rebuck, A.S. (1990): Effects of oxygen withdrawal on catecholamine release in patients on home oxygen therapy. Clin. Sci. 79, 155-159.

Blair, D., Habicht, J.P., Sims, E.A.H., Sylvester, D. and Abraham, S. (1984): Evidence for an increased risk for hypertension with centrally located body fat and the effect of race and sex on this risk. Am. J. Epidemiol. 119, 526-540.

Bloom, J.W., Kaltenborn, W.T. and Quan, S.F. (1988): Risk factors in a general population for snoring. Importance of cigarette smoking and obesity. Chest. 93, 678-683.

Boudoulas, H., Schmidt, H., Gelens, P., Clark, R.W. and Lewis, R.P. (1983): Case reports on deterioration of sleep apnea during therapy with propranolol - preliminary studies. Res. Commun. Chem. Pathol. Pharmacol. 39, 3-10.

Clark, R.W., Boudoulas, H., Schaal, S.F. and Schmidt, H.S. (1980): Adrenergic hyperactivity and cardiac abnormality in primary disorder of sleep. Neurology. 30, 113-119.

Davies, R.J.O. and Stradling, J.R. (1990): The relationship between neck circumference, radiographic pharyngeal anatomy, and the obstructive sleep apnoea syndrome. Eur Respir J. 3, 505-514.

Escourrou, P., Jirani, A., Nedelcoux, H., Duroux, P. and Gaultier, C. (1990): Systemic hypertension in sleep apnea syndrome. Chest. 98, 1362-1365.

Fletcher, E.C., De Behnke, R.D., Lovoi, M.S. and Gorin, A.B. (1985): Undiagnosed sleep apnoea in patients with essential hypertension. Ann. Intern. Med. 103, 190-195.

Fletcher, E.C., Miller, J., Schaaf, J.W. and Fletcher, J. (1987): Urinary catecholamines before and after tracheostomy in patients with obstructive sleep apnoea and hypertension. Sleep. 10, 35-44.

Fletcher, E., Lovoi, M. and Miller, J. (1985): Propranalol and sleep apnea. Suppl. Am. Rev. Respir. Dis. 131, 103-103.

Freidman, M., Rosenman, R. and Carroll, V. (1958): Changes in the serum cholesterol and blood clotting time in men subjected to cyclic variations of occupational stress. Circulation. 17, 852-861.

Gislason, T., Aberg, H. and Taube, A. (1987): Snoring and systemic hypertension - an epidemiological study. Acta Med Scand. 222, 415-421.

Gislason, T., Almqvist, M., Eriksson, G., Taube, A. and Boman, G. (1988): Prevalence of sleep apnea syndrome among Swedish men - an epidemiological study. J. Clin. Epidemiol. 41, 571-576.

Goldstein, D.S. (1983): Plasma catecholamines and essential hypertension. Hypertension. 5, 86-99.

Gonzalez-Rothi, R.J., Foresman, G.A. and Block, A.J. (1988): Do patients with sleep apnea die in their sleep? Chest. 94, 531-538.

Guilleminault, C., Connolly, S.J. and Winkle, R.A. (1983): Cardiac arrhythmias and conduction disturbances during sleep in 400 patients with sleep apnea syndrome. Am. J. Cardiol. 52, 490-494.

Guilleminault, C., Cummiskey, J. and Dement, W.C. (1980): Sleep apnea syndrome: recent advances. Adv. Int. Med. 26, 347-372.

Guilleminault, C., Tilkian, A., and Dement, W.C. (1976): The sleep apnea syndromes. Annu. Rev. Med. 27, 465-484.

Hanly, P.J., Millar, T.W., Steljes, D.G., Baert, R., Frais, M.A. and Kryger, M.H. (1989): Respiration and abnormal sleep in patients with congestive heart failure. Chest. 96, 480-488.

He, J., Kryger, M.H., Zorick, F.J., Conway, W. and Roth, T. (1988): Mortality and apnea index in obstructive sleep apnea. Chest. 94, 9-14.

Hedner, J., Ejnell, H., Sellgren, J., Hedner, T. and Wallin, G. (1988): Is high and fluctuating muscle nerve sympathetic activity in the sleep apnoea syndrome of pathogenetic importance for the development of hypertension. J. Hypertens. 6 (suppl 4), 529-531.

Hedner, J., Ejnell, H., Wallin, G., Carlsson, J., Caidahl, K. and (1990): Consequences of increased sympathetic activity in sleep apnea. A pathogenetic mechanism for cardiovascular complications? In: Sleep 90, ed. J. Horne, pp. 435-439. Bochum: Pontenagel Press

Hirshkowitz, M., Karacan, I., Gurakar, A. and Williams, R.L. (1989): Hypertension, erectile dysfunction, and occult sleep apnea. Sleep. 12, 223-232.

Hoffstein, V., Rubinstein, I., Mateika, S. and Slutsky, A.S. (1988): Determinants of blood pressure in snorers. Lancet. 2, 992-994.

Kales, A., Bixler, E.D., Cadieux, R.J. et al (1984): Sleep apnoea in a hypertensive population. Lancet. 2, 1005-1008.

Katz, I., Stradling, J.R., Slutsky, A.S., Zamel, N. and Hoffstein, V. (1990): Do patients with obstructive sleep apnea have fat necks?. Am. Rev. Respir. Dis. 141, 1228-1231.

Khatri, I.M. and Freis, E.D. (1967): Hemodynamic changes during sleep. J. Appl. Physiol. 23, 964-970.

Knight, I. (1984): The Heights and Weights of Adults in Great Britain. London: H.M.S.O.

Lahive, K.C., Weiss, J.W. and Weinberger, S.E. (1988): Alpha-methyldopa selectively reduces alae nasi activity. Clin. Sci. 74, 547-551.

Larsson, B., Svardsudd, K., Welin, L., Wilhelmsen, L., Bjorntorp, P. and Tibblin, G. (1984): Abdominal adipose distribution, obesity and risk of cardiovascular disease and death: 13 year follow-up of participants in the study of men born in 1913. Br. Med. J. 288, 1401-1404.

Lavie, P., Ben Yosef, R. and Rubin, A. (1984): Prevalence of sleep apnoea syndrome among patients with hypertension. Am. Heart J. 168, 373-376.

Lea, S., Ali, N.J., Goldman, M., Loh, L., Fleetham, J. and Stradling, J.R. (1990): Systolic blood pressure swings reflect inspiratory effort during simulated obstructive sleep apnoea. In: Sleep 90, ed. J. Horne, pp. 178-181. Bochum: Pontenagel Press

Lugaresi, E., Cirignotta, F., Coccagna, G. and Piana, C. (1980): Some epidemiological data on snoring and cardiocirculatory disturbances. Sleep. 3, 221-224.

Norton, P.G. and Dunn, E.V. (1985): Snoring as a risk factor for disease. Br. Med. J. 291, 630-632.

Oparil, S. (1986): The sympathetic nervous system in clinical and experimental hypertension. Kidney Internat. 30, 437-452.

Partinen, M. and Guilleminault, C. (1990): Daytime sleepiness and vascular morbidity at seven year follow-up in obstructive sleep apnea patients. Chest. 97, 27-32.

Partinen, M., Jamieson, A. and Guilleminault, C. (1988): Long-term outcome for obstructive sleep apnea syndrome patients. Chest. 94, 1201-1204.

Podzus, T.E. (1990): Hemodynamics in sleep apnea. In: Sleep and Respiration, ed. F.G.Issa, P.M.Suratt and J.E.Remmers, pp. 353-361. New York: Wiley-Liss.

Prybylski, J., Sabbah, H.N. and Stein, P.D. (1980): Why do patients with essential hypertension experience sleep apnoea syndrome? Medical Hypothesis. 20, 173-177.

Reite, M., Jackson, D., Cahoon, R.L. and Weil, J.V. (1975): Sleep physiology at high altitude.. Electroencephalog. Clin. Neurophysiol. 38, 463-471.

Schmidt-Nowara, W.W., Coultas, D.B., Wiggins, C., Skipper, B.E. and Samet, J.M. (1990): Snoring in a Hispanic-American population. Risk factors and association with hypertension and other morbidity. Arch. Int. Med. 150, 597-601.

Shepard, J.W. (1985): Gas exchange and hemodynamics during sleep. Med. Clin. North Am. 69,

1243-1263.

Shimizu, T., Kogawa, S., Tashiro, T. et al (1990): Mechanisms of transient marked elevations of arterial pressure in patients with sleep apnea syndrome. In: Sleep 90, ed. J. Horne, pp. 182-184. Bochum: Pontenagel Press.

Somers, V.K., Mark, A.L. and Abboud, F.M. (1988): Sympathetic activation by hypoxia and hypercapnia - implications for sleep apnea. Clin. and Exper. - Theory and Practice. A10 (suppl 1), 413-422.

Stradling, J.R. (1989): Sleep apnoea and hypertension. Thorax. 44, 984-989.

Stradling, J.R. and Crosby, J.H. (1990): Relation between systemic hypertension and sleep hypoxaemia or snoring: analysis in 748 men drawn from general practice. Br. Med. J. 300, 75-78.

Stradling, J.R., Crosby, J. (1991): Predictors and prevalence of obstructive sleep apnoea and snoring in 1001 middle-aged men. Thorax. in press.

Sullivan, C.E., Kozar, L.F., Murphy, E. and Phillipson, E.A. (1985): Primary role of respiratory afferents in sustaining breathing rhythm. J. Appl. Physiol. 45, 11-17.

Thorpy, M.J. and Ledereich, P.S. (1988): Follow-up of patients with obstructive sleep apnoea. European Congress of Sleep Research, Jerusalem.

Tolle, F.A., Judy, W.V., Yu, P.L. and Markand, O.N. (1983): Reduced stroke volumes related to pleural pressure in obstructive sleep apnea. J. Appl. Physiol. 55, 1718-1724.

Verdecchia, P., Schillaci, G., Guerrieri, M. et al (1990): Circadian blood pressure changes and left ventricular hypertrophy in essential hypertension. Circulation. 81, 528-536.

Vlachogianni, E.D., Sandhagen, B., Gislason, T. and Stalenheim, G. (1989): High ventilatory response to hypoxia in hypertensive patients with sleep apnea. Upsala J. Med. Sci. 94, 89-94.

Warley, A.R.H., Mitchell, A.H. and Stradling, J.R. (1988): Prevalence of nocturnal hypoxaemia in men with and without hypertension. Quart. J. Med. 68, 637-644.

Weinsier, R.L., Norris, D.J., Birch, R. et al (1985): The relative contribution of body fat and fat patterns to blood pressure level. Am J Trop Med Hyg. 7, 578-585.

Welin, L., Svardsudd, K., Wilhelmsen, L., Larsson, B. and Tibblin, G. (1987): Analysis of risk factors for stroke in a cohort of men born in 1913. New. Eng. J. Med. 317, 521-526.

Williams, A.J., Houston, D., Finberg, S., Lam, C., Kinney, J.L. and Santiago, S. (1985): Sleep apnoea syndromes and essential hypertension. Am. J. Cardiol. 55, 1019-1022.

Zwillich, C., Devlin, T., White, D., Douglas, N., Weil, J. and Martin, R. (1982): Bradycardia during sleep apnea: characteristics and mechanism. J. Clin. Invest. 69, 1286-1292.

Regulation of body fluid compartments in obstructive sleep apnea syndrome

Jean Krieger

Clinique Neurologique, Centre Hospitalier Universitaire, 67091 Strasbourg Cedex, France

SUMMARY

The observation that increased urine and sodium excretion in obstructive sleep apnea syndrome was corrected by continuous positive airway pressure (CPAP) treatment has stimulated the investigation of hormonal systems regulating body fluid compartments. Atrial natriuretic peptide release was increased in 2/3 of our patients, whereas renin and plasma aldosterone levels were decreased in all patients. CPAP treatment corrected all these shifts. Arginine vasopressin levels showed the widest variations. CPAP treatment also results in a decreased hematocrit indicative of a hemodilution which does not seem to be explained reduced diuresis alone. The mechanisms underlying these hormonal changes remain poorly understood.

INTRODUCTION

The regulation of body fluid compartments in obstructive sleep apnea has been only recently, and actually very little, investigated. Attention has been drawn to possible changes in body fluid compartments when an increased urine excretion has been reported (Krieger *et al.*, 1988, Warley & Stradling, 1988), which has led to investigations of the hormonal systems involved in the regulation of body fluids and of vascular tone, since these two functions are intimately coregulated. However, little is known concerning actual changes in body fluid content and distribution. The rationale for these studies is of course the investigation of the possible mechanisms of the hypertension which is often present in obstructive sleep apnea patients.

RENAL FUNCTION IN OBSTRUCTIVE SLEEP APNEA SYNDROME

In 1988, two reports from two separate groups (Krieger *et al.*, 1988, Warley & Stradling, 1988), showed an increased urine and sodium excretion in obstructive sleep apnea patients, when compared to normal subjects. Treatment with nasal CPAP reduced the urine and sodium excretion to a level not different from that of controls.

Further analysis of the changes in renal function associated with these changes in urine flow and sodium excretion demonstrated no significant change in creatinine clearance; this indicated that glomerular filtration was not changed, and thus that an alteration in renal perfusion was probably not the primary mechanism of the observed changes (Krieger *et al.*, 1988).

Similarly, free water clearance was not modified, which suggested that changes in antidiuretic hormone did not play a major role. Finally, no change was observed in aldosterone excretion (Krieger *et al.*, 1988).

The observed correlation between the decrease in esophageal pressure swings and the decrease in urine excretion with CPAP suggested that atrial natriuretic peptide might be involved in the observed changes.

HORMONAL SYSTEMS INVOLVED IN BODY FLUID AND VASCULAR TONE REGULATION

Atrial Natriuretic Peptide (ANP)

ANP appears to play a major role in the regulation of body sodium content, and hence water content and blood pressure.

ANP is a recently discovered 28 amino-acid peptidic hormone released from granules in cardiomyocytes, in response to a multitude of stimuli. These include acute sodium or volume loading; central volume shift (as results from lying down or from water immersion); acute increases in blood pressure; dynamic exercise; increased heart rate; hypoxemia; AVP infusion; *et cetera*. The factor common to these stimuli is atrial stretch (and not simply increased atrial pressure, as demonstrated by the absence of an increase in ANP during cardiac tamponade).

Its vascular effects are observed only at high (supraphysiological ?) levels and seem to result from a direct relaxing effect on the vascular smooth musculature through an activation of the particulate guanylate cyclase resulting in an inhibition of Ca^{++} entry. Its renal effects seem to result both from its vascular effect, via increased glomerular filtration, and from its effects on membrane permeability to sodium leading to an increased sodium excretion at the level of the collecting ducts. The increased permeability to sodium also results in a fluid shift from the plasmatic to the extracellular space.

ANP thus decreases blood pressure and blood volume and increases diuresis and natriuresis through a combination of these mechanisms. It also interacts with other hormonal systems: it inhibits adrenal steroidogenesis (decreasing aldosterone and cortisol); it inhibits renal renin release; and it inhibits angiotensin II-induced vasoconstriction and AVP-mediated water reabsorption.

Independent of the effects of centrally synthesized ANP, peripheral ANP also has central effects by acting upon receptors located in the circumventricular organs (subfornical organ, area postrema, median eminence, and organum vasculosum lamina terminalis). The respective role in body volume regulation of peripheral and central ANP, and of brain natriuretic peptide, (whose structure is close to that of ANP and which appears to be more widespread in the central nervous system than ANP), are currently under investigation.

The circulatory half-life of ANP is short, lasting about 3 minutes, but its effects are longer, lasting about 30 minutes.

In obstructive sleep apnea patients, analysis of the excretion of cyclic guanosine monophosphate (cGMP, Krieger *et al.*, 1989 b), the putative second messenger in atrial natriuretic peptide effects, whose urinary excretion reflects atrial natriuretic peptide secretion, showed a decrease with nasal continuous positive airway pressure treatment, further supporting the role of ANP; however, this was contradicted by the absence of a change in plasma ANP reported in a study where ANP was assayed in the venous blood (Warley *et al.*, 1988). This study, however, was based on 6 patients in whom 3 blood samples were taken, of which only one was taken during sleep, while the other two were taken before the patient rose and at noon.

In contrast, four studies demonstrated increased ANP plasma levels in OSA patients.

One was based (Krieger *et al.*, 1989 a) on 7 patients in whom about 8 to 10 blood samples were taken during the same night repeatedly either off- or on-CPAP. The mean plasma ANP level off CPAP during sleep was higher than during wake; it decreased when apneas were eliminated with CPAP. However, this effect was significant in pulmonary arterial blood, but not in peripheral venous blood, due to a wide inter-subject variability.

In another study, a 10-minute sampling rate of venous blood was used during 2 nights 2 weeks apart either off- or on-CPAP (Krieger *et al.*, 1991). The results showed that ANP levels during sleep were increased in 6 of the 9 OSA patients. This increased ANP release was corrected with CPAP treatment. The mean ANP level was correlated with the mean lowest SaO2 and with the mean end-apneic esophageal pressure swings during sleep, suggesting that the severity of the sleep hypoxemia and the degree of increase in respiratory effort against the occluded upper airway play a role. Furthermore, intranight cross-correlation analysis showed correlations between plasma ANP and mean end-apneic SaO_2 and/or mean end-apneic esophageal pressure swings. These observations are in keeping with the hypothesis that ANP is released in response to the atrial distension induced by the ventricular afterload due to increased arterial pulmonary resistance caused by hypoxemic vasoconstriction, or its preload due to increased venous return caused by increased (more negative) intrathoracic pressures. The role of increased intrathoracic pressure swings is not supported by the lack of an increase in plasma ANP in normal volunteers breathing through an inspiratory threshold load (Warley *et al.*, 1990); however, the inspiratory intrathoracic pressures of

-30 cm H_2O achieved in this study were far from the average -60 cm H_2O mean maximal apneic esophageal pressure swings observed in OSA patients (Krieger et al., 1991).

Another study of 8 patients, 3 of whom were reevaluated on CPAP (sampling rate not specified), also showed increased plasma ANP in the untreated condition, especially when the patients had heart failure, and their decrease with CPAP (Ehlenz et al., 1988). The number of patients in whom ANP was actually increased was not specified in the abstract reporting this study.

Finally, another recent study (Baruzzi et al., 1991) in 6 patients with an hourly sampling rate also showed a decrease in mean plasma ANP concentrations with CPAP. In this study, it was not specified either whether this effect was observed in every patient.

It is also noteworthy that ANP levels measured 30 minutes after awakening decreased with CPAP treatment (Jamieson et al., 1989). If this finding were confirmed, it would suggest, given the short half-life of ANP, that non-apneic mechanisms play a role in the changes in ANP.

Although ANP is probably not the only hormonal system involved in the increased urine excretion in OSA (see below), the demonstration of a significant correlation between the decrease in cGMP excretion and the decrease in sodium excretion with CPAP in 80 OSA patients ($r = 0.60$, $p < 0.0001$, Krieger, unpublished observation, Fig. 1) strongly suggests that it plays a role.

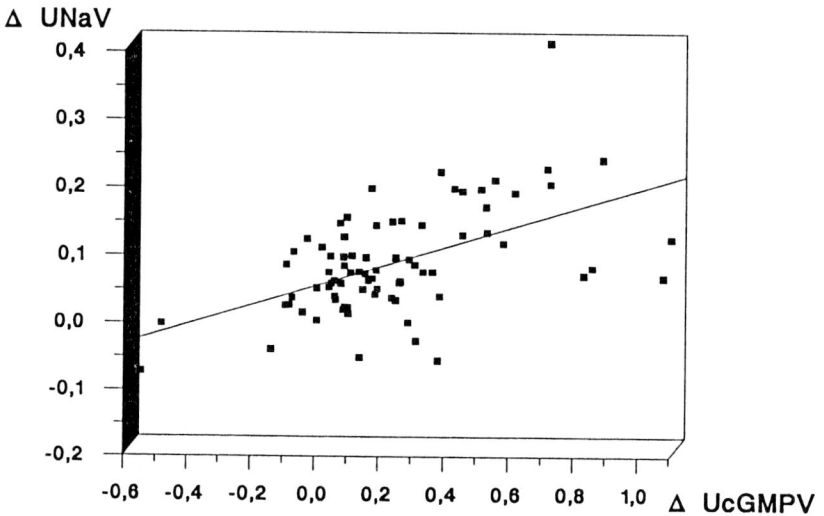

Fig. 1. Change in urinary sodium excretion during sleep (UNaV, in mMol/min) vs change in urinary cyclic guanosine monophosphate excretion during sleep (UcGMPV, in umol/min) with CPAP treatment in 80 obstructive sleep apnea patients.

Renin-Angiotensin-Aldosterone

Renin is a proteolytic enzyme which is released into the bloodstream by the juxtaglomerular cells of the kidney; it converts a protein synthesized by the liver, angiotensinogen, into angiotensin I which is in turn converted by a circulating angiotensin-converting-enzyme (ACE, synthesized in the lungs) into angiotensin II. While neither angiotensinogen nor ACE seem to be under physiological control, the plasma concentration of renin is regulated by a multitude of factors (i.e., activated by beta-adrenergic stimulation and reduced stretch of the afferent glomerular arteriole, as induced by lower plasma volume, reduced effective circulating volume, or pooling of blood in lower extremities; inhibited by somatostatin, angiotensin and ANP, or by an increased tubular load of chloride). Recently, it has been shown that renin release also depended upon central mechanisms, since it closely parallels the rapid eye movement (REM)-non-REM sleep cycle, with a decrease in plasma renin coinciding with the onset of REM sleep (Brandenberger et al., 1988).

Angiotensin II has potent vasoconstrictive effects and plays a crucial role in the re-establishment of blood pressure in emergency situations. It also acts on the kidney, directly and by activating the release of aldosterone from the adrenal zona glomerulosa. Aldosterone is the main mineralocorticosteroid. It acts on the kidney by promoting sodium (and hence water) reabsorption and potassium excretion at the tubular level.

Early studies failed to demonstrate a significant change in plasma renin activity, when it was measured in the morning, before the patients got up. No change in urine aldosterone excretion was found either (Krieger et al., 1989).

Recent results (Follenius et al., in Press) obtained using the 10-minute sampling rate technique in 7 OSA patients studied either off- or on-CPAP 2 weeks apart showed that aldosterone and plasma renin activity (PRA) profiles were flat in untreated patients. The mean plasma aldosterone and PRA doubled with CPAP treatment, which also restored the normal secretory bursts related to the REM non-REM sleep cycles.

An increase in PRA with CPAP has also been demonstrated in a study of 6 patients (Ehlenz et al., 1990) in whom blood samples were taken every 10 minutes, but averaged on a one hour basis, thus smoothing out the possible short-term sleep-state-related changes in PRA.

Arginine-Vasopressin (AVP)

Like the thirst center, the AVP system is based in the hypothalamus and responds to many of the stimuli that trigger or inhibit thirst. AVP is an octapeptide synthesized in the suprachiasmatic cells which migrates to the posterior pituitary (axonal transport), where it is released.

The primary stimulus for AVP release is an increase in plasmatic osmolality detected by hypothalamic and hepatic osmoreceptors; stretch receptors (left atrium) and aortic pressure receptors play an accessory role, which may become predominant in case of hypovolemia. Angiotensin II also stimulates AVP release.

AVP increases the permeability to water of the epithelial cell membrane in the collecting ducts of the kidney; when AVP is present the reabsorption of water following the osmotic gradient is possible, resulting in reduced water output.

AVP has also been found in many other areas of the CNS, and seems to be involved in central mechanisms of stress, as well as in the regulation of appetite and mechanisms of memory.

In OSA, mean AVP levels during sleep varied widely between patients (from 0.2 to 2.7 pg/ml); it increased in 6, decreased in 1 and did not change in 2 of the 9 patients investigated (Krieger *et al.*, 1991). The reasons for this heterogeneity have not been investigated; given the role of AVP in stress mechanisms, it may be postulated that they express a variability in the central reactivity to the aggression represented by sleep apneas. Therefore, they might play a key role in individual susceptibility to sleep apnea.

BODY FLUID REGULATION

The above described changes (increased ANP, decreased renin and aldosterone) concur to promote water and sodium loss. The stimulus behind these changes is not clearly established. We have postulated that the hemodynamic changes induced by obstructive sleep apneas could increase the intra-thoracic volume, by sucking blood into the thorax, and thus result in a state of pseudo-hyperinflation which would distend the atria and increase ANP release (Krieger *et al.*, 1989). A similar mechanism has been proposed for the increased renin activity (Ehlenz *et al.*, 1990). However, the restoration of a PRA pattern related to the REM-non-REM sleep cyclicity clearly demonstrates that central mechanisms do play a role.

The extent to which these mechanisms alter body fluid distribution is not well established, in so far as no study has actually measured body fluid compartments directly. The only evidence is indirect, resulting from observed decreases in hematocrit, red cell count (RCC) and hemoglobin after a single treatment night with CPAP (Krieger *et al.*, 1990), which can only be explained by a hemodilution.

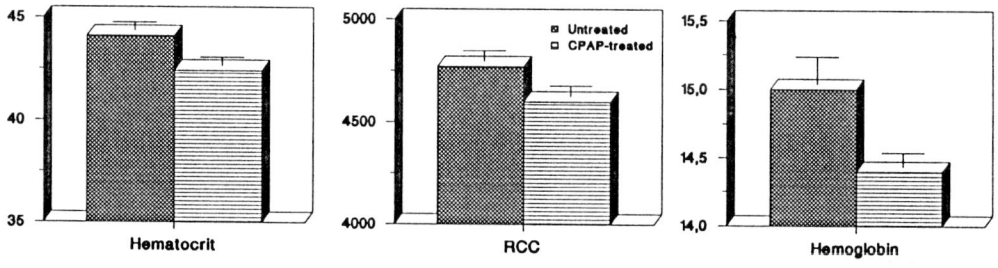

Fig. 2. Immediate effects of a single treatment night with CPAP on Hematocrit (%), Red Cell Count (RCC, 10^3 cells/mm^3 and Hemoglobin (g/100 ml) in 80 obstructive sleep apnea patients.

In the 80 above-mentioned patients (Krieger, unpublished observation), urine excretion during sleep decreased from 1.23 ± 0.07 to 0.855 ± 0.06 ml/min ($p < 0.00001$) with CPAP treatment, the hematocrit decreased from 44.1 ± 0.4 % to 42.4 ± 0.4 %, the RCC from $4,769.6 \pm 51.2 \times 10^3$ /mm^3 to $4,597.6 \pm 52.3 \times 10^3$ /mm^3 and the hemoglobin concentration from 15.0 ± 0.2 to 14.4 ± 0.1 g/100 ml (means $\pm$ sem, $p < 0.00001$ for the 3 variables, paired t test, Fig. 2). The corresponding increase in blood volume (Dill & Costill, 1974) is one of 4.17 %, i.e., 208 ml (assuming a 5 liter blood volume); this is in the same order of magnitude as the decrease in urine volume during sleep, which was 199 ml in these 80 patients. However, there was no significant correlation between the change in either hematocrit or RCC and the change in urine volume, suggesting that the observed hemodilution did not simply result from excess fluid not excreted by the kidney.

Given the effects of ANP on vascular membrane permeability promoting a shift of salt and water from the vascular to the interstitial volume, it can be hypothesized that the decreased ANP excretion with CPAP could favor a return of fluid from the extravascular volume to the vascular bed. The effects of ANP on renal function and on vascular permeability could explain the paradox of decreased urine excretion concomitant with a reduction in peripheral edemas which is commonly observed when CPAP is initiated.

The above described changes all result in increased salt excretion and decreased vascular tone, which obviously cannot explain the development of hypertension in OSA. They rather appear as defense mechanisms against a process which would tend to increase blood volume and/or vascular tone. The nature of this process remains to be established. It might be the recently described (Krieger *et al.*, in Press) altered prostanoid release, indicated by a decreased prostacycline (vasodilator) to thromboxane (vasoconstrictive) urinary ratio.

REFERENCES

Baruzzi, A., Riva, R., Cirignotta, F., Zucconi, M., Capelli, M., & Lugaresi, E. (1991): Atrial natriuretic peptide and catecholamines in obstructive sleep apnea syndrome. Sleep 14, 83-86.

Brandenberger, G., Follenius, M., & Muzet, A. (1988): Nocturnal oscillations in plasma renin activity and REM-NREM sleep cycles in humans: a common regulatory mechanism. Sleep 11, 242-250.

Dill, D. B., & Costill, D. L. (1974): Calculation of percentage changes in volumes of blood, plasma, and red cells in dehydration. J Appl Physiol 37, 247-248.

Ehlenz, K., Peter, J. H., Schneider, H., Elle, T., Scheele, B., Wichert, P. v. & Kaffarnik, H. (1990): Renin secretion is substantially influenced by obstructive sleep apnea syndrome. In Sleep '90, ed. J. Horne, pp. 193-195. Bochum: Pontenagel Press.

Ehlenz, K., Schmidt, P., Podszus, T., Becker, H., Peter, H., Wichert, P. von, & Kaffarnik, H. (1988): Plasma levels of atrial natriuretic factor in patients with sleep apnea syndrome (Abstr). Acta Endocrinol Suppl 287, 234-235.

Follenius, M., Krieger, J., Krauth, M. O., Sforza, E., & Brandenberger, G. (1991): Obstructive sleep apnea: peripheral and central effects on plasma renin activity and aldosterone. Sleep, in Press.

Jamieson, A. O., Fuchs, I. E., Becker, P. M., Brown, D., & Roffwarg, H. P. (1989): Atrial natriuretic peptide (ANP) in obstructive sleep apnea; changes with nasal CPAP - A pilot study (Abstr). Sleep Res 18, 93.

Krieger, J., Benzoni, D., Sforza, E., & Sassard, J. Urinary excretion of prostanoids during sleep in obstructive sleep apnea patients. Clin Exp Pharmacol Physiol, in Press.

Krieger, J., Follenius, M., Sforza, E., Brandenberger, G., Peter, & J. D. (1991): Effects of treatment with nasal continuous positive airway pressure on atrial natriuretic peptide and arginine vasopressin release during sleep in obstructive sleep apnea. Clin Sci 80, 443-449.

Krieger, J., Imbs, J. L., Schmidt, M., & Kurtz, D. (1988): Renal function in patients with obstructive sleep apnea. Effects of nasal continuous positive airway pressure. Arch Intern Med 148, 1337-1340.

Krieger, J., Laks, L., Wilcox, I., Grunstein, R. R., Costas, L. J. V., Mcdougall, J. G., & Sullivan, C. E. (1989 a): Atrial Natriuretic Peptide Release During Sleep in Patients with Obstructive Sleep Apnoea Before and During Treatment with Nasal Continuous Positive Airway Pressure. Clinical Science 77, 407-411.

Krieger, J., Schmidt, M., Sforza, E., Lehr, L., Imbs, J. L., Coumaros, G., & Kurtz, D. (1989 b): Urinary excretion of 3'-5'-cyclic guanosine monophosphate during sleep in obstructive sleep apnea patients with and without nasal continuous positive airway pressure treatment. Clin Sci 76, 31-37.

Krieger, J., Sforza, E., Barthelmebs, M., Imbs, J. L., & Kurtz, D. (1990): Overnight decrease in hematocrit after nasal CPAP treatment in patients with OSA. Chest 97, 729-730.

Warley, A. R. H., & Stradling, J. R. (1988): Abnormal diurnal variation in salt and water excretion in patients with obstructive sleep apnea. Clin Sci 74, 183-185.

Warley, A. R. H., Fontes, F., Raine, A. E. G., & Stradling J.R. (1990): Lack of effect of an inspiratory threshold load on plasma natriuretic peptide levels. Clin Sci 78, 311-313.

Warley, A. R. H., Morice, A., & Stradling, J. R. (1988): Plasma levels of atrial natriuretic peptide (ANP) in obstructive sleep apnoea (OSA)(Abstr). Thorax 43, 253p-254p.

Résumé

La description au cours du syndrome d'apnées du sommeil d'une augmentation de la diurèse et de la natriurèse corrigée par le traitement par la pression positive continue a conduit à explorer les systèmes hormonaux régulant les compartiments hydriques de l'organisme. La sécrétion de peptide natriurétique auriculaire est augmentée chez 2/3 des malades, alors que l'activité rénine et le taux d'aldostérone plasmatique sont diminués dans tous les cas examinés. Le traitement par la pression positive continue corrige ces anomalies. Les modifications des taux d'arginine vasopressine sont plus dispersées. Ce traitement s'accompagne également d'une diminution de l'hématocrite témoignant d'une hémodilution qui ne semble pas s'expliquer par la seule diminution de la diurèse. Les processus sous-tendant ces modifications hormonales restent mal connus.

Cardiorespiratory mechanisms implicated in sudden infant death syndrome : a possible role for the autonomic nervous system

A. Kahn, E. Rebuffat, M. Sottiaux, J.J. Grosswasser and D. Michel

Pediatric Sleep and Development Unit, University Children Hospital, Free University of Brussels, Av. J.J. Crocq 15, B-1020 Brussels, Belgium

AUTONOMIC NERVOUS SYSTEM DYSREGULATIONS AND SIDS

Epidemiological, as well as clinical, and laboratory experience indicate that infants victims of Sudden Infant Death syndrome (SIDS) form an heterogeneous entity. It was suggested that the in utero environment, and the postneonatal care of SIDS infants were less than optimal. Subtle differences in symptoms could indicate that the SIDS infants are since birth different from control infants (Valdes-Dapena, 1980). Among many other potential causes, the autonomic nervous system could contribute to some SIDS cases. The following notes will explore the potential role of autonomic system dysregulations on heart rate changes, and on respiratory controls in sleeping infants.

HEART RATE CONTROLS AND SIDS.

Studies done in infants who subsequently died of SIDS occasionally disclosed the presence of cardiac rythm abnormalities, possibly associated with autonomic nervous system dysregulations. In SIDS victims both excessive sympathetic and vagal abnormalities have been suggested to account for reports of elevated tachycardia index (Southall et al.,1983), excessive heart rate slowing (Guilleminault et al., 1981), decreased heart rate variability (Leistner et al.,1980), and prolonged Q-Tc index (Schwartz, 1976). Other cardiac abnormalities include Wolff-Parkinson-White syndrome (Keeton et al.,1977), and isolated ventricular extrasystoles (Southall et al.,1982). Prospective studies have yet failed to confirm that these heart rate manifestations significantly characterise infants at higher risk for SIDS (Southall et al., 1982, 1983).

Cardiac rythm and auditory stress during sleep

Exaggerated autonomic cardiac responses can be evidenced by imposed stressful stimulations. In some infants with a sleep apnea, or an apparent life-threatening event (A.L.T.E.), oculocardiac stimulations induce exaggerated cardioinhibitory responses (Kahn et al.,1983). Another example of enhanced autonomic response is based on the animal litterature. An infant rodent exposed to a sudden and unfamiliar noise, while sleeping in REM sleep may develop a "fear-paralysis reflex", with an abrupt and profound bradycardia, asystole and fatal cardiac arrythmia (Kaada, 1987). The acute cardiac stress is associated with vagal discharge, and are significantly enhanced by the restraint of the animal's movements. It has been postulated that in infants, acute bradycardia and sudden death could also be related to similar stressful stimulations imposed during sleep. To investigate this potential cause for SIDS, we studied 22 infants with a median age of 12 weeks. Seven had been admitted after an unexplained A.L.T.E. during sleep, and 15 were asymptomatic. The infants were monitored polygraphically during one night. During REM sleep they were presented a 100 dB (A) white-noise tone for 10 seconds, via an earpiece. Each child was tested twice: once lying "unrestrained", free to move, and once in body movements "restrained" condition, the head, body and limbs tightly wrapped in bed sheets and sand bags. The two series of stimulations were given in alternate order. In the "restrained" condition, when no body movement was allowed, the minimal heart rates were significantly lower than that measured when lying "unrestrained" (Table I). The "restrained" condition was also related to an earlier bradycardic response, with the heart rate dropping before the onset of a reflex tachycardic response. The ALTE and the control infants could not be diffrentiated by their response to auditory stress. The lower and earlier bradycardic reponse shown during conditions of movement-restriction lends support to the contribution of the autonomic nervous system to sudden bradycardia during sleep.

TABLE I

Variables	HEART RATE CHANGES DURING AUDITORY STIMULATION		P
	UNRESTRAINED CONDITION	RESTRAINED CONDITION	
Heart rates (b.p.m.)			
Basal	140 (110-148)	134 (110-148)	NS
Minimal	135 (95-144)	112 (98-138)	.008
Early bradycardia (at onset of stimulation)	1/22	8/22	.010

TABLE I: Changes in heart rate during auditory stimulation, the same infants lying either "unrestrained", or their body movements "restrained". Figures represent absolute values, median values and ranges. Statistical analysis was done with the Fisher exact test, and Wilcoxon rank test, with P value under .05.

II. RESPIRATORY CONTROLS AND SIDS

In some infants who eventually died of SIDS, respiratory monitoring occasionally disclosed prolonged sleep apnea (Steinschneider,1972; Kelly et al.,1986), greater frequency of short-lasting apneas (Steinschneider et al.,1982), or increased periodic breathing (Steinschneider et al.,1982; Kelly et al.,1986). Still, the statistical significance of these respiratory manifestations have been questioned by prospective population-based studies (Southall et al., 1982, 1983).

In most of these studies, the information was derived from chest wall breathing movements and recorded on tape. Investigations performed with more sophisticated polysomnographic techniques occasionally documented evidence of obstructive apneas in some infants who later were victims of SIDS (Guilleminault et al.,1979).

In a preliminary study, we confirmed the presence of obstructed breathing events in some infants who eventually died of SIDS (Kahn et al.,1988). In this study, 11 future SIDS victims were compared to 22 matched control infants. Controls were matched for sex, gestational age, postnatal age, and weight at birth with the SIDS victims. Their polygraphic recordings had been performed in similar conditions at a mean age of 12 weeks. Obstructive and mixed sleep apneas were seen in 8 of 11 SIDS victims and in only 3 of 22 control infants. Three future SIDS infants had 20 or more obstructive episodes in one night. Obstructive apneas were significantly more frequent (total number of episodes: 89 in the SIDS group, and 3 in the control group), and lasted longer in the SIDS victims than in the control group. The obstructed breathing episodes were accompanied by heart rate decreases, and falls in oxygen pressure, or oxygen saturation measurments. The study also showed that future SIDS victims had no central apnea longer than 14 seconds. The observation thus confirmed the presence of breathing control abnormalities in infants who eventually die of SIDS.

To confirm the findings of this preliminary report, we analysed a new group of 19 SIDS victims and 19 pairs of control infants. The data were collected from various centers in Europe. The clinical characteristics of these new groups of infants were similar to the ones arleady described (Table II).

TABLE II

CLINICAL CHARACTERISTICS OF THE INFANTS

Variables	SIDS VICTIMS	CONTROLS	P
No.	30	60	-
Gender (M/F)	19/11	38/22	-
Gestational age (wks)	39 (31-40)	39 (31-40)	-
Age at study (wks)	9.2 (4.5-20)	9.2 (4.5-20)	-
Birth weight (gm)	3113 (1260-4390)	3132 (2540-5200)	-
Apgar	10 (8-10)	9 (6-10)	NS
Rank Order in Family	2 (1-3)	1 (1-5)	NS
Age at death (wks)	17 (8.5-36)	-	-
Delay between study and death	10.2 (1.5-27)	-	-
History of the infants:			
Siblings of SIDS	5	0	-
A.L.T.E.	9	0	-

TABLE II: Clinical characteristics of the SIDS and control infants. Figures represent absolute values, median values and ranges. Statistical analysis was done with the Fisher exact test, and Wilcoxon rank test, with P value under .05.

The analysis of the recordings was again done without knowledge of the infants' indentity. For the total group 30 SIDS victims, and 60 matched control infants, the only variables that significantly characterized the SIDS cases were the presence of obstructed breathing events, corresponding to either obstructive, or mixed apneas (Table III).

TABLE III
POLYSOMNOGRAPHIC STATISTICALLY SIGNIFICANT DIFFERENCES

Variables	SIDS		CONTROL 1	P	CONTROL 2	P
Obstructive apneas						
No. infants	21/30		4/30	.0001	2/30	.0001
No. apneas per infant	2	(0-25)	0 (0-7)	.0003	0 (0-1)	.0001
Duration (sec.)	6	(0-14)	0 (0-5)	.001	0 (0-6)	.001
Mixed apneas						
No. infants	18/30		4/30	.0005	0/30	.0001
No. apneas per infant	1	(0-11)	0 (0-10)	.004	0 (0-3)	.001
Duration (sec.)	6	(0-15)	0 (0-8)	.0002	0 (0-12)	.0006
All obstructed breathing events						
No. infants	25/30		7/30	.0001	2/30	.0010
No. episodes per infant	5	(0-32)	0 (0-10)	.0002	0 (0-2)	.0001

TABLE III: Polysomnographic characteristics of the SIDS and control infants. The significant findings are shown only. Figures represent absolute values, median values and ranges. Statistical analysis was done with the use of Fisher exact test, and Wilcoxon rank test, with P value under .05.

Obstructive sleep apneas were seen in 21 of the 30 SIDS victims, but in only 6 of the 60 control infants. Eleven of the 30 SIDS victims had at least five obstructive apneas per night. Only 1 of 60 control infants had 7 obstructive apneas per night. Mixed apneas were seen in 18 of 30 SIDS, and 4 of 60 control infants. All together, obstructed breathing events were seen in 25 of 30 SIDS infants, and in 9 of 60 control infants. When present, the obstructed events were more frequent, and were longer in the SIDS than in the control infants. In 5 SIDS victims no obstructed breathing event was seen. This finding does not appear to be due to a night-to-night variability in breathing monitoring. When two consecutive nights were recorded in a group of 20 infants studied at a mean age of 12±3 weeks, the variability in obstructed breathing events occcurence was less than 8%. We failed to see any heart rate difference between the SIDS and the control infants.

Although these observations do not establish risk prediction for infants who eventually become victims of SIDS, they add further indirect evidence for a possible sleep-related impairment of respiratory controls in some of these infants.

Potential causes for obstructive sleep apneas in infants.

The causes of obstructed breathing during sleep in infants are still poorly understood. Airway obstructions have been associated with the presence of anatomical, or functional abnormalities of the airways, such as craniofacial abnormalities, micrognathia, cleft palate, adenotonsillar hypertrophy, laryngomalacia, subglottic stenosis, or neck tumor (Guilleminault et al.,1981; Kahn et al.,1988). The obstructions may also be enhanced by factors such as excess body weight, body position, infections, or the use of sedatives (Kahn et al.1985, 1989; Abreu et al.,1986; Cartwright,1984).

Acid esophageal reflux as a precipitating factor

We reported that while episodes of apnea can occur during regurgitations or vomiting, acid reflux in the distal portion of the esophagus does not play a significant role in the development of cardiorespiratory changes during sleep (Kahn et al.,1990). We also studied sleeping infants to investigate whether a temporal relation exists between acid reflux extending to the proximal portion of the esophagus and cardiorespiratory events. One hundred infants with occasional regurgitations were studied: 50 infants admitted after an apparently life-threatening event ("ALTE") that occurred during sleep and that remained unexplained despite medical investigation, and 50 asymptomatic infants ("Non-ALTE") . The infants had a median age of 8 weeks (range 4-26 weeks); 54 were boys. In each child a pH probe was placed in the proximal portion of the thoracic esophagus, under radiological control. Polygraphic monitoring of state of alertness, cardiorespiratory activity, and proximal esophageal pH changes was conducted continuously during one night. The data were analysed blind. In 80 infants a total of 186 drops in esophageal pH below 4 units were seen; 37 % occurred during wakefulness, and 40 % during REM sleep. A total of 7029 central and 61 obstructive apneas were monitored, mainly during REM sleep. Within 5 minutes before, and 5 minutes after the pH drops, there was no difference in the number, or the duration of bradycardia, central, mixed, or obstructive apnea. The infants with an ALTE could not be differentiated from the Non-ALTE infants for any of the variables studied. We concluded that within the limits of this study, spontaneous acid reflux extending to the proximal portion of the esophagus during sleep is usually not temporally related with the development of apneas or bradycardias.

Potential contribution of the autonomic nervous system in upper airway controls

We have investigated whether infants' upper airways could at least partly be controlled by the autonomic nervous system. The hypothesis was based on the literature (Matsumoto et al.,1985; Widdicombe, 1986), as well as on our clinical experience. Obstructed sleep apneas were reported in children and adults suffering from various autonomic nervous system disorders, including familial dysautonomia, diabetes, ganglioneuroma, Shy-Drager syndrome, or olivopontocerbellar degeneration (Guilleminault et al.,1981; Lehrman et al.,1978; Frank et al.,1981; Chokroverty et al.,1984). In infants, the administration of atropine has occasionally been reported to prevent obstructive sleep apneas (Kelly & Shannon,1981), while in adults, tricyclic antidepressants with anticholinergic actions reduce the frequency of obstructive apneas (Brownell et al.,1982). In animal models, such as monkeys, electrical stimulation of the superior laryngeal nerve induces glottal closure (Sutton et al.,1978).

Sleep airway obstructions in infants with breath holding spells

During their sleep, infants with breathholding spells may show repeated upper airway obstructions (Kahn et al.,1990). We studied 71 breath holders with a median age of 14 weeks: 34 infants without loss of consciousness, and 37 with loss of consciousness (16 with pallid spells, 21 with cyanotic spells). For each breath holder, one control infant without a history of breath holding was chosen. All infants were selected in a well babies clinic. The infants were studied during a one-night monitoring session, and the 142 sleep recordings were analyzed without knowledge of the history. While central apneas were evenly distributed in the two groups, airway obstructions were found in 41 of the 71 breath holders, but in only 6 of the 71 control infants. The obstructions had a median duration of 6 seconds (range 4 to 12 seconds) in the breath holders, but only 3 seconds (range 3 to 6 seconds) in the control infants (p= .025). 80% of the obstructed breathing occurred during REM sleep, and 20% during NREM stage I or II sleep. The obstructive episodes were accompanied by a median drop in heart rate of 8% (range 0 to 47%), and in oxygen saturation of 1.7 % (range 0 to 9%). The infants with airway obstruction during sleep snored more often (p= .023), and sweated more (p= .035) during sleep than those without obstruction. Profuse night sweats had also been reported in 21% of future SIDS victims, were measured in infants with unexplained A.L.T.E. events, and were attributed to autonomic stimulation (Kahn et al., 1987). We concluded that the obstructed breathing seen during both wakefulness and sleep in breath holders could be related to a common immature breathing control. Indeed if breathholding spells may be favored by psychogenic factors (Abe et al.,1984), it has also been shown to be related to an underlying dysfunction of the autonomic nervous system (Lombroso & Lerman, 1967; Gastaut

& Gastaut, 1958), and atropinic drugs have been advocated for the treatment of the most severe cases (Laxdal et al.,1969).

Belladonna for obstructed breathing in sleeping infants

The discovery of obstructed apneas in breath holding infants prompted us to investigate the possibility that the abnormal breathing patterns could be regulated by autonomic controls. We therefore studied 20 breath holding infants with a median age of 12 weeks (range 4 to 46 weeks). In every infant, a double-blind crossover challenge was conducted. It included the oral administration of tincture of belladonna, equivalent to 0.01 mg/kg weight of atropine, and placebo syrup containing no belladonna. The belladonna, or the placebo, was administred bedtime for 7 days, followed by a 7-day washout period. Another 7-day series of syrup administration was then undertaken. A night-time polygraphic recording was made after each 7-day series. It was the belladonna, and not the placebo that induced the disappearence of the obstructions in 10 infants; these were called "drug responsive" (Table IV).

TABLE IV

SLEEP STUDIES IN BREATH HOLDERS TREATED WITH BELLADONNA

	Initial recording (no drug treatment)	Sleep studies After the placebo	After belladonna	P
Central apneas:				
No. of infants	20/20	19/19	19/19	-
No. of apneas/8 hr	41 (34-129)	46 (29-134)	40 (33-132)	NS
Duration (sec)	9 (4-12)	8 (3-11)	9 (3-13)	NS
Obstructed breathing events:				
No. of infants	20/20	18/19	5/19	.001
No. of episodes/8 hr	6 (3-16)	6 (4-14)	7 (3-14)	NS
Duration (sec)	8 (4-12)	7 (3-13)	8 (3-11)	NS
Asystoles with ocular compression:				
Duration (sec.)	8 (4-14)	10 (4-13)	3.6 (1.4-8)	.012

TABLE IV
Results of sleep studies performed in infants breath holders after the oral administration of either placebo, or belladonna. The asystole values represent longer R-R intervals measured during manual ocular compression. The figures represent absolute, median and range values. Statistical analysis was done with the use of Wilcoxon signed Rank test for paired sets of data, and the Fisher test for two-by-two tables, with P value under .05.

In 5 children no drug effect was observed after either the placebo or belladonna; these infants were defined as "drug unresponsive". In 4 subjects the obstructions disappeared after both belladonna and the placebo; the children were considered to have an "inconclusive response". One infant was excluded from the study because he developed an airway infection. Ocular compression was done following a standard protocol (Kahn et al., 1983). Compared to the longest R-R intervals measured before any drug was administred, the R-R intervals were unchanged during placebo administration, and were significantly reduced during belladonna treatment ($p= .012$). The reduced asystole could reflect the inhibitory effect of atropine on the vagally-mediated oculo-cardiac stimulation. Likewise, measurements of sweating activity from the skin returned to nomal values after the administration of atropine. It was concluded from this study that in some breath holding infants, obstructed breathing episodes during sleep disappear after the administration of an atropinic drug. We can only speculate as to how atropine prevents the development of obstructed breathing during sleep. The atropinic may have increased the permeability of the nasal passages (White et al.,1985), could have acted upon the oropharyngeal dilator muscles (Block et al.,1984), or on the central medullary parasympathetic neurons (Sullivan et al.,1979).

Our observations thus suggest that in some infants with breath holding spells, obstructed breathing during sleep could be regulated by the autonomic nervous system. If at present, belladonna should not be recommended for the treatment of obstructive sleep apneas in infants, potential development of appropriate treatment strategies may be considered in some specific cases.

CONCLUSIONS

Some infants at risk for SIDS could thus present an autonomic dysfunction of respiratory and/or cardiovascular controls. It remains to be established whether abnormalities of the autonomic regulation of respiratory and/or cardiovascular function may lead to significant symptomatology, or even death. Such evidence could contribute to a better understanding of some of the causes of a sudden death in infants, and eventually lead to new therapeutic approaches.

REFERENCES

Abe K, Oda N, et al. (1984): Natural history and predictive significance of head-banging, head-rolling and breath-holding spells. Dev. Med. Child. Neurol. 26:6 648.

Abreu E Silva FA, Macfayden UM, et al. (1986): Sleep apnoea during upper respiratory infection and metabolic alkalosis in infancy. Arch. Dis. Child. 61:1056-1062.

Block AJ, Faulkner JA, et al. (1984): Factors influencing upper airway closure. Chest 86:114-122.

Brownell LG, West P, et al. (1982): Protriptyline in obstructive sleep apnea: a double-blind trial. N. Engl. J. Med. 307:1037-1042.

Cartwright RD (1984): Effects of sleep position on sleep apnea severity. Sleep 7:110-114

Chokroverty S, Sachdeo R, et al. (1984): Autonomic dysfunction and sleep apnea olivopontocerebellar degeneration. Arch. Neurol. 41:926-931.

Frank Y, Kravath RE, et al. (1981): Sleep apnea and hypoventilation syndrome associated with acquired nonprogressive dysautonomia: clinical and pathological studies in a child. Ann. Neurol.10:18-27.

Gastaut H, Gastaut Y (1958): Electroencephalographic and clinical study of ano: convulsions in children; their location within the group of infantile convulsions and their differentiation from epilepsy. Electroenceph. Clin. Neurophysiol. 10:607-620.

Guilleminault C, Ariagno RI, et al. (1979): Obstructive sleep apnea and near miss SIDS: I. Report of an infant with sudden death. Pediatrics 63:837-843.

Guilleminault C, Brisikin JG, et al. (1981): The impact of autonomic nervous system dysfunction on breathing during sleep. Sleep 4:263-278.

Guilleminault C, Korobkin R, et al. (1981): A review of 50 children with obstructive sleep apnea syndrome. Lung 59:275-287.

Kaada B (1987): The sudden infant death syndrome induced by 'fear paralysis reflex'? Medical Hypotheses 22:347-356.

Kahn A, Riazi J, et al. (1983): Oculocardiac reflex in near miss for sudden infant death syndrome infants. Pediatrics 71:49-52.

Kahn A, Hasaerts D, et al. (1985): Phenothiazine-induced sleep apneas in normal infants. Pediatrics 75:844-847.

Kahn A, Van de Merckt C, et al. (1987): Transepidermal water loss during sleep infants at risk for sudden death. Pediatrics 80:245-250.

Kahn A, Rebuffat E, et al. (1988): Problems in management of infants with an apparent life-threatening event. The Sudden Infant Death Syndrome. Annals New York Academy of Sciences 533:78-88.

Kahn A, Blum D, et al. (1988): Polysomnographic studies of infants who subsequently died of sudden infant death syndrome. Pediatrics 82:721-727.

Kahn A, Mozin MJ, et al. (1989): Sleep pattern alterations and brief airway obstructions in overweight infants. Sleep 12:430-438.

Kahn A, Rebuffat E, et al (1990): Brief airway obstructions during sleep in infants with breath-holding spells. J. Pediatr. 117:188-193.

Kahn A, Rebuffat E, et al. (1990): Sleep apneas and acid esophageal reflux in control infants and in infants with an apparent life-threatening event. Biol. Neonate 57:144-149.

Keeton BR, Souhall E, et al. (1977): Cardiac conduction disorders in six infants with "near-miss" sudden infant deaths. Br. Med. J. 2: 600-601.

Kelly DH, Shannon DC (1981): Episodic complete airway obstruction in infants. Pediatrics 67:823-827.

Kelly DH, Golub H, et al. (1986): Pneumograms of infants who subsequently died of sudden infant death syndrome. J. Pediatr 109:249-254.

Laxdal T, Gomez MR, et al. (1969): Cyanotic and pallid syncopal attacks in children (Breath-holding spells). Develop. Med. Child. Neurol. 11:755-763.

Lehrman KL, Guilleminault C, et al. (1978): Sleep apnea syndrome in a patient with Shy- Drager syndrome. Arch. Intern. Med. 138:206-209.

Leistner HL, Haddad GG, et al. (1980): Heart rate and heart rate variability during sleep in aborted sudden infant death syndrome. J Pediatr 97:51-55.

Lombroso CT, Lerman P (1967): Breathholding spells (cyanotic and pallid infantile syncope). Pediatrics 39:563-581.

Matsumoto N, Inoue H, etal (1985): Effective sites by sympathetic beta-adrenergic and vagal nonadrenergic inhibitory stimulation in constricted airways. Am. Rev. Respir. Dis. 132:1113-1117

Schwartz PJ (1976): Cardiac sympathetic innervation and the sudden infant death syndrome: a possible pathological link. Am. J. Med. 60:167-172.

Southall DP, Richards JM, et al. (1982): Prolongeed apnea and cardiac arrythmias in infants discharged from neonatal intensive care units: failure to predict an increased risk for sudden infant death syndrome. Pediatrics 70: 844-851.

Southall DP, Richards JM, et al. (1983): Prospective population-based studies into heart rate and breathing patterns in newborn infants: Prediction of infants at risk of SIDS ? In *Sudden Infant Death Syndrome*. ed. Tildon T, Roeder LM, Steinschneider A, pp 621-652. New York Academic Press.

Steinschneider A (1972): Prolonged apnea and the sudden infant death syndrome: clinical and laboratory observations. Pediatrics 50: 646-654.

Steinschneider A, Weinstein SL, et al. (1982): The sudden infant death syndrome and apnea/obstruction during neonatal sleep and feeding. Pediatrics 70:858-863.

Sullivan CE, Zamel N, et al. (1979): Regulation of airway smooth muscle tone in sleeping dogs. Am. Rev. Resp. Dis. 119:87-97.

Sutton D, Taylor EM, et al. (1978): Prolonged apnea in infant monkeys resulting from stimulation of superior laryngeal nerve. Pediatrics 61:519-527.
Valdes-Dapena (1980): Sudden infant death syndrome: a review of the medical literature 1974-1979. Pediatrics 66:597-614.
White DP, Cadieux RJ, et al. (1985): The effects of nasal anesthesia on breathing during sleep. Am. Rev. Respir. Dis.132:972-975.
Widdicombe JG (1986): Role of the parasympathetic cholinergic system in normal and obstructed airways. Respiration 50:1-8.

Acknowledgments

We thank Professor H.L. Vis for constant encouragement. The study was supported by the Fondation Nationale de la Recherche Scientifique (Grant 9.4524.87).

Cardiac and respiratory vagal reactivity in infants

J. Ramet, M. Dehan* and C. Gaultier*

*Department of Pediatrics, AZ-Vrije Universiteit, 101 Laarbeeklaan, 1090 Brussels, Belgium and *Laboratoire de Physiologie, Hôpital Antoine Béclère, 92141 Clamart, France*

Our knowledge of the autonomic nervous system balance and of the autonomic regulation of heart rate is incomplete. It is assumed that a prominence of vagal tone exists in premature infants. The understanding of factors controlling heart rate is rendered more complex by the known impact of the different states of alertness (wakefulness, "active" REM and "quiet" NREM sleep) on the autonomic nervous balance in human infants. It is hazardous to extrapolate from observations during wakefulness to sleep and from animal data to human infants as sleep-state maturation may be species related. The purpose of this review is to evoke the cardiac and respiratory responses to various vagal stimulation tests in infants. We successively studied the responses to standardized ocular compression test, to trigeminal airstream stimulation test, to esophageal dilatation and to esophageal acid infusion in healthy preterm and term infants. We demonstrated that these tests are not only age but also sleep-state related. Moreover, normative data for the cardiac responses to a standardized ocular compression test in healthy infants and children are presented. Our works emphasize the need to standardize the procedures during vagal stimulation tests in order to obtain reproducible and representative results.

Supported by grants from INSERM CJF 8909, INSERM CFB, the AZ-VUB Brussels and NFWO-grant n° 3.0033.91.

THE OCULAR COMPRESSION TEST

a) Preterm and term infants

In 1908, Aschner and Dagnini published early descriptions of the oculocardiac reflex and reported cardiac rhythm slowing secondary to eyeball pressure on humans and experimental animals. This reflex involves an afferent pathway through the ophthalmic branch of the trigeminal nerve and an efferent pathway involving the motor nucleus of the vagus nerve and its cardiac efferents. Several authors proposed to assess the cardiac reactivity to vagal stimuli by evaluation of the amplitude of the cardiac response to ocular pressure. Philips et al. showed that such pressure evoked severe cardiac slowing in premature infants.

To appreciate the effect of maturation on this well-known reflex involving the autonomic nervous system, we performed controlled ocular compression during polygraphically documented REM sleep to evaluate the heart rate response as a function of maturation in premature infants.

The ocular compression tests were performed in a standardized manner, between 09.00 and 13.00 h. Infants were asleep on their backs. All were in active (REM) sleep just before and during the testing period as documented by polygraphic monitoring of ECG, respiration, electroencephalogram potentials and by continuous behavioral observation. The ECG was recorded using bipolar chest leads (DI lead). Biologic variables were monitored on an ALVAR 16 channels polygraph at 15 mm/s speed.

To perform the ocular compression, a water-filled pressure sensor (external diameter : 18 mm) was gently placed on each infant's eyelid just before testing. Each pressure sensor was connected to a pressure transducer ; the applied pressure to each sensor was recorded on the polygraph. The mean and SD of the manually applied pressure, recorded via the water-filled sensors, was 103 ± 9 mmHg. The pressure applied to each sensor was identical for each eye and was maintained without change during 10 sec. ; a square wave stimulation was, thus, performed with an identical pressure applied on both eyes during a constant stimulation period.

Data analysis included following parameters : 1) the control RR interval defined as the mean RR interval determined from measurement of each RR interval recorded during the 60 s before the ocular compression ; 2) the longest RR interval, in milliseconds noted just after eyelid pressure, the percent RR maximum was defined as the longest RR interval in milliseconds just after eyelid pressure divided by mean control RR, in milliseconds, multiplied by 100, i.e. %RR maximum ; 3) the latency from applied eyelid pressure to the first measurable RR interval increase compared to mean control RR + 1 SD, expressed in milliseconds.

Results were analyzed relative to gestational age, postnatal age, and postconceptional age. There was a clear effect of maturation on mean control RR, on the longest RR interval secondary to ocular compression, and on the latency variables. When multiplicative analyses were performed for these variables, mean control RR, longest RR interval, and latency were significantly influenced by postconceptional age. Not too surprisingly "%RR maximum" which had a high correlation coefficient with longest RR interval, was also statistically influenced by postconceptional age.

Stepwise linear regression analyses performed after determination of the statistical independence of the selected variables confirmed the effect of maturation on the ocular compression variables.

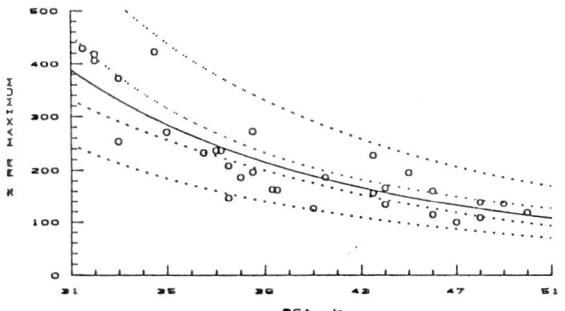

Fig. 1. %RR maximum in function of postconceptional age (PCA) in weeks. %RR = longest RR interval divided by mean control RR interval multiplied by 100. There was a significant decrease in %RR with increasing PCA when the ocular compression test was performed during "active" REM sleep ($p < 0.0001$).

Conclusion : Our results indicate that during rapid eye movement sleep, "baseline heart rate" decreases with maturation, an effect supposedly related to increased vagal activity, whereas the heart rate response on ocular pressure stimulus, a vagally mediated reflex, is significantly influenced and blunted with maturation.

b) Influence of the sleep states

In a second study, we evaluated the strength of the cardiac responses to an ocular compression test in various states of alertness : "active" REM sleep, "quiet" NREM sleep and wakefulness. An example of an ocular compression test during "active" REM is illustrated : CTG = cardiotachogram, EOG = electro-oculogram, Th Mvts and Abd Mvts : thoracic and abdominal movements measured by strain gauges ; P_1 and P_2 indicate the pressures on both eyes during the ocular compression test.

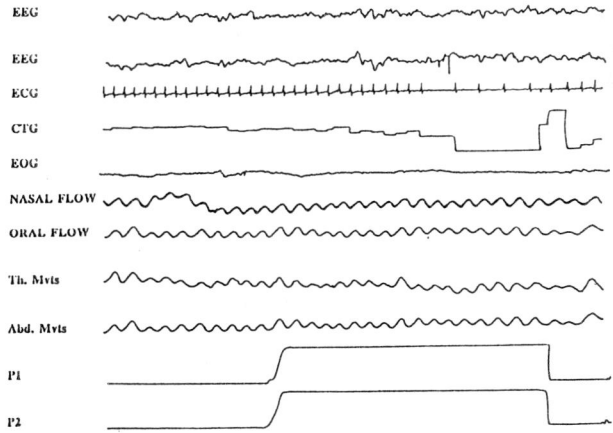

Illustration of an ocular compression test during "active" REM sleep. As a response to the ocular compression test (P_1, P_2) there was a marked prolongation of the RR interval.

Moreover, we performed a "control" non-vagally mediated cutaneous leg compression, using the same pressure sensors as for the eyes, during the 3 states of alertness. The respective responses of the ocular compression test and of the cutaneous compression test are indicated in table 1.

	OCULAR COMPRESSION TEST		
	Quiet sleep	Active sleep	Wakefulness
RR control (msec)	420 ± 34	402 ± 41	380 ± 39
Longest RR (msec)	538 ± 60	939 ± 360*	623 ± 355
%RR	129 ± 16	236 ± 91*	164 ± 89

	CUTANEOUS COMPRESSION TEST		
	Quiet sleep	Active sleep	Wakefulness
%RR	104 ± 11	102 ± 7	99 ± 11

The cutaneous compression did not provoke any significant prolongation of the RR interval in either state of alertness. The cardiac responses to the ocular compression test were significantly greater in "active" REM sleep when compared to "quiet" NREM sleep and wakefulness ($p < 0.001$ and $p < 0.05$). We thus can conclude that the cardiac responses to a standardized ocular compression test are significantly dependent on the state of alertness in which the test is performed.

c) The longitudinal children study

To expand our knowledge concerning the cardiac responses to the ocular compression test (OCT) in children, we performed, between 1982 and 1991, a longitudinal study including 37 healthy children. The purpose of this prospective study was to determine normative data of the oculocardiac reflex during quiet wakefulness. The first OCT was performed at 6 weeks followed by controls at 6 and 18 months and at 4, 6 and 8 years. Only children with at least 3 OCT-tests at different ages were retained for this study. None of the investigated infant, child or adolescent had signs of an underlying cardiac disease and had a normal ECG investigation, absence of heart murmur and for most of them normal findings on the 24-hours electrocardiographic holter recording.

The individual results of the longest RR interval during OCT or maximal prolongation of the RR interval in msec in function of age are indicated in the figure.

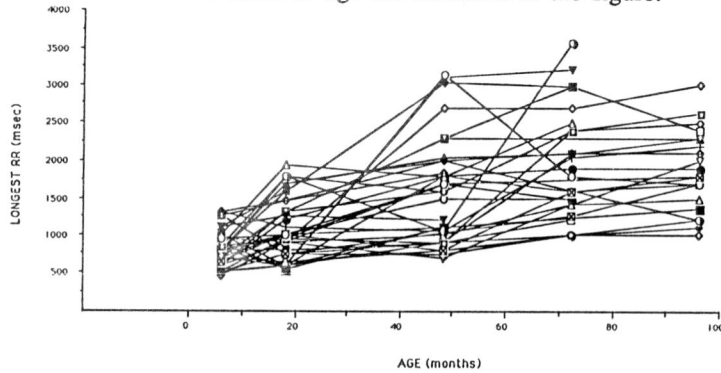

Cardiorespiratory variability and development of sleep state organization

Lilia Curzi-Dascalova, Jean Clairambault*, François Kauffmann**, Claire Médigue* and P. Peirano

*INSERM, CJF 89-09, Laboratoire de Physiologie, Hôpital Antoine Béclère, 92141 Clamart; *INRIA, Rocquencourt, and **Université de Caen, Département de Mathématiques, France*

To assess the influence of sleep state and conceptional age (CA) on heart rate (measured in RR intervals) and heart rate variability, we performed polygraphic recordings in three groups of normal newborns: 8 premature (31-36w CA), 8 near-term (37-38w CA) and 8 full-term (39-41wCA) infants. Using Short-Time Fourrier Transform, total tracings (2 to 3 hours duration) were analysed by 512 heartbeat epochs.

At all ages studied, RR intervals were shorter and low frequency heart rate variability (LF=30 to 100 heartbeats/period) was higher during active sleep (AS) than during quiet sleep (QS). High frequency variability (HF=3 to 8 heartbeats/period) was significantly higher during QS than during AS near-term and full-term newborns.

In all age groups, we found significant correlations between mean RR intervals and LF heart rate variability during AS and QS.

In general, all variables increased with age but rate of modifications varied with sleep state and with the parameter studied. During AS, age-related modifications were more gradual, without significant between-age differences. During QS, the largest modifications in RR and HF occurred between premature and near-term age groups.

There was no parallelism between previously described age related modifications of respiratory rate and the modifications of RR and heart rate variability described herein.

<u>In conclusion,</u> data obtained are additional evidence that between-state differentiation of vital functions control occurs early during human ontogenesis, before subsequent modulating by CA factors.1

° Supported by Grant RGR62 INSERM-CNAMTS (CRAMIF) and INSERM CJF 89-09.
 Aknowledgements to Dr. A. Wolfe for reviewing the English manuscript.

INTRODUCTION.

Differences in autonomic nervous system control during the various wakefulness and sleep states have been demonstrated early during human ontogenesis. Beyond 31 weeks conceptional age (wCA), spontaneous skin potential responses (4), under sympathetic control, prevail during periods of continuous EEG tracing characteristic of active, REM sleep (AS), as compared with periods of discontinuous EEG tracing characteristic of quiet NREM sleep (QS). As far as respiratory control is concerned, significant between state differences in thoraco-abdominal phase shift and apnea index are observed beyond 31w CA (AS>QS), while respiratory rate becomes significantly higher in AS as compared with QS beyond 35 w CA (6).

Between-state differences in cardiac control have been described in full-term newborns and in infants during the first months of life (2, 9, 11). Studies in premature infants are scant and most evaluated QS only (1); others investigated both QS and AS but used total heart rate variability (HRV) as the only studied parameter (13).

The purpose of the present work was to investigate development of heart rate (HR) and HRV in normal premature and full-term newborns. Data obtained will be discussed in the light of our previous investigations on sleep states and respiratory control development in these ages.

METHODS.

The study was carried out in 24 physically and neurologically normal newborns of postnatal age of less than 10 days, grouped according to CA in weeks on the day of recording, as follows: a) premature infants, 31-36 w CA (n=8); b) near-term infants, 37-38w CA (n=8); c) and full-term infants 39-41w CA (n=8). Criteria used to define CA and normality have been previously described (5). Polygraphic recordings included EEG, rapid eye movements (REMs) and body movements, chin and diaphragmatic inspiratory surface EMG, respiratory movements, and ECG (ref. in 5).

Tracings, performed during the morning between two feedings, lasted 2 to 4 hours. Data were simultaneously recorded on paper and on analog magnetic tape. Sleep states were coded according to: 1) EEG patterns (7) and 2) REMs (present in AS, absent in QS). Each tracing included one or more complete sleep cycles. Only pure AS and QS states were analyzed.

Automatic analysis of total tracings was performed off line, using methods elaborated by Kauffmann et al. (14) and detailed in a separate paper in this book. After digitalization of the ECG at 282 Hz, R-R intervals were detected with 7 milliseconds accuracy and stored in 512-point epochs. All epochs including > 10% artefact time were rejected. Every raw RR serie was processed by Short-Time Fourier Transform, a non-stationary spectral analysis method, which yields spectral amplitude signals in given frequency bands. RR intervals and three types of HRV were studied as follows: a) High Frequency (HF) with 3 to 8 heartbeat/period; b)

Mid Frequncy (MF) with 10 to 25 heartbeat/period and c) Low Frequency (LF) with 30 to 100 heartbeat/period. Means of data per infant and sleep state were statistically analyzed by ANOVA, t-test and correlation coefficient computing.

RESULTS.

Between-state differentiation.

All but MF parameters were relevant for sleep state distinction in all age groups. Degree of between-state differences varied with age and parameters studied (Fig.1). Differences were greater in full-term newborns than in premature infants. LF was the best parameter for state discrimination in premature infants.

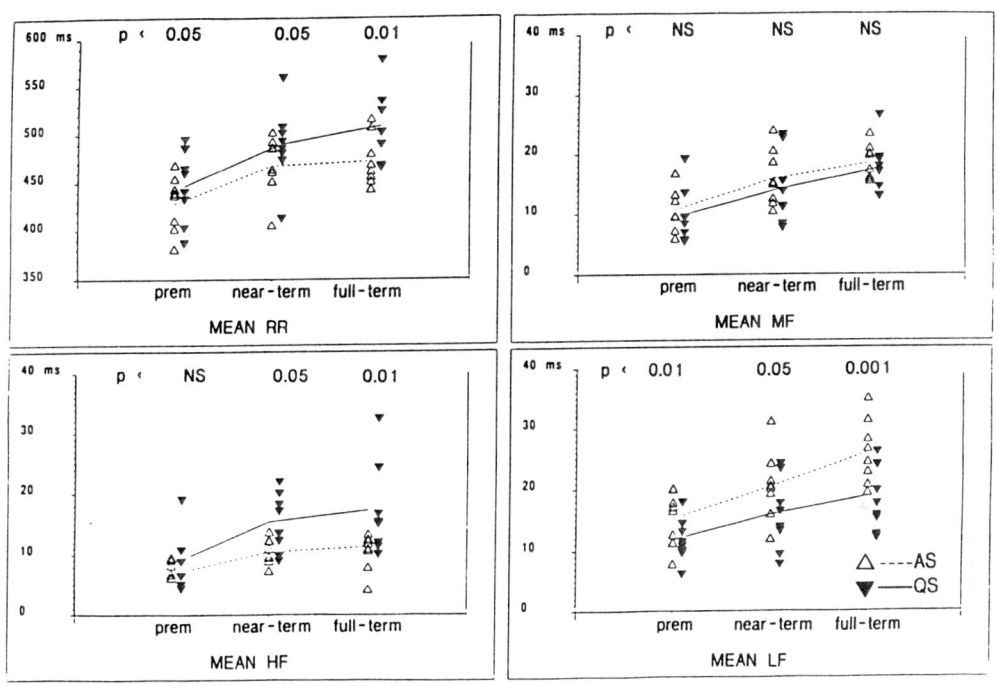

Figure 1. Mean RR intervals and different heart rate variabilities in active (AS) and quiet (QS) sleep states according to conceptional age (CA), in normal newborn infants.
Legend: p<-for between AS and QS differences; and -individual values in the given state; prem.=premature infants of 31-36w CA; near-term=37-38w CA; full-term=39-41w CA. For HF, MF and LF definition and for between-age differences, see text.

Modifications with age.

RR intervals, as well as different HRV parameters increased with age. The slope of this increase varied with the state and parameter studied (Fig. 1).

During <u>AS</u>, all parameters increased significantly from the premature to the near-term group ($p < 0.05$ for RR intervals and MF, $p < 0.01$ for HF), except LF for which the increase did not reach statistical significance ($p < 0.06$). The increase observed from the near term to the full-term groups, although not statistically significant, increased the significant difference between premature and full-term newborns ($p < 0.01$ for RR and HF, $p < 0.001$ for MF and LF).

During <u>QS</u>, age-related modifications were less marked. RR and HF increased only from the premature to the near-term groups ($p < 0.05$), while no significant differences between near-term and full-term groups were found. However, gradual increases in all parameters resulted in significant differences between premature and full-term infants ($p < 0.05$ for HF and LF, $p < 0.01$ for RR and MF).

<u>Correlations between values obtained during AS and QS.</u>

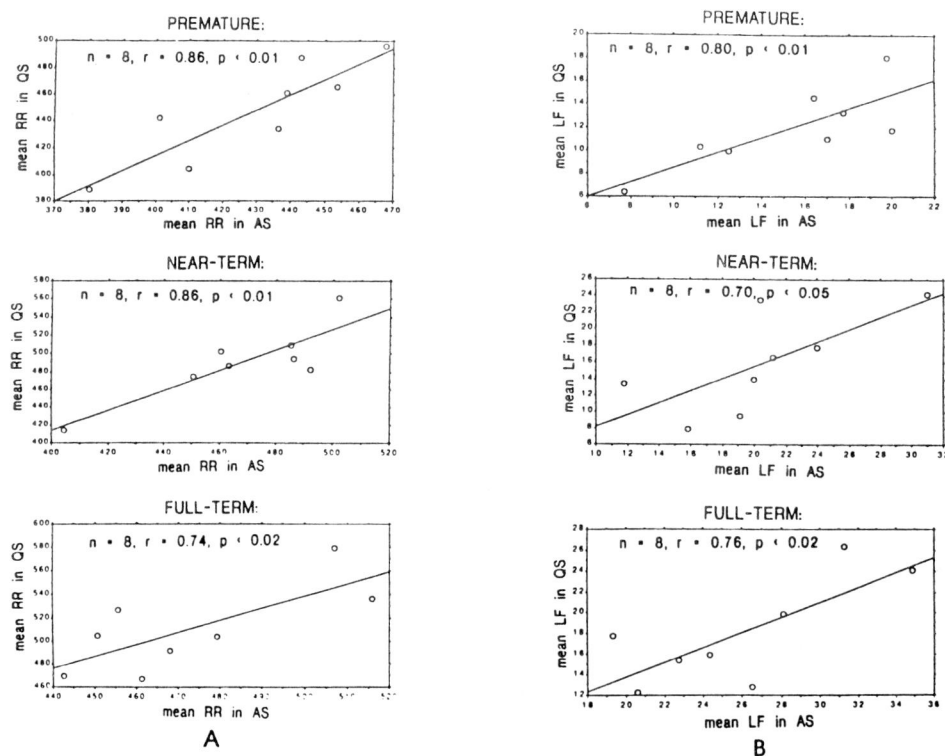

<u>Figure 2.</u> Correlations between individual RR intervals (in A) and LF heart rate variability (in B) at different ages. For Legend, see fig.1.

Figure 1 shows the high dispersion of mean values obtained in different subjects for given ages and states.

To assess relationships between data obtained during AS and QS, correlations between values in both states were computed.

Strong correlations between RR intervals during AS and QS were demonstrated (Fig.2.A) At all ages studied, infants with higher heart rate during AS also had higher heart rates during QS, and vice versa. Similar between-state correlations were found when LF was analyzed (Fig. 2-B).

No between-states correlations were obtained for HF at any age. MF showed significant correlations in full-term infants only ($p < 0.01$).

DISCUSSION.

The present study demonstrated the presence of between-state differences in heart rate control early in human ontogenesis. Beyond 31 w CA, AS can be distinguished from QS by shorter RR intervals and higher LF heart rate variability. To the best of our knowledge, there are no data in the literature describing similar between-state differences in premature infants. Our results demonstrate that the differences in heart rate control during AS and QS, previously described in full-term newborns (11, 12) and older infants (10, 17, 18), are also present earlier in human ontogenesis.

Beyond 31w CA, AS and QS can be distinguished by EEG and REM criteria (5). The present data demonstrate that the control of HRV continues to mature in both states.

The study of age-related modifications showed that the most significant increase in RR intervals and HRV occurred from the premature to the near-term groups of newborns. Increase in all parameters from near-term (37-38w CA) to full-term (39-41w CA) were not statistically significant. Thus, according to heart rate and HRV criteria, near-term 37-38w CA newborns were near similar to full-term newborns and significantly different from premature infants. In general, age-related modifications were greater during AS than during QS. Thus, maturation as evaluated by heart rate and HRV occurred faster for AS than for QS. Finally, values obtained in our group of full-term newborns tended to approach values obtained by Harper et al. (9) for heart rate and Schechtman et al. (17, 18) for HRV in normal infants less than one month of postnatal age.

It was surprising that the best parameter allowing state discrimination in premature infants was LF variability. LF is presumed to be related to thermoregulation (15). However, defective thermoregulation is well-known clinical finding in premature infants (ref. in 8, 19). This discrepancy between defective thermoregulation and well-organized LF between-state differentiation in premature infants suggests that other factors influence HRV at this age. Especially, relationships with motor activity must be taken into account.

In all age groups, important differences were observed between data obtained in individual infants. In spite of this between-subject variability, highly significant correlations between RR and LF in both sleep states were observed. Thus, heart rate and LF variability seem to be an individual characteristic, present as soon as 31w CA.

parameters	premature/ near-term		near-term/ full-term		premature/ full-term	
	AS	QS	AS	QS	AS	QS
RR intervals	0.05	0.05	NS	NS	0.01	0.01
HF variability	0.01	0.05	NS	NS	0.01	0.05
Respiratory rate	NS	NS	0.001	0.001	0.001	0.001

Table 1. Degree of significance of between-age differences (p<) in mean RR intervals, HF heart rate variability, and respiratory rate during active sleep (AS) and quiet sleep (QS).
For HF and age group definitions, see text.

The close linkage between respiratory and heart rate control by the central nervous system have been well documented. A marked effect of breathing patterns on heart rate and HFV has been described in full-term newborns (ref. in 12, 16). However, our data show that age-related modifications of heart rate and HRV on the one hand and of respiratory rate on the other are not closely parallel.

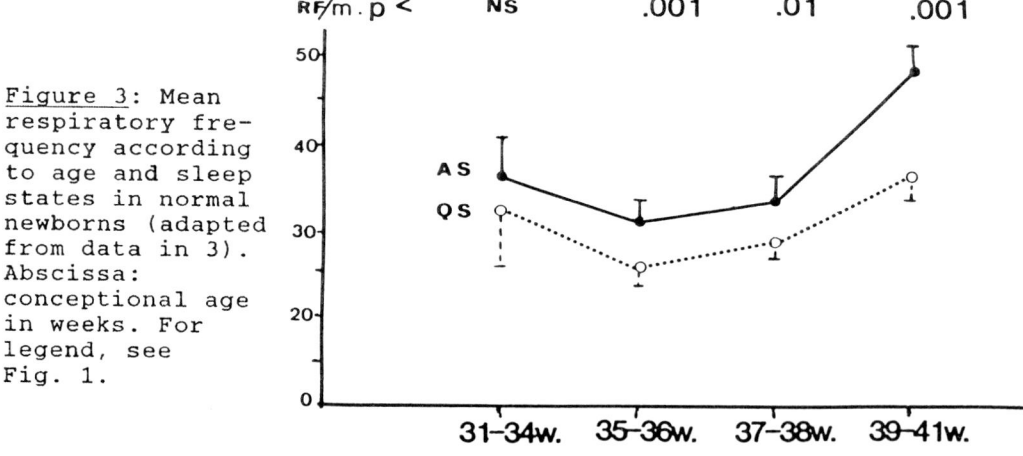

Figure 3: Mean respiratory frequency according to age and sleep states in normal newborns (adapted from data in 3). Abscissa: conceptional age in weeks. For legend, see Fig. 1.

The comparison between age-related modifications of RR and HF shown in Fig. 1 and respiratory frequency modifications presented on Fig 3. illustrates the absence of such a parallelism (see also table 1). On the one hand, respiratory rate remained similar from 31 to 38w CA before to increase significantly in 39-41w CA infants (3). On the other hand, heart rate diminished significantly at 37-38 CA as compared to premature infants and was very similar in 37-38 and in 39-41w CA newborns. These findings suggest that there is no fixed relationship between respiratory rate on the one hand and heart rate and HF (sinusal arrhythmia) on the other. This agrees with the findings of Hathorn (12) in full term newborns and those of Harper et al. (10) in infants. Correlations between heart rate and respiratory variability are probably influenced by different physiological mechanisms, mainly sleep-state-related modulations of cardiac and respiratory control.

In conclusion, data on heart rate and HRV presented herein are additional evidence that between-state differentiation of vital functions control occurs early in human ontogenesis. As previously described for respiratory and motor functions (ref. in 5), between-states differences are later improved and modulated by age-dependent factors.

REFERENCES.

1. Äärimaa T., , Oja, R., Antila, K., Välimaki, I. (1988):Interaction of heart rate and respiration in newborn babies. Pediatr. Res. 24: 745-750.
2. Baldzer, K., Dykes, F.D., Jones, S.A., Brogan, T.A., Carrigan, T.A., and Giddens, D.P. (1989): Heart rate variability analysis in full-term infants: spectral indices for study of neonatal cardiorespiratory control. Pediatr. Res. 26: 188-195.
3. Curzi-Dascalova, L., Lebrun,F., and Korn, G. (1983): Respiratory frequency according to sleep state and age in normal premature infants. A comparison with full-term infants. Pediatr. Res., 27: 152-156.
4. Curzi-Dascalova, L., Pajot, N., and Dreyfus-Brisac, C. (1973): Spontaneous skin potential responses in sleeping infants between 24 and 41 weeks of conceptional age. Psychophysiology, 10: 478-487.
5. Curzi-Dascalova, L., Peirano, P., and Morel-Kahn, F. (1988): Developmental aspect of sleep states in normal premature and full-term newborns. Develop.Psychobiol., 21: 431-444.
6. Curzi-Dascalova, L. (1990): Sleep and respiratory control development during the first months of life. In "Ergebh. exp. Med.", H. Schwartze and P. Schwartze eds, Verlag Gesundheit, Berlin, 53: 137-152.
7. Dreyfus-Brisac, C. (1979) Neonatal electroencephalography. In: *Reviews in Perinatal Medecine,* eds E.M. Scarpelli, and V. Cosmi, pp. 397-472. Raven Press: New York.
8. Green, M., and Behrendt, H. (1969): Sweating capacity in neonates. Amer. J. Dis. Child. 118: 725-732.
9. Harper, R.M., Leake, B., Hoppenbrouwers, T., Sterman, M.B., McGinty, D.J., and Hodgman, J. (1978): Polygraphic studies of normal infants and infants at risk for sudden infant death syndrome: heart rate and variability as a function of state. Pediatr. Res. 12: 778-785.
10. Harper, R.M., Walter, D.O., Leake, ., Hoffman, H.J., Sieck,

G.C., Sterman, M.B., Hoppenbrouwers, T., and Hodgman, J. (1978) Development of sinus arrhythmia during sleeping and waking states. Sleep 1: 33-48.
11. Hathorn, M.K.S. (1987): Respiratory sinus arrhythmia in newborn infants. J. Physiol. (London) 385: 1-12.
12. Hathorn, M.K.S. (1989): Respiratory modulation of heart rate in newborn infants. Early Hum. Dev. 20: 81-99.
13. Katona, P.G., Frasz, A., and Egbert, J. (1980): Maturation of cardiac control in full-term and preterm infants during sleep. Early Hum. Dev. 4: 145-159.
14. Kauffmann, F., Clairambault, J., and Médigue, C. (1991): Un système d'analyse des signaux biomédicaux. Bull. de Liaison de la Recherche en Informatique et en Automatique (INRIA), 131: 38-41.
15. Lindqvist, A., Oja, R., Hellman, O., and Välimäki, I. (1983): Impact of thermal vasomotor control on the heart rate variability of newborn infants. Early Hum. Dev. 8: 37-47.
16. Rother, M., Zwiener, U., Witte, H., Eiselt, M., and Frenzel, J. (1988): Objective characterization and differentiation of sleep states in healthy newborns and newborns-at-risk by spectral analysis of heart rate and respiratory rhythms. Acta Physiol. Hung. 71: 383-393.
17. Schechtman, V.L., Harper, R.M., and Kluge, K.A. (1989): Development of heart rate variation over the first 6 months of life in normal infants. Pediatr. Res. 26: 343-346.
18. Schechtman, V.L., Harper, R.M., Kluge, K.A., Wilson, A.J., Hoffman, H.J., and Southall, D.P. (1989): Heart rate variation in normal infants and victims of the sudden infant death syndrome. Early Hum. Dev. 19: 167-181.
19. Stothers, J.K., and Warner, R.M. (1984): Thermal balance and sleep state in the newborn. Early Hum. Dev. 9: 313-322.

Résumé

Les modifications des intervalles RR et de la variabilité cardiaque en fonction de l'âge et des stades de sommeil ont été étudiées, à l'aide d'enregistrements polygraphiques, chez trois groupes de nouveau-nés normaux: 8 prématurés de 31 à 36 semaines d'âge conceptionnel (s. d'AC), 8 près-du-terme de 37 à 38s d'AC et 8 nouveau-nés à terme de 39 à 41s d'AC. La durée totale des enregistrements a été analysée par blocs de 512 battements cardiaques, à l'aide d'une Transformé de Fourier à Court Terme.

A tous les âges étudiés, les intervalles RR étaient significativement plus courts et la variabilité cardiaque lente (périodes de 30 à 100 battements cardiaques) plus élevée en sommeil agité (SA) qu'en sommeil calme (SC). La variabilité cardiaque rapide (périodes de 3 à 8 battements) devenait significativement plus élevée en SC qu'en SA à partir de 37-38s d'AC.

A tous les âges nous avons constaté une corrélation significative entre les moyennes des intervalles RR et la variabilité cardiaque lente observées en SA et SC.

Dans l'ensemble, toutes les variables ont augmenté avec l'âge, mais la rapidité des modifications dépendait des stades du sommeil et du paramètre étudié. En SA, les modifications étaient moins importantes, sans différences statistiquement significatives entre les différents groupes d'âge. Par contre, en SC, les principales modifications sont intervenues entre les prématurés et les pré-terme de 37-38s d'AC.

Les modifications avec l'âge des intervalles RR et de la variabilité cardiaque rapide n'étaient pas parallèles aux modifications de la fréquence respiratoire.

En conclusion, les résultats obtenus sont une nouvelle preuve d'une différenciation précoce du contrôle des fonctions vitales au cours de l'ontogenèse. Ces modifications sont modulées par des facteurs liés à l'âge conceptionnel.

Circadian rhythms of cardiorespiratory controls in preterm infants

Majid Mirmiran, Yolanda Maas* and Joke Kok*

Netherlands Institute for Brain Research, Meibergdreef 33, 1105 AZ Amsterdam and *Department of Neonatology, Academic Hospital of the University of Amsterdam (AMC), Meibergdreef 9, 1105 AZ Amsterdam, The Netherlands

SUMMARY

Preterm babies show circadian rhythms in heart rate variability and temperature rhythms as early as 29 weeks of conceptional age. Animal studies have shown that circadian rhythms are solely induced by the hypothalamus (Rusak and Zucker, 1979). The presence or absence of circadian rhythms might be an easy but precise indicator for normal/abnormal brain maturation in preterm infants.

"Circadian" rhythms, i.e. rhythms with a periodicity of around 24 h are present in all physiological variables studied so far (Moore-Ede et al., 1982). These endogenous rhythms are entrained to 24 h light-dark cycle inducing "diurnal" rhythms with a periodicity of exactly 24 h. Diurnal rhythms of heart rate variability has been recorded as early as by 22 weeks of gestation in human fetuses (Patrick et al., 1982; De Vries et al., 1987; for review see Mirmiran et al., 1989). The fetal heart rate rhythm is controlled by the maternal circadian system, with low fetal heart rate variability during the night (maternal sleep) and high variability during the day (De Vries et al., 1987).

We have studied circadian rhythms of different physiological functions in preterm infants. We have developed an on-line computer controlled system that was coupled with the Hewlett Packard neonatal intensive care monitor. Data, including heart rate and respiratory rate variabilities, body temperature, incubator temperature, transcutaneous pO_2 and pCO_2, and rest-activity cycles were analysed and fed every minute into a personal computer. We have studied a group of twelve low-risk preterm infants with gestational age between 25 and 32 weeks under a fairly constant undisturbed condition over a long period of time (1-2 weeks) continuously.

A circadian rhythm was present in heart rate and body temperature in more than fifty per cent of these infants (for previously published data see Mirmiran et al., 1990a, b; Mirmiran and Kok, 1991). Figure 1 illustrates 24 h continous recordings of heart rate, respiratory rate and body temperature variabilities in an infant of 29 weeks gestational age, recorded 1-2 weeks post delivery. A clear circadian rhythm is visible in the heart rate variability, which was almost in phase with the infant's body temperature rhythm. However, no concomitant circadian variation was present in respiratory rate.

In conclusion, our preliminary data demonstrate the presence of circadian rhythms in heart rate variability in preterm infants. Two significances can be given at present to these observations. First of all, in evaluation of cardiorespiratory functions in preterm infants circadian fluctuations ought to be taken into account. Secondly, and more importantly, the presence or absence of circadian rhythms in heart rate variability might soon become an indicator for the degree of central (brain) control of cardiorespiratory function. Decrease of heart rate, increase of its variability and appearance of its circadian rhythms could not only be related to sympathetic and parasympathetic controls, but could also be used as indicators for normal brain maturation in preterm infants.

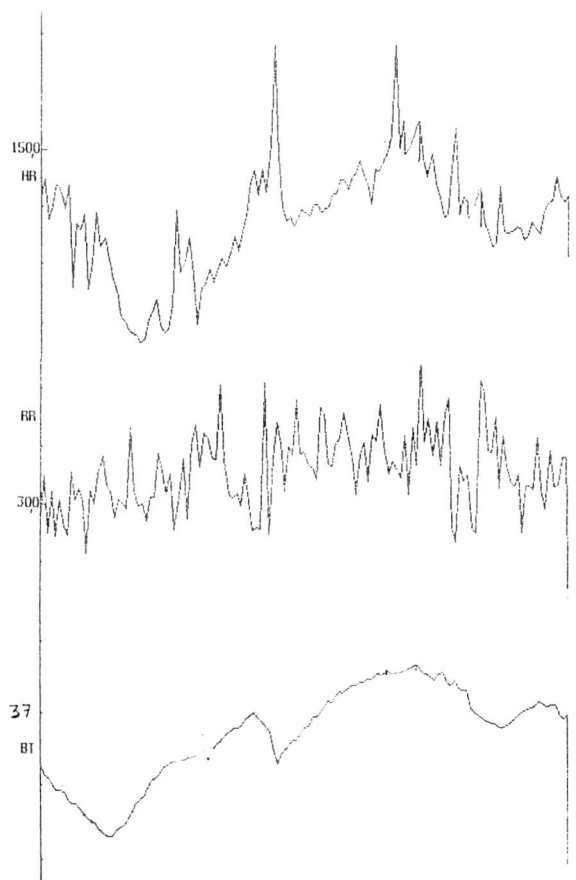

Fig. 1

From top to bottom: 24 h continuous recordings of heart rate (HR), respiratory rate (RR) and body temperature (BT) in an infant of 29 weeks of gestational age. Note periods of high and low levels of heart rate and body temperature during the 24 h period indicative of a presence of circadian rhythmicity. In contrast, no circadian rhythm was found in respiratory rate.

REFERENCES

Davis, F.C. (1981): Ontogeny of circadian rhythms. In *Biological Rhythms*, ed. J. Asschoff, pp. 257-274. New York: Plenum Press.

De Vries, J.I.P., Visser, G.H.A., Mulder, E.J.H., and Prechtl, H.F.R. (1987): Diurnal and other variations in fetal movement and heart rate patterns at 20 to 22 weeks. *Earl. Hum. Dev.* 15: 333-348.

Mirmiran, M., and Kok, J.H. (1991): Circadian rhythms in early human development. *Sleep Res.* 20: 106.

Mirmiran, M., Kok, J.H., de Kleine, M.J.K., Koppe, J.G., Overdijk, J., and Witting, W. (1990a): Circadian rhythms in preterm infants: a preliminary study. *Earl. Hum. Dev.* 23: 139-146.

Mirmiran, M., Kok, J.H., and Koppe, J.G. (1990b): Emergence of circadian rhythms in early human development. In *Sleep 90*, ed. J. Horne, pp. 26-28. Bochum: Pontenagel Press.

Mirmiran, M., Swaab, D.F., Witting, W., Honnebier, M.B.O.M., Van Gool, W.A., and Eikelenboom, P. (1989): Biological clocks during development, aging and in Alzheimer's disease. *Brain Dysfunction* 2: 57-66.

Moore-Ede, M.C., Sulzman, F.M., and Fuller, C.A. (1982) *The Clocks that Time Us.* Cambridge: Harvard University Press.

Patrick, J., Campbell, K., Carmichael, L., Natale, K., and Richardson, B. (1982): Patterns of gross fetal body movements over 24 hour observation during the last 10 weeks of pregnancy. *Am. J. Obstet. Gynecol.* 142: 363-371.

Rusak, B., and Zucker, I. (1979): Neural regulation of circadian rhythms. *Physiol. Rev.* 59: 449-526.

Postnatal organization of cardiorespiratory interaction in neonates during quiet sleep

Ilkka Välimäki, Jarmo Jalonen and Tuula Äärimaa

Cardiorespiratory Research Unit and Department of Paediatrics, University of Turku, SF-20520 Turku, Finland

Irregularities of normal sinus rhythm have been termed sinus arrhythmia and in adults a considerable part of heart-rate variability (HRV) is related to respiration. Heart rate increases during inspiration and decreases during expiration; this phenomenon has been called respiratory sinus arrhythmia (RSA). In neonates RSA can hardly been visually detected from the ECG or arterial blood pressure or even instantaneous heart-rate signal. However, if heart rate is examined in frequency domain using power-spectral analysis, a peak of HRV corresponding to the simultaneously recorded respiratory activity can be demonstrated (Äärimaa et al. 1988, Kitney et al 1985). HRV is smaller in preterm than in fullterm babies, in particular when the preterm baby has respiratory problems (Rudolph et al. 1965, Äärimaa et al. 1988, Anttila 1989). As the respiratory activity is often attenuated in immature neonates and in respiratory distress it would be interesting to look whether the limited HRV in these babies is caused by decreased RSA.
In this study we examined the magnitude of RSA during quiet sleep in newborn babies using spectral analysis of HRV and respiratory waveform. In addition, we compared the magnitude of RSA with statistical indices of beat-to-beat HRV, the reason being that these are considerably easier to be computed than the spectral density of RSA.

SUBJECTS AND METHODS

A total of 22 healthy term babies (gestational age 37-41 wks), 21 healthy preterm babies (27-36 wks) and 11 preterm babies (27-34 wks) with respiratory distress syndrome (RDS) were studied during the days 1, 3 and 5 postnatally. As the babies were in quiet sleep according to the criteria of Prechtl (1974), 5 min. records of ECG and transthoracic electrical impedance respirogram (RESP) were obtained on magnetic tape using a Corometrics 512 Neonatal Monitor and a Racal instrument recorder.

From each tape recording 200 noise-free successive R-R intervals and the respective segment of RESP signal were digitized by means of a mini computer system (Data General, Southboro, MA). Beat-to-beat indices of HRV were computed for the R-R interval vectors (Välimäki et al. 1974):

$$\mathrm{RMSSD} = (1/(N-1) \mathrm{SUM}(\mathrm{RR}_i - \mathrm{RR}_{i+1})^{**}2)^{**\frac{1}{2}}$$
$$\mathrm{CVS} = 100 * \mathrm{RMSSD}/\mathrm{meanRR},$$

where RR_i is the ith interval and N is the number of RR intervals (=200)

The R-R intervals were converted to instantaneous HR and made continuous by linear interpolation, sampled at 2.2 Hz, and filtered (cut-off frequency 0.025 Hz). The RESP signal variability was examined around a zero mean and filtered using a Hanning window of 99 data points (cut-off frequency 0.02 Hz). Autocovariance function was computed for the HR and RESP signals and this was used to compute the respective autospectra (Fig 1) by means of an FFT algorithm (for detailed description see Äärimaa et al. 1988).

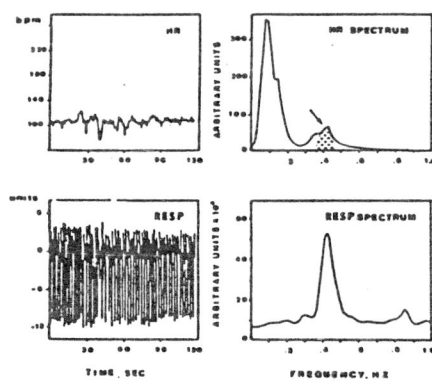

Fig. 1. Source signals of heart rate and respiratory waveform and the respective power spectra. RSA indicated by arrow.

For the examination of RSA the maximum peak between 0.1 Hz and 1.0 Hz of the RESP autospectrum for each record was identified. Thereafter a 0.1 Hz wide band of the HR spectrum was integrated over the frequency around the maximum respiratory power spectral peak. This was considered an estimate of the RSA. Also a ratio of this estimate over the total power under the HR spectral curve was computed to assess the relative respiratory sinus arrhythmia, i.e. RSA% = 100*RSA/HRVtot. These as well as the indices RMSSD and CVS for the groups of term, preterm and RDS babies were compared on each day using descriptive and linear correlation statistics.

RESULTS

The indices of beat-to-beat HRV increased with age in all

groups. The RMSSD was lowest in the babies with RDS and highest in the healthy term babies (Table 1). The CVS behaved similarily (data not shown).

Table 1 Beat-to-beat HRV in healthy term and preterm babies, and in preterm babies with RDS during quiet sleep

Group	RMSSD (msec)		
	Day1	Day3	Day5
Term	8.88	14.82*	17.75*
Preterm	4.95	11.51*	9.65**
RDS	2.85	3.97	5.00*

Difference to Day1 significant *p<0.05, **p<0.01

In all records of HR most of the HRV power was at the lower frequencies ($\leq$ 0.1 Hz). These low-frequency oscillations increased with age in all groups, most in the term babies and least in the babies with RDS.

The percentage of respiratory sinus arrhythmia (RSA%) was rather small in all groups (Table 2). It varied between 4 and 11 %.

Table 2 The percentage of respiratory sinus arrhythmia of the total HRV power in healthy term and preterm infants, and in preterm infants with RDS during quiet sleep

Group	RSA (%)		
	Day1	Day3	Day5
Term	4.22	7.33	9.63
Preterm	6.30	7.46	6.17
RDS	5.18	11.14	4.92

The linear correlation between the indices of beat-to-beat HRV and spectral estimates of RSA was in general low (Table 3). On day-by-day basis significant correlation was found on day 1 and day 3 in the term babies and on day 5 in preterm babies. Beat-to-beat HRV does not seem to be related to RSA in our groups of

Table 3 Significant correlation coefficients between statistical indices of HRV and spectral estimates of RSA in healthy term and preterm babies and in babies with RDS during quiet sleep.

	Beat-to-beat heart-rate variability					
	Term babies		Preterm		RDS	
	RMSSD	CVS	RMSSD	CVS	RMSSD	CVS
RSA	.28*	.31*	.41**	.44**	-	-
RSA%	-	-	-	-	-	-

$* p < 0.05$, $** p < 0.01$

DISCUSSION

One of the criteria for the behavioural state of quiet sleep is regular respiration (Prechtl 1974). Therefore we assumed that if respiratory sinus arrhythmia can be detected in neonates it would appear during quiet sleep. Also heart rate is lower and HRV greater in quiet sleep than in active sleep indicating dominance of vagal tone (Radvanyi & Morel-Kahn 1976, Siassi et al 1979, Anttila 1989). It was therefore expected that both of the signals studied would be stationary, which is a prerequisite for meaningful spectral analysis.

It was found that a major part of HRV was caused by slow changes and there was an increase of these slow oscillations with age. This is in agreement with previous reports (Välimäki et al 1980, Giddens & Kitney 1985, Äärimaa et al. 1988, Anttila 1989). These oscillations are considered to represent control systems related to vasomotor thermoregulation and baroreflex. Although heart rate is mainly controlled by the vagal division of the autonomic nervous system, also beta-adrenergic system plays a major role, mediating the low-frequency changes of heart rate and arterial blood pressure in the neonatal period (Siimes et al.1990).

Respiratory sinus arrhythmia appeared fairly small in our study, less than 11% of the total HRV power. It did not have any clear cut relation to the maturity. Only in the term babies the RSA% showed an increasing trend with age. Giddens and Kitney (1985) have explained that the magnitude of RSA increases when the respiratory rate approaches the frequency of 0.1 Hz and entrains there the natural oscillation of baroreflex. The rate of breathing in neonates is mostly much greater and this kind of entrainment does not take place in normal conditions. On the other hand common periodicities in respiratory and cardiac activity may be occasionally detected at frequencies of 0.1-0.2 Hz. These are probably caused by periodic respiration (Äärimaa et al. 1988).

Although RSA and beat-to-beat control of heart rate are considered to be mediated by the vagal system, our study failed to show linear correlation between the indices of beat-to-beat HRV and spectral estimates of RSA. It may well be that these variables display different phenomena in cardiac control. Also, one has to remember that spectral analysis has been originally designed for the detection of oscillatory components in pure sinusoidal signals. Most bio-signals are far from sinusoidal and also their stationarity is not ideal. Therefore, one has to be careful in explaining the results of power spectral estimates of heart rate.

We conclude that respiratory sinus arrhythmia is small in magnitude in neonates. It does not explain the differences of heart rate variability between term and preterm babies. Beat-to-beat variability represents an entity different from respiratory sinus arrhythmia.

Acknowledgement
The support from the Academy of Finland is cordially acknowledged.

REFERENCES

Äärimaa, T., Oja, R., Antila, K. and Välimäki, I. (1988): Interaction of heart rate and respiration in newborn babies. Pediatr. Res. 24: 745-750.
Anttila,H.(1989): Analysis of neonatal heart rate variability. MD thesis. Ann.Univers.Turkuensis D37 Univ. of Turku, Finland.
Giddens, D.P. and Kitney, R.I.(1985): Neonatal heart rate variability and its relation to respiration. J.Theor. Biol. 113:795-780.
Kitney, R.I., Fulton, T., McDonald, A.H. and Linkens, D.A. (1985): Transient interactions between blood pressure, respiration and heart rate in man. J. Biomed. Engin. 7:217-224.
Prechtl, H.F.R. (1974): The behavioural states of the newborn infant. (A review). Brain Res. 76:185-212
Radvanyi, M.F. and Morel-Kahn, F. (1976): Sleep and heart rate variations in premature and full-term babies. Neuropädiatrie 7: 302-312.
Rudolph, A.J., Vallbona, C. and Desmond, M.M. (1965): Cardiodynamic studies of the newborn III. Heart rate patterns in infants with idiopathic respiratory distress syndrome. Pediatrics 36:551-559.
Siassi, B., Hodgman J.E., Cabal, L., Hon, E.H.(1979): Cardiac and respiratory activity in relation to gestation and sleep states in newborn infants. Pediatr.Res. 13:1163-1166.
Siimes, A.S.I., Välimäki, I.A.T.,Antila, K.J., Julkunen, M.K.A., Metsälä, T.H., Halkola, L.T., Sarajas, H.S.S. (1990): Regulation of heart rate variation by the autonomic nervous system in lambs Pediatr.Res. 27:383-391.
Välimäki, I., Anttila, H., Antila,K. and Kero, P.(1980): Spectral analysis of neonatal heart rate. A preliminary report. In P.Rolfe (ed.): Fetal and Neonatal Physiological Measurements. Pitman Press, Bath. pp. 104-109.
Välimäki, I., Rautaharju, P.M., Roy, S.B. and Scott, K.E.(1974): Heart rate patterns in healthy term and premature infants and in respiratory distress syndrome. Eur. J. Cardiol. 4:411-419.

IV. Pathophysiology of cardiorespiratory control. Clinical aspects and treatment

IV. *Physiopathologie du contrôle cardio-respiratoire. Aspects cliniques et thérapeutiques*

Cardiovascular risk in sleep-related breathing disorders

Thomas Podszus, Ole Feddersen, J. Hermann Peter and Peter von Wichert

Medizinische Poliklinik, Philipps-Universität, 3550 Marburg, Deutschland

Sleep-related breathing disorders (SRBD) can be classified into disorders with and without upper airway obstruction (17). Out of the disorders with extrathoracic airway obstruction, obstructive sleep apnea (complete occlusion of extrathoracic airways) and snoring (partial obtruction) are of outstanding importance. These two clinical syndromes are found in the vast majority of patients with sleep-related breathing disorders, and for the last twenty years, especially obstructive sleep apnea has been subject to intense research activity.

In the sixties already, Jung and Kuhlo (11) could show that patients suffering from the Pickwickian syndrome, an extreme variant of obstructive sleep apnea, developed excessive rises in pulmonary arterial blood pressure (6) and, in the long term cor pulmonale. Additionally, it was shown that effective treatment with tracheostomy normalized respiration and hemodynamic sequelae (12,13).

Since the beginning seventies, several teams have worked with the problems of pathological changes in the pulmonary and systemic circulation in patients with SRBD. Several investigators (2,5,8,16,24,26) correspondingly found that systemic arterial and pulmonary arterial blood pressure rise during obstructive sleep apnea and can reach threateningly high values. Even development of a lung edema at sleep during the obstructive apnea (4) was described as one sequel of apnea. Most of the authors (5,8,14,16) attributed these hemodynamic changes to hypoxia and hypercapnia induced by the apnea. This has its origin in the mechanism of hypoxic vasoconstriction described by von Euler and Liljestrand (27). These authors reported that under hypoxic breathing cats show a rise in pulmonary arterial blood pressure on the ground of vasoconstriction of the precapillary pulmonary arteries. In patients with sleep apnea, however, evidence for hypoxic vasoconstriction has not yet been provided.

Looking at blood pressures in the pulmonary and systemic circulation during obstructive apnea or during snoring, marked blood pressure oscillations which are primarily associated to breathing efforts are striking. These pressure swings are strictly linked to respiration. Therefore, paying due attention to the mechanics to be of special importance for the explanation of these blood pressure swings. Certainly, hypoxic vasoconstriction can have additional influences on the hemodynamics of heart and circulation (7) when simultaneaously hypoxia plus an individual predisposition occurs. In the continuation, we will therefore primarily present the mechanical influences which become active and have an effect on the hemodynamics of heart and circulation during snoring or obstructive apnea.

RESPIRATION

From a physical point of view, the extrathoracic airways can be compared with a Starling-Resistor (25). In such a system, the effective flow does not only depend on the up- and downstream pressure gradient but is also determined by the pressure gradient between the pressure surrounding the collapsible segment and the intraluminal pressure. The oropharyngeal and hypopharyngeal regions represent the collapsible segment in the human body relevant for airway obstruction. When muscle tone in this segment declines tissue pressure rises and can assimilate to or even exceed the actual intraluminal pressure. In proportion to that extent, partial obstruction (obstructive snoring) or, in case of a further rise in pressure gradient, complete occlusion in the shape of obstructive apnea arises. The relations of pressure and flow in the extrathoracic airways can be measured and quantified with the help of appropriate measuring procedures. Normally, effective flow is measured by means of a pneumotachograph and intrathoracic pressure by means of the intraesophageal pressure which reflects pleural pressure.

Figure 1

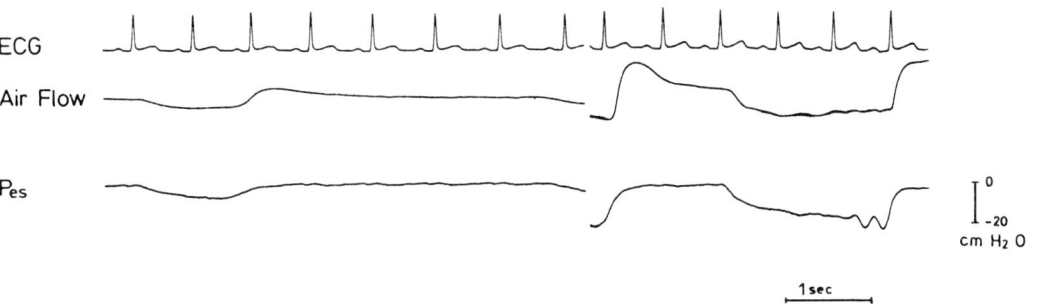

Fig. 1: Recording example of quiet breathing (left) and snoring (right). Shown are ECG, esophageal pressure, air flow, and arterial oxygen saturation. Besides inspiratory breathing activity (P_{es}), an unrestrained airflow is recognizable at the pneumotachograph. During upper airway obstruction a peak negative intrathoracic pressure swing and flow limitation are visible.

Figure 1 shows a recording example for unimpeded and obstructed respiration. Besides ECG registration, an unrestrained airflow is recognizable (left), as well as negative inspiratory esophageal pressures which are usually regarded as the expression of pleural pressure. Arterial oxygen saturation remains stable in such a situation. On the right side an obstructed breath (snoring) is shown. Inspiration is characterized by marked inspiratory pressure swings; at the same time, limitation of airflow is recognizable due to extrathoracic airway obstruction.

RIGHT HEART

Physiologically, a negative intrathoracic pressure during inspiration with simultaneous rise in abdominal pressure leads to an increase in venous return to the right heart (10). This effect is limited, however, because of a collaps of the inferior and superior venae cavae which implies a limitation of venous return and thus protects the heart from volume overload. Since during snoring or obstructive sleep apnea, in contrast to normal respiration, much more distinct negative inspiratory intrathoracic pressure swings are measurable, the question may be raised to what extent this may cause changes in venous return to the right heart. In an earlier study (22), we could already show that during obstructive sleep apnea, blood pressure in the right atrium rises. Since right atrial pressure (relative to pleural pressure) is primarily the expression of right heart filling and compliance, a rise in venous return to the right heart during the apneic period can be deducted. Via Frank-Starling mechanism, this results in an elevated right ventricular stroke volume, as was shown by Mahlo (15). Since during the inspiratory phase of the obstructed breathing maneuver, pulmonary arteries are unable to carry through an appropriate blood pooling (1), volume displacement into the pulmonary circulation leads directly to a rise in blood pressure in pulmonary circulation.

Figure 2

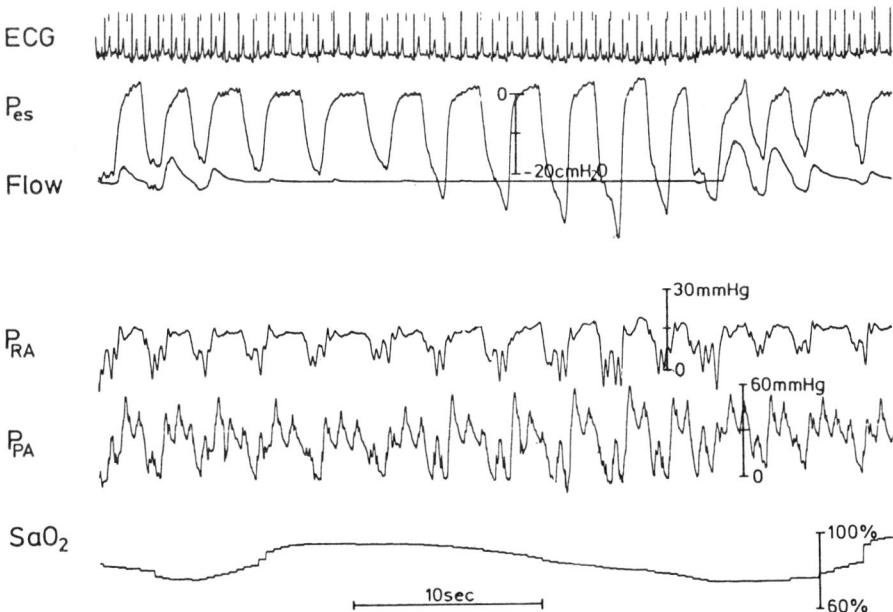

Fig. 2: Recording example of an obstructive apnea. Shown are: ECG, esophageal pressure (P_{es}), air flow, right atrial – (P_{RA}), and pulmonary arterial pressure (P_{PA}), arterial oxygen saturation.

The increase in right heart filling volume during inspiration is also responsible for a rise in systolic wall tension of the right ventricle. The latter plus pulmonary arterial blood pressure (relative to pleural pressure) represent the decisive parameters of right ventricular afterload, the force against which the right ventricle has to work. It is most likely that by an increase in systolic wall tension and a possible increase in pulmonary vascular resistance (on the basis of the von Euler und Liljestrand mechanism) due to apnea induced hypoxia, right ventricular afterload is increased during the inspiratory phases in obstructive apnea. Further investigations are required dealing with the questions of pre- and afterload and the contractile state of the right heart during obstructive apnea. At present, it can be stated that extrathoracic airway obstruction or obstructive sleep apnea results in an increase in right ventricular pre- and afterload although no studies have been presented in literature about the behaviour of right heart contractile state. Fig. 2 shows a recording of an obstructive apnea, and parallel right atrial and pulmonary arterial pressure (P_{PA}). The calculation of transmural P_{PA} results in pathologically high values during the apnea. Transmural P_{PA} values shows no significant differences between the beginning and the end of the apnea. Note that P_{RA} (relative to atmosphere) increases up to values of 17 torr at the end of the apnea during expiration. The calculation of transmural P_{RA} again shows pathologically high values in this situation (14 torr).

Pulmonary vascular resistance (PVR) is composed of two compartments which act parallel as well as serial (3). Under the condition that respiration is above functional residual capacity, a rise in alveolar pressure during inspiration can cause a mechanical constriction of intra-alveolar vessels and thus, mechanically, a pressure rise in this compartment as well as a rise in pulmonary vascular resistance. Parallel to this, the extra-alveolar (intra-parenchymal) pulmonary arterial vessels are stretched and lengthened and cause an additional rise in pulmonary vascular resistance. The consequences for the pulmonary vascular resistance are determined by lung volume. Below functional residual capacity, the intraparenchymal vessels take a winding course so that under normal inspiration, stretching and elastic extension of these vessels result in a decrease in PVR. Only when lung volume rises above functional residual capacity, the mechanical forces on the contrary cause an increase in PVR. The parallel component of the pulmonary vascular resistance has its origin in the model of lung circulation described by West. A rise in intrapulmonary blood volume allows the assumption that the lungs change from zone 2 to zone 3. Under the condition that respiration at rest is at the level of functional residual capacity, we can deduce from above that the right heart's stroke volume which is elevated during obstructive apnea entails a pressure increase in the pulmonary circulation. Future studies will have to take the specific proportions of these different aspects into consideration; especially about the question of pulmonary vascular resistance during obstructive apnea, no detailed investigations are present.

Measurements of blood pressure in the pulmonary circulation have shown that during habitual snoring already, i. e. partial extrathoracic airway obstruction, pulmonary arterial blood pressure rises. Pathologically elevated values can be reached hereat without a decrease of arterial oxygen saturation (23). The mechanism of hypoxic vasoconstriction is therefore not considered the decisive part in the explanation of elevated blood pressures in the pulmonary circulation of these patients, but it can, provided that there is an individual predisposition, aggravate additionally existing and mechanically determined problems.

LEFT HEART

During normal respiration, the hemodynamic changes during inspiration are characterized by a decrease in left ventricular stroke volume as well as a fall in systolic arterial blood pressure. The left ventricular stroke volume is determined by changes in pre- and afterload and by the state of myocardial contractility and compliance. As to the evaluation of left ventricular preload, no studies are at hand about the influence of venous return on the left heart during obstructive apnea. Indirect examinations of preload in the shape of measurements of pulmonary capillary wedge pressure - which under certain conditions reflects left ventricular enddiastolic pressure - have shown that pulmonary capillary wedge pressure can rise continuously and pathologically high during inspiration as well as in the course of the apnea (2,19).

Figure 3 shows a registration example of pulmonary capillary wedge pressure duringr obstructive apnea. It is remarkable that pulmonary capillary wedge pressure also shows marked pressure swings associated to respiration.

Figure 3

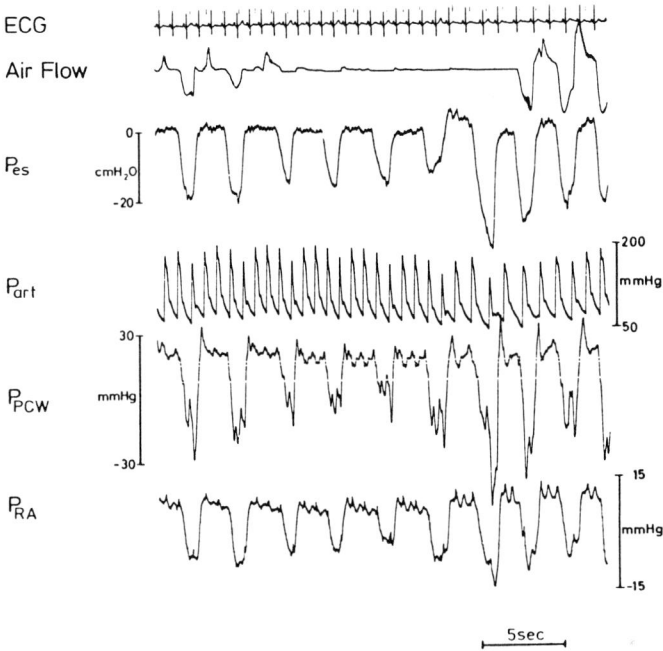

Fig. 3: Obstructive apnea episode showing pathologoically elevated pulmonary capillary wedge pressure (P$_{PCW}$) values.

In the presented episode, a pressure of 30 torr was measured expiratorily. Here pressure values measured relative to atmosphere as well as transmural pressures are pathologically elevated. It can be assumed that such values can be regarded as an expression of a left ventricular dysfunction during obstructive apnea. Investigations of stroke volume of the left ventricle are methodically very difficult to carry through under obstructive apnea and can only be of limited explanatory value. The investigations carried through so far (9,21), however, correspondingly found a decrease of left ventricular stroke volume during obstructive apnea. This decrease in stroke volume, together with a simultaneous rise in left ventricular enddiastolic filling pressures, represents left ventricular dysfunction during obstructive apnea, so that this seems possibly to be an explanation for the observed phenomenon of lung edema (4) during obstructive apnea.

In contrast to normal breathing, arterial blood pressure shows a decrease of systolic as well as diastolic pressure in the inspiratory phases during obstructive apnea, i.e. pulsus paradoxus occurs. Additionally, continuous pressure rises during the obstructive apneas are usually found. For the determination of left ventricular afterload, it is also necessary, however, that during negative intrathoracic pressure transmural arterial blood pressure has to be calculated. Compared to intravasally measured values (18), correction of intravasally measured arterial blood pressure values displays even higher transmural arterial pressure values. Recording of intravasal values thus results in an underestimation of transmural arterial pressure values and thus of left ventricular afterload.

Figure 4 presents a recording example of an obstructive apnea phase; additionally, arterial blood pressure (relative to atmospheric pressure) is displayed, which shows a continuous rise in the course of the apnea phase and parallel pressure oscillations associated to the obstructive breathing efforts.

Figure 4

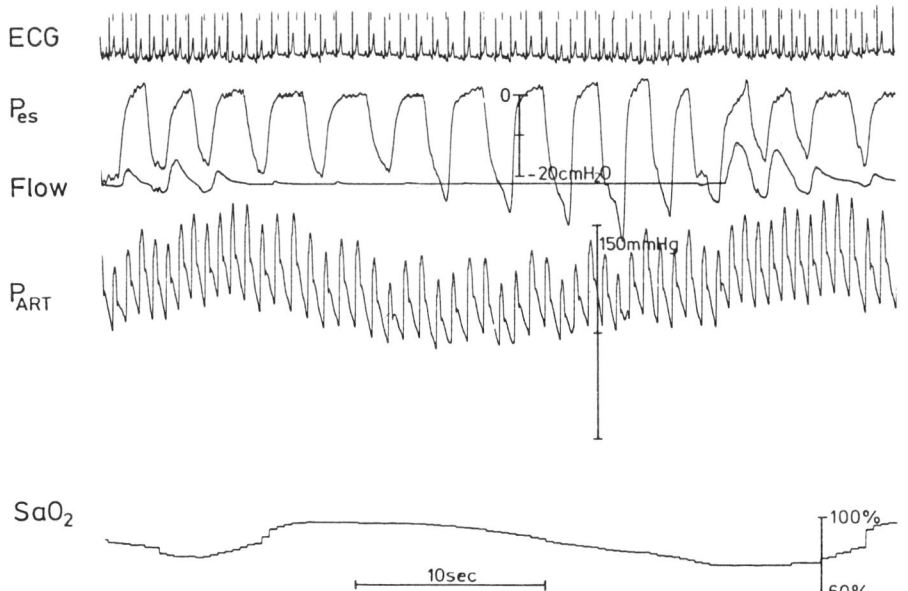

Fig. 4: Arterial blood pressure during obstructive apnea. Note that during postapneic ventilation a further increase of P_{ART} can be recorded so that a maximum of P_{ART} can be measured here and not in the apnea.

As to the entire function of the left ventricle, it may be assumed that during obstructive apnea, not only a rise in left ventricular preload takes place but also a rise in left ventricular afterload. In how far the acute hemodynamic changes occuring during extrathoracic airway obstruction during sleep in the long term favour the development of left heart insufficiency in the patients with sleep apnea or to what extent manifestation of hypertension is hereby supported has not yet been clarified.

An additional risk is faced by patients with obstructive sleep apnea because of the fact that also decreases in arterial blood pressure can occur (20) in the course of single obstructive apneas. It could be shown that arterial blood pressure can decrease continuously towards the end of an obstructive apnea. In own studies, values below 60 to 40 mmHG were measured at the end of long apneas.

Even if at present, the pathophysiological fundamentals of such changes have to be considered unclear, from the clinical point of view, a mechanism could be viewed here which is coresponsible for sleep apnea patients' elevated risk of developping cerebral ischemia during sleep. It is remarkable that in situations with falling arterial blood pressure only moderate intrathoracic pressure swings occur during the apnea, which are reflected in the small fluctuations of right atrial pressure. Probably, the crucial aspect of an explanation of such changes during apneas with blood pressure decrease is not the merely mechanically induced effects of disturbed breathing on heart and circulation but possibly decreases in left ventricular stroke volume. However, further studies are needed to explain such hemodynamic abnormalities. Especially, studies of cardiac output and volumes are of interest.

SUMMARY

Sleep related extrathoracic airway obstruction (obstructive snoring) or occlusion (obstructive sleep apnea) produces a variety of hemodynamic changes in heart and circulation. On the respiratory side, mainly changes in lung volume as well as in intrathoracic pressure are responsible for these changes. During snoring or obstructive sleep apnea, venous return to the right heart rises and consequently, preload is increased. Furthermore, via Frank-Starling mechanism, stroke volume is increased and thus, blood volume in the pulmonary circulation is elevated, which is expressed by a rise in pulumonary arterial blood pressure. Changes in pulmonary vascular resistance, which become effective mechanically on the one hand and by changes in blood volume in the lungs as well as on the ground of hypoxic vasoconstriction on the other hand, seem to be of outstanding importance and should be subject to further investigation. The most striking hemodynamic changes concerning the left heart are presented by a rise in left ventricular enddiastolic pressure and thus preload, as well as an increase in transmural arterial blood pressures and thus afterload. Additionally, left ventricular stroke volume decreases. These changes reflect a reduced left ventricular function which may possibly favour the occurrence of left heart insufficiency or even lung edema during obstructive sleep apnea. Additionally, in the course of obstructive apnea, grave blood pressure drops and even situations which are responsible for a low perfusion of the organism can occur.

From the pathophysiological point of view, many details of these hemodynamic changes still have to be considered unclear at present. Decisive influences seem to emanate from the mechanical changes becoming active in the course of airway obstruction or -occlusion. In addition, the hemodynamics of heart and circulation already pathologically impaired hereby can then be further deteriorated by hypoxia, hypercapnia und acidosis. It seems to be of special necessity to take interest in the problems of disturbed respiratory mechanics and its effects on the hemodynamics of heart and circulation in the future.

REFERENCES

1) Brecher, G.A. (1956): Venous Return. Grune & Stratton, New York London.
2) Buda, A.J., Schroeder, J.S., and Guilleminault, C. (1981): Abnormalities of pulmonary artery wedge pressures in sleep-induced apnea. Int. J. Cardiol. 1: 67-74.
3) Cassidy, S.S., Robertson, C.H., Pierce, A.K., and Johnson Jr., R.L. (1978): Cardiovascular effects of positive end-expiratory pressure in dogs. J. Appl. Physiol. 44: 743-750.
4) Chaudhary, B.A., Ferguson, D.S., and Speir, W.A. (1982): Pulmonary edema as a presenting feature of sleep apnea syndrome. Chest 82:122-124.
5) Coccagna, G., Mantovani, M., Brignani, F., Parchi,C., and Lugaresi, E. (1972a): Continuous recording of the pulmonary and systemic arterial pressure during sleep in syndromes of hypersomnia with periodic breathing. Bull. Physiopatho. Resp. 8:1159-1172.
6) Doll, E., Kuhlo, W., Steim, H., and Keul, J. (1968): Zur Genese des Cor pulmonale beim Pickwick-Syndrom. Dtsch. Med. WSchr. 49: 2361-2365.
7) Fishman, A.P. (1976): Hypoxia on the pulmonary circulation. Circ. Res. 38: 221-231.
8) Guilleminault, C., Eldridge, F.L., Simmon, F.B., and Dement, W.C. (1975): Sleep apnea syndrome. Can it induce hemodynamic changes? West. J. Med. 123: 7-16.
9) Guilleminault, C., Motta, J., Mihm, F., and Melvin, K. (1986): Obstructive sleep apnea and cardiac index. Chest 89:331-334.
10) Guyton, A.C., and Adkins, J.H. (1954): Quantitative aspects of the collapse factor in relation to venous return. Am. J. Physiol. 177:523-527.
11) Jung, R., and Kuhlo, W. (1965): Neurophysiological studies of abnormal night sleep and the pickwickian syndrome. In: Progress in Brain Research. Vol. 18, edited by K. Ackert and C. Bally. Elsevier, Amsterdam, pp. 140-159.
12) Kuhlo, W., Doll, E., and Franck, M.C. (1969). Erfolgreiche Behandlung eines Pickwick-Syndroms durch eine Dauertrachelkanüle. Deutsche Medizinische Wochenschrift 94: 1286-1290.
13) Kuhlo, W., and Doll, E. (1972): Pulmonary hypertension and the effect of tracheotomy in a case of Pickwickian syndrome. Bull. Physio.-path. Resp. 8: 1205 - 1216.
14) Lugaresi, E., Coccagna, G., Cirignotta, F., and Montagna, P. (1987): Sleep-related hemodynamic changes in health and respiratory disorders. Interdiscipl. Topics Geront. 22: 37-46.
15) Mahlo, H.R., Podszus, T., Penzel, T., Peter, J.H., and von Wichert, P. (1990): Right ventricular stroke volume at the end of obstructive apneas. Sleep Research 19: 250
16) Motta, J., Guilleminault, C., Schroeder, J.S., and Dement, W.C. (1978): Tracheostomy and hemodynamic changes in sleep-induced apnea. Ann. Intern. Med. 89: 454-458.
17) Peter, J.H., Becker, H., Blanke, J., Clarenbach, P., Mayer, G., Raschke, F., Rühle, K.-H., Rüther, E., Schläfke, M., Schönbrunn, E., Sieb, J.P., Stumpner, J., and Weis, R. (1991): Empfehlungen zur Diagnostik, Therapie und Langzeitbetreuung bei Schlafapnoe. Medizinische Klinik 86: 46-50.
18) Peter, J.H. (1990): Transmural systemic pressure in obstructive apnea. 10th Congress of the European Sleep Research Society Abstract Book: 85.
19) Podszus, T., Köhler, U., Mayer, J., Penzel, T., Peter, J.H., and von Wichert, P. (1986): Veränderungen des pulmonal-capillären Verschlußdruckes im Schlaf bei obstruktiver Schlaf-Apnoe. Kli.Wo. 64: 246-247.

20) Podszus, T., Köhler, U., Mayer, J., Penzel, T., Peter, J.H., and von Wichert, P. (1986): Systemic Arterial Blood Pressure Decreases during Obstructive Sleep Apnea. Sleep Research 15: 155.
21) Podzus, T., Mayer, J., Penzel, T., Peter, J.H., and von Wichert, P. (1986): Nocturnal hemodynamics in patients with obstructive sleep apnea. Eur. J. Respir. Dis. 69(Suppl 146): 435-442.
22) Podszus, T., Köhler, U., Mayer, J., Penzel, T., Peter, J.H., and von Wichert, P. (1987): Right and left atrial blood pressure changes during sleep apnea. 5th International Congress of Sleep Research Abstracts: 10.
23) Podszus, T., Peter, J.H., Ploch, T., Schneider, H., von Wichert, P. (1991): Pulmonalarterieller Blutdruck und Schnarchen. Praxis und Klinik der Pneumologie 45: 233-238.
24) Scharf, S.M. (1984): Influence of sleep state and breathing on cardiovascular function. In: Saunders, N.A., Sullivan, C.E. (Eds.) Sleep and Breathing. Marcel Dekker Inc, New York Basel, pp 221-240.
25) Smith, P.L., Wise, R.A., Gold, A.R., Schwartz, A.R., and Permutt, S. (1988): Upper airway pressure-flow relationships in obstructive sleep apnea. J. Appl. Physiol. 64:789-795.
26) Tilkian, A.G., Guilleminault, C., Schroeder, J.S., Lehrman, K.L., Simmons, F.B., and Dement, W.C. (1976): Hemodynamics in sleep induced apnea. Ann. Int. Med. 85: 714-719.
27) von Euler, U.S., Liljestrand, G. (1946): Observations on the pulmonary arterial blood pressure in the cat. Acta Physiol Scand 12: 301 - 320.

Résumé

Au cours du sommeil l'obstruction des voies aériennes extrathoraciques (ronflement obstructif) ou l'occlusion (apnée obstructive du sommeil) entraînent de nombreuses modifications de l'hémodynamique cardiaque et artérielle. Sur le plan respiratoire, les variations de volume pulmonaire et de pression intrathoracique sont les principaux responsables de ces modifications. Pendant le ronflement ou l'apnée obstructive, le retour veineux au coeur droit augmente et la précharge est accrue. De plus, grâce au mécanisme de Frank Starling, le volume d'éjection systolique augmente et donc aussi le volume sanguin intrapulmonaire ; ce qui entraîne une augmentation de la pression artérielle pulmonaire. Les modifications de la résistance vasculaire pulmonaire, par voie mécanique d'une part, par augmentation du volume sanguin et par la vasoconstriction hypoxique d'autre part, semblent avoir une importance considérable et méritent de plus amples recherches. Les modifications hémodynamiques les plus notables concernant le coeur gauche sont une augmentation de la pression télédiastolique du ventricule gauche et donc de la précharge, ainsi qu'une augmentation de la pression artérielle transmurale et donc de la post-charge. De plus, le volume d'éjection systolique du ventricule gauche diminue. Ces modifications reflètent une diminution de la fonction ventriculaire gauche qui peut être responsable d'une insuffisance cardiaque gauche ou même d'oedème pulmonaire pendant l'apnée obstructive. Egalement pendant les apnées obstructives peuvent survenir d'importantes chutes de pression et même des situations responsables d'une baisse de perfusion de l'organisme. Sur le plan physiopathologique, de nombreux détails de ces modifications hémodynamiques doivent être encore considérés comme peu clairs. Des influences majeures semblent venir des modifications mécaniques mises en jeu lors de l'obstruction ou l'occlusion des voies aériennes. De plus, les conditions hémodynamiques du coeur et de la circulation déjà pathologiques peuvent être encore détériorées par l'hypoxie, l'hypercapnie et l'acidose. Il semble particulièrement nécessaire dans le futur de s'intéresser aux problèmes des anomalies de la mécanique respiratoire et de ses effets sur l'hémodynamique cardio-circulatoire.

Pulmonary hemodynamics and sleep apnea syndrome

Emmanuel Weitzenblum, Jean Krieger, Monique Oswald and Michel Apprill

Service de Pneumologie, Centre Hospitalier Régional et Universitaire, 67098 Strasbourg Cedex, France

SUMMARY

The pulmonary hemodynamic consequences of obstructive sleep apneas have been investigated by several groups during the last twenty years. The earlier data have been obtained by measuring the intravascular pulmonary arterial pressure (PAP) and have shown a rise of PAP during apneas, the highest PAP being observed at the end of apneas. Actually, during obstructive apneas the only reliable measurements are those of transmural PAP which increases throughout the apneas, as a consequence of hypoxic vasoconstriction, and decreases after ventilation has resumed. The link between episodic (night-time) and permanent (daytime) pulmonary hypertension is poorly understood. Recent studies have clearly indicated that daytime hypoxemia, generally due to an associated chronic airflow obstruction, is the major determinant of permanent pulmonary hypertension and cor pulmonale, and that severe nocturnal hypoxemia is not sufficient per se.

In recent years, with the development of sleep laboratories and polysomnography, a great number of studies have been devoted to sleep apnea syndrome (SAS). Since alveolar hypoxia induces pulmonary vasoconstriction, it can be expected that sleep-related episodes of hypoxemia will be accompanied by peaks of pulmonary hypertension (PH). In fact, there have been few hemodynamic investigations during sleep in SAS patients and the number of patients who could be investigated was rather restricted in all the published studies. This is probably accounted for by the fact that hemodynamic investigations are not easily performed during sleep.
Another important question is that of the development of permanent (diurnal) PH in patients with SAS : does sleep-related (episodical) PH lead to daytime (permanent) PH and later to right heart failure which dominates the clinical picture of the "Pickwickian" syndrome ? What is the real incidence of permanent PH in a population of SAS subjects and what are the mechanisms leading to permanent PH ? We will try to answer these questions in this short review.

1. Pulmonary hemodynamics during sleep in SAS patients

Coccagna et al. (1972) and Lonsdorfer et al. (1972) were probably the first to measure continuously pulmonary artery mean pressure during sleep in SAS patients. They used small Grandjean catheters and these investigations were combined with polysomnography. Both groups of authors observed an increase of PAP during

apneic episodes, particularly when the latter occurred during REM sleep. PAP increased with the deepening of sleep from stage 1 to 4, the highest values being recorded during REM sleep (Coccagna et al., 1972) but returned to baseline values with awakening in the morning. There was a concomitant rise in systemic arterial pressure (Coccagna et al., 1972).
These results have been confirmed by the Stanford group (Tilkian et al., 1976 ; Schroeder et al., 1978) : ten out of twelve patients developed rises in PAP which were severe in five of them. PAP returned to control levels if several minutes of normal ventilation occurred, but conversely PAP gradually increased in the case of repeated apnea episodes in close sequence. Buda et al. (1981), from the same group, found in addition that in those patients in whom they could be recorded pulmonary artery wedge pressures were also increased, but to a lesser degree. There is an agreement on the fact that the highest pulmonary artery pressures are observed in the immediate post apnea period (Coccagna et al., 1972 ; Lonsdorfer et al., 1972 ; Schroeder et al., 1978 ; Shepard, 1985).
In fact the measurements of intravascular pressures, related to the atmospheric pressure, are not reliable during apneas because of the considerable variations of intrathoracic pressure. Obstructive apneas can be assimilated to a Müller manoeuvre (inspiratory effort against a closed glottis) and the pulmonary artery pressure reflects the changes in intrathoracic pressure ; the latter may decrease by as much as 30mmHg during an obstructive apnea, with a subsequent fall of PAP which decreases to negative values (Shepard, 1986). In this instance the only significant variable is the transmural pressure (intravascular minus intrathoracic pressure) which can be obtained by simultaneously measuring PAP and intrathoracic pressure. The transmural pressure represents the effective pressure against which the right ventricle must work. It is possible to substract electronically the oesophageal pressure, obtained from an oesophageal balloon, from the intravascular PAP by means of a differential amplifier (Krieger and Weitzenblum, 1990). Marrone et al. (1989) have observed that pulmonary transmural pressures show a trend to increase throughout the apneas and to decrease after ventilation has resumed, while pressures referenced to atmosphere had an opposite behaviour. In most of their patients (5/7) there was a significant negative correlation between transmural PAP and SaO_2.
We have observed (Krieger and Weitzenblum, 1990) that in a sample of apneas randomly chosen among the longest ones, transmural PAP followed a biphasic evolution with an initial decrease and a final increase. Transmural PAP was correlated SaO_2, heart rate and oesophageal pressure. We therefore suggested that transmural PAP decreases during the initial part of an obstructive apnea, due to the decrease in cardiac output and heart rate and increases during the final part due to hypoxic vasoconstriction. Even if rather good correlations have been observed between SaO_2 and transmural PAP, markedly hypertensive values of PAP are not the rule in SAS patients during sleep (Marrone et al., 1989 ; Krieger and Weitzenblum, 1990). Guilleminault et al. (1986) have measured the cardiac index, by the thermodilution method, in 17 SAS patients and have found it to decrease regularly during apneas, by 35 % of its baseline value as a mean, and to increase at the resumption of ventilation. On the other hand, Marrone et al. (1989) have not found significant trends in the changes in cardiac output during obstructive apneas.
These factors are obviously not the only ones that may play a role. An increased pulmonary artery wedge pressure has been observed by Buda et al. (1981), suggesting that an impaired left ventricular function could play a role in the increased pulmonary artery pressure. Actually, indirect measurement of the left ventriculars stroke volume has shown a decrease which was correlated with the decrease in pleural pressure (Tolle et al., 1983) : through ventricular interdependence mechanisms, the increased venous return to the right ventricle could reduce left ventricular preload and hence left ventricular output.
Thus, it seems that the changes in PAP during obstructive apneas are the consequences of the interaction of multiple factors including changes in intrathoracic pressure, hypoxic vasoconstriction and variations in heart rate, cardiac output

and, possibly left heart filling pressures.

2. From nocturnal to daytime pulmonary hypertension

Cor pulmonale is a classical feature of the "Pickwickian" syndrome which was described more than thirty years ago (Burwell et al., 1956 ; Gastaut et al., 1965). The sleep apnea syndrome was described later (Guilleminault et al., 1976). Early studies by the Stanford group (Schroeder et al., 1978) have found a high incidence (near 60 %) of awake resting PH defined as a mean $PAP \geq 20mmHg$. However this figure was obtained in a small group (n = 22) of SAS patients selected from a larger population, which could have introduced a bias. Since 1985 four studies on large series of unselected patients (Bradley et al., 1985 ; Podszus et al., 1986 ; Weitzenblum et al., 1988 ; Krieger et al., 1989) have clearly indicated that the occurrence of cor pulmonale or PH was not high, ranging from 12 % to 20 %, which was rather different from the earlier studies mentioned above which included smaller numbers of patients.

Bradley et al. (1985) found that clinical cor pulmonale was present in 6/50 patients (12 %). Podszus et al. (1986) have observed the presence of daytime PH in 13/65 patients (20 %) but only 11 of their 65 patients underwent a conventional polysomnography. In the first study of our group (Weitzenblum et al., 1988) daytime PH, defined by a resting mean $PAP \geq 20mmHg$, was present in 9/46 patients (20 %) and these data have been confirmed in a more recent study (Krieger et al., 1989) showing that 19/100 SAS patients had resting PH. The occurrence of exercising PH was more common : 40 % of the patients without resting PH (Weitzenblum et al., 1988) in agreement with the results of earlier studies (Tilkian et al., 1976 ; Podszus et al., 1986). A higher incidence of resting PH has been reported by Fletcher et al. (1987) but in selected patients with associated lung disease ("overlap syndrome"). Thus, resting PH is far from being the rule in SAS patients, but exercising hemodynamic abnormalities are more frequent.

Why do some patients develop daytime PH whereas the majority of SAS patients do not ? Bradley et al. (1985) have observed that their cor pulmonale patients had a markedly lower daytime PaO_2 (52 ± 4 vs $75 \pm 2mmHg$ for SAS patients without cor pulmonale, $p<0.001$) and a similar difference was found for $PaCO_2$ (51 ± 2 vs $36 \pm 1mmHg$, $p<0.001$) while the apnea index and the apnea-hypopnea index were identical in the two groups (Table 1). All patients with cor pulmonale had evidence of mild to moderate obstructive airway disease (Table 1) and they were more overweight than the others ($p<0.05$). Another study from the same group (Bradley et al., 1986) has clearly shown that in these patients, hypercapnia (and to some degree hypoxemia) could be attributed to diffuse airway obstruction.

	Patients without RHF (n = 44)	Patients with RHF (n = 6)	p value
Age (years)	49 ± 2	49 ± 3	NS
Weight (% ideal)	147 ± 7	186 ± 12	0.05
PaO_2 (mmHg)	75 ± 2	52 ± 4	0.001
$PaCO_2$ (mmHg)	36 ± 1	51 ± 2	0.001
FVC (% pred.)	105 ± 3	75 ± 7	0.001
FEV1 (l)	3.3 ± 0.1	1.8 ± 0.3	0.001
FEV1/FVC (%)	76 ± 1	56 ± 5	0.001
TLC (% pred.)	110 ± 2	111 ± 8	NS
CO_2 response (l/min/mmHg)	2.4 ± 0.2	1.2 ± 0.3	0.01

Table 1
Awake data in patients with and without right heart failure (RHF).
From Bradley et al. (1985). (Values are means $\pm$ standard error of the mean).

The data of Leech et al. (1985) somewhat contradicted those of Bradley et al. since they observed that in 64 SAS patients the occurrence of signs of right ventricular dysfunction (right ventricular failure or right ventricular hypertrophy or dilation) was linked to the severity of sleep induced respiratory disorders assessed by an index combining the frequency and degree of nocturnal desaturation. However clinical, ECG and echocardiographic signs of cor pulmonale are probably not very sensitive and may be late complications of SAS, and the measurement of PAP gives an earlier and more precise indication of the consequences of the disease on the pulmonary circulation.

Our results (Weitzenblum et al., 1988) complete and confirm those of Bradley et al. (1985) by including precise data obtained from hemodynamic investigations. When comparing the two groups with (n = 9) and without (n = 37) PH, it appeared that PH was related to the presence of daytime hypoxemia, hypercapnia and bronchial obstruction (Table 2) but not to the severity of respiratory events during sleep. Daytime hypoxemia was significantly lower ($p<0.001$) in the group with PH and there was a highly significant correlation between daytime PaO_2 ($r = -0.61$, $p<0.001$), $PaCO_2$ ($r = 0.55$, $p<0.001$), FEV_1 ($r = -0.52$, $p<0.001$) and PAP, but not significant correlations between the apnea index or the apnea + hypopnea index or the lowest sleep transcutaneous SaO_2 and diurnal PAP.

	Patients with PH (n = 9)	Patients without PH (n = 37)	p value
FVC (% pred.)	72 + 12	97 + 14	0.001
FEV1 (ml)	1560 + 420	2750 + 660	0.001
FEV1/FVC (%)	59 + 11	73 + 8	0.001
PaO2 (mmHg)	61 + 8	76 + 9	0.001
PaCO2 (mmHg)	45 + 4	38 + 4	0.001
Lowest sleep StcO2 (%)	58 + 21	66 + 18	NS
Apnea index (/hour)	62 + 31	65 + 40	NS
Apnea + hypopnea index (/hour)	102 + 33	86 + 36	NS

Table 2
Pulmonary volumes, daytime arterial blood gases and sleep variables in SAS patients subdivided into two groups according to the presence or not of daytime pulmonary hypertension (PH).
From Weitzenblum et al. (1988). (Values are means + standard deviation of the mean).

These data have been confirmed by a more recent study (Krieger et al., 1989) where 114 SAS patients could be included. Pulmonary hypertensive patients (19/100) were more hypoxemic ($p<0.001$) more hypercapnic ($p<0.001$), and had lower lung volumes ($p<0.001$) than pulmonary normotensive patients. But they had higher apnea ($p<0.01$) and apnea + hypopnea indices than the remainder, and lower mean ($p < 0.001$) and minimal ($p<0.01$) transcutaneous SaO_2 during sleep, which was somewhat different from our first study (Weitzenblum et al., 1988). A multiple regression analysis showed that FEV1 and daytime PaO2 contributed the most to the model for PAP. However the r2 value for the model was of only 0.44. Nighttime hypoxemia did not appear to contribute at all once the contribution of FEV1 and daytime PaO2 had been taken into account. These results demonstrate the primary role of diffuse airway obstruction and of hypoxemia in the development of PH in SAS patients.
That PH requires the presence of daytime hypoxemia in SAS patients is still confirmed by the study of Fletcher et al. (1987) whose patients with SAS and a associated lung disease exhibited PH and had markedly lower PaO2 than those without "overlap syndrome" in whom PH was rather rare.
The major cause of daytime hypoxemia in SAS patients seems to be an associated obstructive airway disease (Bradley et al., 1985 ; Weitzenblum et al., 1988). This associated airway disease is not necessarily severe (Table 3) and may be cli-

nically silent. When chronic airflow obstruction is not present, the role of (major) obesity and, possibly, of a diminished chemosensitivity must be considered.

no.	Age yrs	Actual/ideal weight %	FVC pred. %	FEV1 ml	FEV1/FVC %	PaO2 mmHg	PaCO2 mmHg	Apnea index /hour
1	69	146	84	1825	69	62	42	5
2	69	144	79	1100	43	60	46	44
3	53	155	76	1620	62	47	46	82
4	66	125	70	1360	59	55	54	109
5	55	214	50	1100	76	60	40	75
6	39	234	75	2425	70	72	43	65
7	58	164	56	1400	58	57	47	87
8	58	125	84	1820	51	65	42	38
9	50	133	72	1375	46	69	42	50

Table 3
Individual data in patients with SAS and daytime pulmonary hypertension.
From Weitzenblum et al. (1988).

REFERENCES

Bradley, T.D., Rutherford, A., Grossmann, R.F., Lue, F., Zamel, R., Moldofsky, H., Phillipson, E.A. (1985) : Role of daytime hypoxemia in the pathogenesis of right heart failure in the obstructive sleep apnea syndrome. Am. Rev. Respir. Dis. 131: 835-893.
Bradley, T.D., Rutherford, A., Lue, F., Moldofsky, H., Grossman, R., Zamel, N., Phillipson, E.A. (1986) : Role of diffuse airway obstruction in the hypercapnia of obstructive sleep apnea. Am. Rev. Respir. Dis. 134: 920-924.
Buda, A.J., Schroeder, J.S., Guilleminault, C. (1981) : Abnormalities of pulmonary artery wedge pressure in sleep-induced apnea. Int. J. Cardiol. 1: 67-74.
Burwell, C.S., Robin, E.D., Whaley, R.D., Bickelmann A.G. (1956) : Extreme obesity associated with alveolar hypoventilation. A Pickwickian syndrome. Am. J. Med. 21: 811-818.
Coccagna, G., Mantovani, M., Brignani, F., Parchi, C., Lugaresi, E. (1972) : Continuous recording of the pulmonary and systemic arterial pressure during sleep and syndromes of hypersomnia with periodic breathing. Bull. Physiopathol. Respir. 8: 1159-1172.
Fletcher, E.C., Schaaf, J.M., Miller, J., Fletcher, J.G. (1987) : Long-term cardiopulmonary sequelae in patients with sleep apnea and chronic lung disease. Am. Rev. Respir. Dis. 135: 525-533.
Gastaut, H., Tassinari, C.A., Duron, B. (1965) : Etude polygraphique des manifestations épisodiques (hypniques et respiratoires) du syndrome de Pickwick. Rev. Neurol. 112: 568-579.
Guilleminault, C., Motta, J., Minh, F., Melvin, K. (1986) : Obstructive sleep apnea and cardiac index. Chest 89: 331-334.
Krieger, J., Sforza, E., Apprill, M., Lampert, E., Weitzenblum, E., Ratamaharo, J. (1989) : Pulmonary hypertension, hypoxemia and hypercapnia in obstructive sleep apnoea patients. Chest 96: 729-737.
Krieger, J., Weitzenblum, E. : Pulmonary hemodynamics in the obstructive sleep apnoea syndrome. Proceedings of the Marburg meeting (1989) on Sleep Disordered Breathing, In Press.
Leech, J.A., Onal, E., Givan, V., Gallestegui, J., Lopata, H. (1985) : Right ventricular dysfunction relates to nocturnal hypoxemia in patients with sleep apnoea syndrome. Am. Rev. Respir. Dis. 131: A104 (Abstr.).

Lonsdorfer, J., Meunier-Carus, J., Lampert-Benignus, E., Kurtz, D., Bapst-Reiter, J., Fletto, R., Micheletti, G. (1972) : Aspects hémodynamiques et respiratoires du syndrome pickwickien. Bull. Physiopathol. Respir. 8: 1181-1192.
Marrone, O., Bellia, U., Ferrara, G., Milone, F., Romano, L., Salvaggio, Stallone, A., Bonsignore, G. (1989) : Transmural pressure measurements : importance in the assessment of pulmonary hypertension in obstructive sleep apnoeas. Chest 95: 338-343.
Podszus, T., Bauer, W., Mayer, J., Penzel, T., Peter, J.H., Wichert, P. (1986) : Sleep apnea and pulmonary hypertension. Klin. Wschr. 64: 131-134.
Schroeder, J.S., Motta, J., Guilleminault, C. (1978) : Hemodynamic studies in sleep apnea. In Sleep Apnea Syndromes. C. Guilleminault, WC Dements eds, Alan Liss, New York, 177-196.
Shepard, J.W. (1985) : Gas exchange and hemodynamics during sleep. Med. Clin. North. Am. 69: 1243-1264.
Shepard, J.W. (1986) : Hemodynamics in obstructive sleep apnoea. In Fletcher EC (ed) Abnormalities of respiration during sleep. Grune and Stratton, Orlando, pp 39-61.
Tilkian, A.G., Guilleminault, C., Schroeder, J.S., Lehrman, K.L., Simmons, F.B., Dement, W.C. (1976) : Hemodynamics in sleep-induced apnea. Ann. Inter. Med. 85: 714-719.
Tolle, F.A., Judy, W.V., Yu, P.L., Markand, O.N. (1983) : Reduced stroke volume related to pleural pressure in obstructive sleep apnoea. J. Appl. Physiol. 55: 1718-1724.
Weitzenblum, E., Krieger, J., Apprill, M., Vallee, E., Ehrhart, M., Ratomaharo, J., Oswald, M., Kurtz, D. (1988) : Daytime pulmonary hypertension in patients with obstructive sleep apnea syndrome. Am. Rev. Respir. Dis. 138: 345-349.

Résumé

Les répercussions hémodynamiques pulmonaires des apnées obstructives, liées au sommeil, ont été étudiées par plusieurs groupes d'auteurs au cours de ces 20 dernières années. Les données initiales ont été obtenues en mesurant la pression artérielle pulmonaire (PAP) intra-vasculaire : les résultats ont indiqué une élévation de la PAP pendant les apnées, les valeurs les plus élevées de PAP étant observées à la fin des apnées. En fait, au cours d'apnées obstructives, les seules mesures hémodynamiques fiables sont celles de la PAP transmurale ; celle-ci augmente tout au long des apnées, probablement du fait de la vasoconstriction pulmonaire hypoxique, et elle diminue après la reprise de la ventilation.
On sait peu de choses sur la relation entre l'hypertension pulmonaire épisodique (liée au sommeil) et l'hypertension pulmonaire permanente (diurne) dans le syndrome d'apnée du sommeil. Plusieurs études récentes ont clairement montré que l'hypoxémie diurne, généralement due à une bronchopneumopathie chronique obstructive associée, est la cause déterminante de l'hypertension pulmonaire permanente et du coeur pulmonaire, et que l'hypoxémie artérielle nocturne isolée (sans hypoxémie diurne) n'est pas suffisante pour induire une hypertension pulmonaire, même si elle est sévère.

Baroreflex control of heart rate in sleep apnea patients. Comparison of normotensive and hypertensive patients and effect of CPAP therapy

P. Escourrou, V. Le Gros and C. Gaultier

Laboratoire de Physiologie, INSERM CJF 89-09, Hôpital Antoine Béclère, 92141 Clamart, France

ABSTRACT :

The sleep apnea syndrome (SAS) is usually characterized by a cyclical bradytachycardia and is often associated with systemic hypertension. Conversely essential hypertension is accompanied by an abnormal baroreflex control of heart rate (HR). The aim of this study was to compare the baroreflex control of HR in 8 normotensive patients with apnea index of 45 ± 18/hour and 6 untreated hypertensive patients of similar age and body mass index with apnea index of 49 ± 18/hour. The cardiac arm of the baroreflex was evaluated by a 100 µg intravenous bolus injection of phenylephrine during wakefulness, at the beginning of apneas and during sleep with nasal CPAP. The results showed that the sensitivity i.e. the slope of the relationship between HR and blood pressure, was normal in normotensive SAS subjects during wakefulness and sleep with CPAP. The sensitivity tended to be lower in hypertensive SAS patients during the same periods. But the sensitivity was increased during apnea to 239 % of wakefulness value in normotensive patients whereas it did not vary significantly in hypertensive patients. Despite this difference in baroreflex sensivity between normotensive and hypertensive patients there was no significant difference between these two groups for absolute and relative variations of heart rate during the bradytachycardia cycles : 28.4 ± 7.8 bpm in normotensive patients and 24.8 ± 11.3 bpm in hypertensive patients. The cardiac baroreflex is not therefore the main factor of the bradycardia during apnea. This bradycardia appears to be predominantly controlled by the arterial chemoreflex and by the lung inflation reflex. It is noteworthy that the hypertensive subjects have a higher pressure reactivity to phenylephrine infusion. But this effect on long term development of hypertension remains to determined.

Supported by INSERM CJF 89-09

INTRODUCTION :

Sleep apnea patients have during sleep cyclical variations of heart rate and blood pressure characterised by bradycardia and lower blood pressure during apnea and tachycardia and surges of blood pressure during resumption of ventilation (Coccagna et al, 1971, Guilleminault et al, 1984). The sleep apnea syndrome (SAS) is accompanied by increased secretion of catecholamines at night (Fletcher et al, 1987). It has been recently shown indeed that apnea are accompanied by an increased activity of muscle sympathetic fibers (Ejnell et al, 1991) and this increase seems to persist even during daytime in sleep apnea patients.

Permanent hypertension is observed in 50 % to 90 % of patients with obstructive SAS (Guilleminault et al 1978 ; Lugaresi et al 1978 ; Jeong et al, 1989). But the causal relationship between both diseases is unclear : the presence of permanent hypertension was not significantly related to respiratory disturbances, nor gross sleep disruptions in 50 patients controlled for age and obesity (Escourrou et al, 1990). Also the reason why a significant proportion of SAS patients do not develop permanent systemic hypertension is unknown.

Permanent hypertension is associated with a resetting of the baroreflex control of heart rate to higher pressure and the sensitivity i.e. the slope of the relationship between blood pressure (BP) and heart rate (HR) is decreased (Bristow et al, 1969). Although the causal relationships of these baroreflex changes in hypertension are unclear, they seem to play a role in the maintenance of hypertension.

The baroreflex control of heart rate during sleep in normal subjects has been addressed by the study of Bristow et al, 1969 who showed no systematic changes in sensitivity of the baroreflex during sleep. There was nevertheless a resetting of HR towards lower BP value and a decreased reactivity to vasoconstrictor agents.

But in patients with SAS the baroreflex control of heart rate during sleep is unknown. Therefore we sought to evaluate the baroreflex control of HR in normotensive and hypertensive patients during wakefulness, during sleep apnea and under CPAP therapy.

POPULATION AND METHODS :

Population : we have studied 14 patients : 8 normotensive (NT) (6 men, 2 women) and 6 hypertensive (HT) (all men) untreated or after 2 weeks cessation of hypertension therapy. Hypertension was defined following the WHO criteria (systolic pressure above 160 mmHg and/or diastolic above 95 mmHg at 3 consecutive measurements) (WHO, 1978). Both groups had similar age (NT : 52.1 $\pm$ 10.9 yrs, HT 50.7 $\pm$ 5.9 yrs), body mass index (NT : 32.6 $\pm$ 9.6 kg/m^2 ; HT 33.5 $\pm$ 4.7) and apnea-hypopnea index (45 $\pm$ 18/hour in NT vs : 49 $\pm$ 18/hour in HT).

Methods : All patients underwent a standard polysomnography including : 2 channels EEG, EOG, submental EMG, oral and nasal flows (thermistors), thoracic and abdominal movements (Respitrace), diaphragmatic EMG, end-tidal PCO_2, EKG, tracheal sounds. Baroreflex control of heart rate was assessed by a bolus i.v. injection of 100 μg phenylephrine through an infusion line placed on the forearm. RR intervals have been measured by a periodmeter triggered by the EKG. Blood pressure was measured non invasively by a Finapres 2300. Baroreflex sensitivity of HR control was assessed by the slope of the relationship between HR and systolic pressure and vascular reactivity was estimated by the rise in pressure following the phenylephrine infusion as shown on Fig 1. Several evaluations of baroreflex activity were averaged at each experimental period. Measurements during sleep apnea and CPAP were made during slow wave sleep. Statistical comparisons have been made by Student-t-tests. Results are given as mean ± 1 SD.

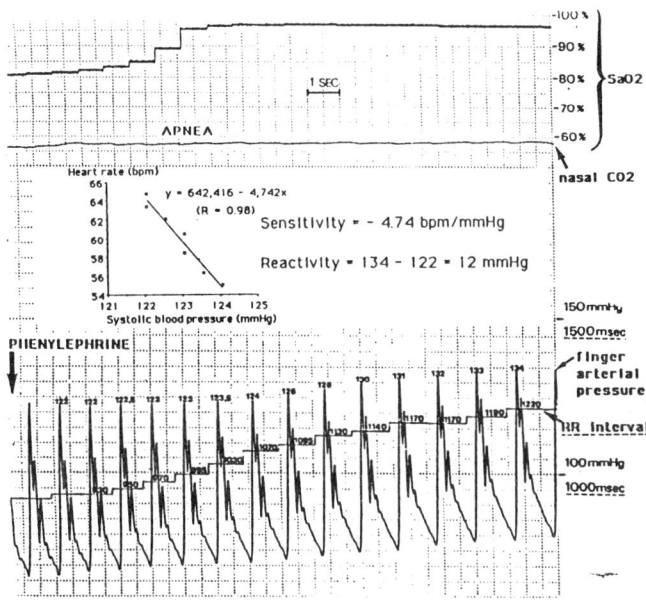

Fig 1 : Effect of an intravenous bolus of 100 microg phenylephrine on finger arterial pressure and RR interval during apnea in a normotensive subject.

RESULTS :

Supine awake average values of HR and BP were significantly higher in the HT than in the NT group : HR was 69 ± 4 bpm in NT and 76 ± 5 bpm in HT (p<0.05), systolic BP : 126 ± 8 mmHg vs. 169 ± 12 mmHg and diastolic BP : 71 ± 9 mmHg vs. 93 ± 2 mmHg respectively.

Changes in HR between apnea and resumption of breathing were not different in NT (28.4 ± 7.8 bpm) vs. HT (24.8 ± 11.3 bpm). Absolute variations of BP from apnea to resumption were also similar in both groups for systolic (NT : 50 ± 11 mmHg ; HT : 48.3 ± 10.9) and for diastolic (NT : 28.2 ± 8.4 mmHg ; HT : 31.0 ± 9.8) as shown on Fig 2. A, B.

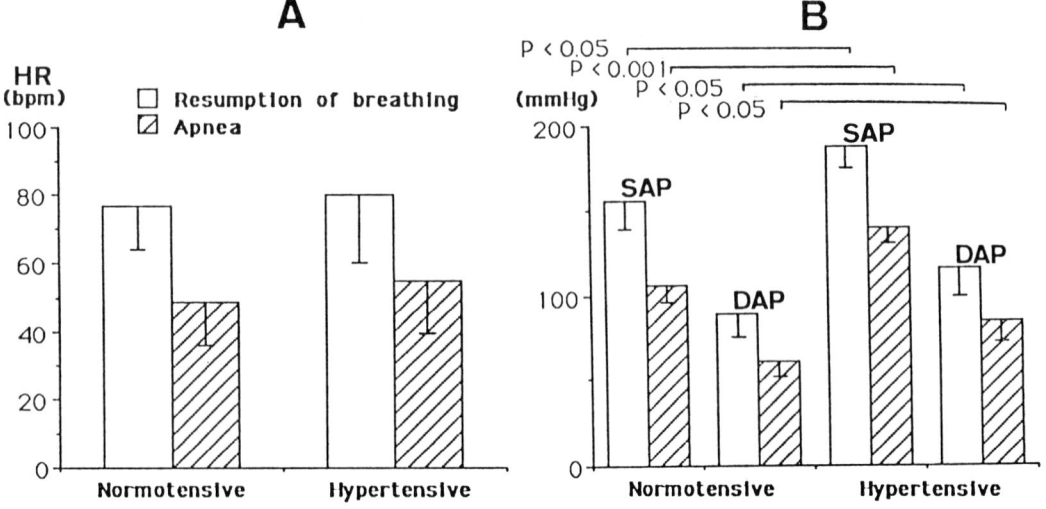

Fig 2 : A : Mean (± 1 SD) extreme values of heart rate in Normotensive and Hypertensive patients during apnea and resumption of breathing. B : Mean (± 1 SD) extreme values of systolic (SAP) and diastolic arterial pressures (DAP) in Normotensive and Hypertensive patients during apnea and resumption of breathing.

Responses to phenylephrine :

Figure 3 shows the mean baroreflex changes in all subjects. Sleep apnea and CPAP were accompanied by a reset of HR to lower BP than during wakefulness in both groups of patients. During wakefulness and sleep with CPAP, sensitivity and reactivity were not significantly different between NT and HT. Compared with wakefulness sensitivity increased significantly during apnea in NT only ($p < 0.05$) and was greater during apnea in NT than in HT ($p = 0.01$).

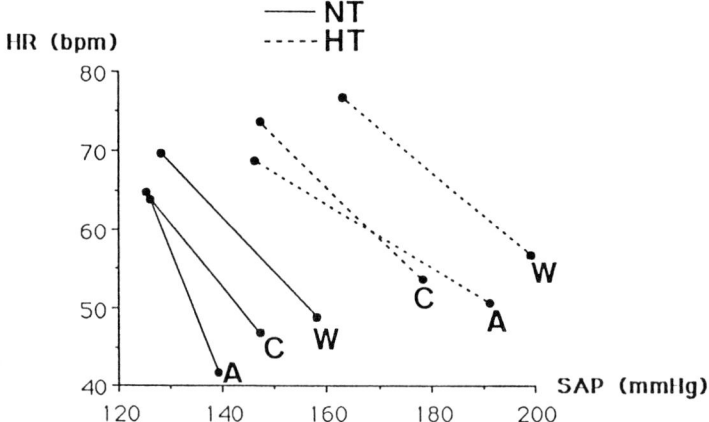

Fig 3 : Average relationships between heart rate (HR) and systolic arterial pressure (SAP) in Normotensive (NT) and Hypertensive (HT) sleep apnea patients. Wakefulness (W), Apnea (A) and CPAP (C) relationships are not different in HT. But in NT patients (A) is different from (W) and (C) ($p < 0.05$).

Reactivity was higher during apnea in HT than in NT (p < 0.05) (Fig 4 A,B). No significant correlation was found between baroreflex sensitivity and changes in HR during the apnea-resumption cycles.

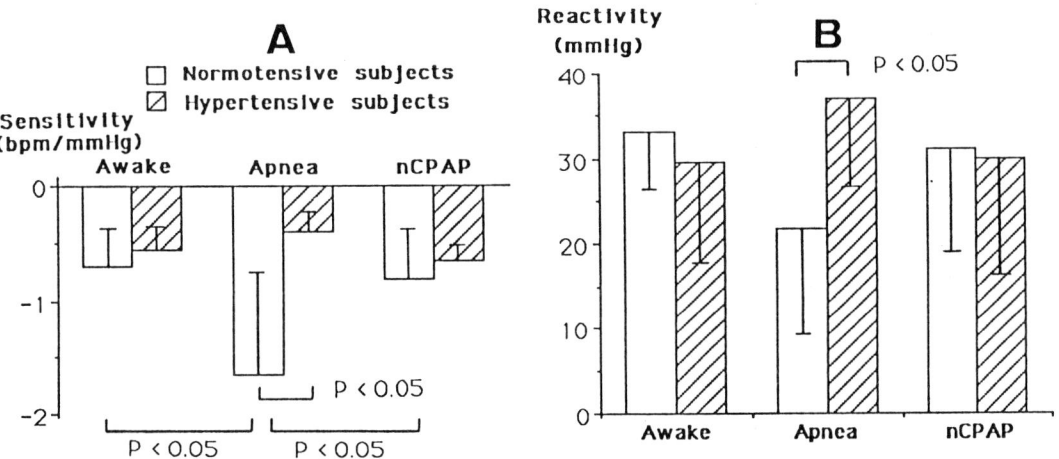

Fig 4 : A : Mean values (± 1 SD) of baroreflex sensitivity during wakefulness, apnea and nasal CPAP. B : Mean values (± 1 SD) of reactivity (rise in systolic pressure after a bolus infusion of 100 microg phenylephrine).

DISCUSSION :

We evaluated the baroreflex control of HR in normotensive and hypertensive patients during wakefulness, during sleep apnea and under CPAP therapy. Our major finding were that 1) the sensitivity of the baroreflex was increased during apnea in normotensive patients and this increase was reversed under CPAP therapy 2) no change in sensitivity was observed in hypertensive patients during apnea, whereas reactivity was higher than in normotensive patients 3) despite this difference in sensitivity there were no significant difference between the two groups for absolute and relative variations in heart rate during the apnea-related bradytachycardia cycles.

Zwillich et al, 1982 have shown that the bradycardia observed during apnea is the result of parasympathetic activation as atropine blocks it. This vagal stimulation presumably results from hypoxemia as it is correlated to desaturation and as O_2 administration inhibits the bradycardia (Zwillich et al, 1982).

Changes in heart period quantitatively reflects changes in vagal cardiac activity (Katona et al, 1970). During apnea, vagal cardiac activity is mainly under the dependance of the arterial chemoreflex and the pulmonary inflation reflex. The chemo-receptors situated in the carotid and aortic bodies (de Burgh Daly, 1975) are stimulated by the changes in PO_2 and PCO_2 secondary to the apnea. Blood pressure is maintained by an increase in peripheral resistance in all vascular beds but coronary and cerebral vessels which are relatively unaffected. There is indeed an increase in sympathetic nerve activity in response to hypoxia (Somers et al, 1989). Vagal tone is also stimulated by a low lung volume which reduces the activity of pulmonary receptors with afferent pathway in the vagus nerves (de Burgh Daly, 1975). This reflex results in bradycardia and vasoconstriction through modulation of both muscle sympathetic and vagal cardiac outflow (D.L. Eckberg, 1985). But cardiac vagal outflow is also under the dependance of the arterial baroreflex which exerts a tonic inhibitory influence at the medullary level. The baroreflex is modulated by interactions with the respiratory activity (Eckberg, 1977) and also with the arterial chemoreflex (Andersen, 1966).

The fact that bradycardia occurs at relatively constant pressure at the beginning of apnea means that the normal relationships between arterial pressure and heart rate are altered.

The aim of the study was therefore to determine the role of the baroreflex on heart rate response during apnea.

Our results show that normotensive patients have baroreflex sensitivity within normal range during wakefulness (Bristow et al, 1969) but the sensitivity of the baroreflex is strikingly increased during apnea. This may result from the peripheral action of acute hypoxia or more likely from a central reflex. This is confirmed during CPAP when the chemoreflex is not activated and the lung inflation vagal inhibitory reflex is functional : the baroreflex sensitivity is restored to awake value. The hypertensive patients have a blunted baroreflex during apnea as already observed during normal sleep and wakefulness (Bristow, 1969). Therefore in these patients chemoreflex and lung inflation reflex do not seem to potentiate the baroreflex control of HR during apnea.

These observed changes in baroreflex sensitivity were not related to sleep stage changes as all sleep measurements were made during slow-wave sleep in the present study.

It has been suggested that patients with obstructive SAS have an impaired ventilatory response to acute hypoxia (Tafil-Klawe et al, 1991). In apnea secondary to high altitude the HR depression was smaller in subjects with lower hypoxic ventilatory drive (Masyama et al, 1990). At the contrary a higher ventilatory drive has been reported in young hypertensive subjects (Trzebski A, 1982). But the ventilatory drive has not been compared between normotensive and hypertensive SAS patients. Therefore the role of the chemosensitivity cannot be ascertained.

During apnea, the phenylephrine induced increase in blood pressure was higher in HT patients. This higher reactivity demonstrates an increased state of peripheral vasoconstriction during apnea in HT subjects. This effect of vasoconstriction on blood pressure may be potentiated by a blunted decrease in HR which does not allow further decrease in cardiac output.

CONCLUSION :

During apnea the sensitivity of the baroreflex control of HR is increased in NT but these baroreflex changes are not accompanied by greater bradycardia in NT subjects. Chemoreflex and lung inflation reflex probably play the major role according to the scheme of cardio-vascular control during apnea on Fig 5.

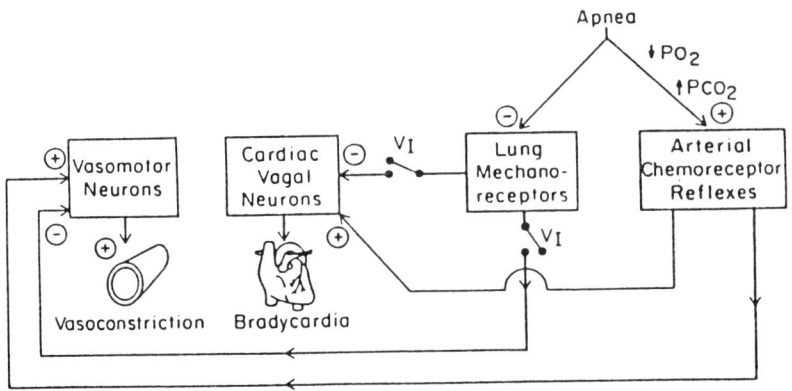

Fig 5 : Schematic representation of interaction among reflexes evoked in apnea. Apnea lowers PO_2 and raises PCO_2, which stimulates chemoreceptors, which in turn triggers arteriolar constriction and bradycardia as long as lung mechanoreceptors are not activated by breathing. When breathing commences, switches labeled V_1 close (lung mechanoreflex) and inhibit both sympathetic outflow to blood vessels and vagal outflow to the heart. Vasoconstriction is reduced and bradycardia is abolished (adapted from Rowell LB, 1986, Human Circulation - Regulation during physical stress, Oxford University Press by permission).

In hypertensive patients pressure reactivity is increased during apnea compared to normotensive patients but this effect on long term development of hypertension remains to be determined.

REFERENCES :

Andersen HT (1966). Physiological adaptations in diving vertebrates. Physiol Rev 46, 212-43.

Bristow JD, Honour AJ, Pickering TG and Sleight P. (1969). Cardiovascular and respiratory changes during sleep in normal and hypertensive subjects. Cardiovasc Res 3, 476-485.

Coccagna G, Mantovani M, Brisnani P, Manzani A, Lugaresi E (1971) : Arterial pressure changes during spontaneous sleep in man. Electroencephalogr Clin Neurophysiol 31 : 277-81.

Daly M de B and Angell James JE (1975). Role of the arterial chemoreceptors in the control of the cardiovascular responses to breath-hold diving. In : The peripheral arterial chemoreceptors. Ed by M.J. Purves. London : Cambridge Univ. Press 384 - 407.

Eckberg DL, Nerhed C and Wallin G. (1985) Respiratory modulation of muscle sympathetic and vagal cardiac outflow in man. J Physiol 365, 181-196.

Eckberg DL and Orshan CR (1977). Respiratory and baroreceptor reflex interactions in man. J Clin Invest 59, 780-785.

Ejnell H, Hedner J, Caidahl K, Sellgren J and Wallin G (1991). Increased sympathetic activity as possible etiology of hypertension and left ventricular hypertrophy in patients with obstructive sleep apnea syndrome.
In : "Sleep and Health risk" ed J.H Peter, T. Penzel, T. Podszus, P von Wichert, Springer - Verlag, Berlin p. 341 - 347.

Escourrou P, Jirani A, Nedelcoux H, Gaultier Cl. (1990). Systemic hypertension in sleep apnea syndrome : Relationship with sleep architecture and breathing abnormalities. Chest 98, 1362-1365.

Fletcher EC, Miller J, Schaaf JW and Fletcher JG (1987). Urinary catecholamines before and after tracheostomy in patients with obstructive sleep apnea and hypertension. Sleep : 10, 35-44.

Guilleminault C, Connolly S, Winkle RA (1984). Cyclical variation of the heart rate in sleep apnea syndrome : mechanisms and usefulness of 24h electrocardiography as a screening technique. Lancet : 2 : 126-131.

Jeong DU, Dimsdale JE (1989) Sleep apnea and essential hypertension : a critical review of the epidemiological evidence for co-morbidity. Clin and Exper. Hyper. : A 11 (7) : 1301-23.

Katona PG, Poitras JW, Barnett GO and Terry BS (1970). Cardiac vagal efferent activity and heart period in the carotid sinus reflex. Am J Physiol 218, 1030-1037.

Lugaresi E, Coccagna G et al (1978). Breathing during sleep in man in normal and pathological conditions. Adv Exp Med Biol ; 99 : 35-45.

Masuyama S, Shinozaki J, Kochchiyama S, Okita S, Kimura H, Honda Y and Kuriyama T (1990). Heart rate depression during sleep apnea depends on hypoxic chemosensitivity. Am Rev Respir Dis 141 : 39-42.

Somers VK, Mark AL, Zavala DC and Abboud FM, (1989). Influence of ventilation and hypocapnia on sympathetic nerve responses to hypoxia in normal humans. J Appl Physiol 67 (5) : 2095 - 2100.

Tafil-Klawe M, Raschke F, Becker H, Hein H, Stoohs R, Kublik A, Peter JH, Penzel T, Podzus T and von Wichert P. (1991). Investigations of Arterial Baro- and Chemoreflexes in patients with arterial hypertension and obstructive sleep apnea syndrome.
In : "Sleep and Health risk" ed J.H. Peter, Penzel T, Podszus T, von Wichert P, Springer-Verlag, Berlin p. 319-334.

Trzebski A, Tafil M, Zoltowski M, Przybylski J (1982). Increased sensitivity of the arterial chemoreceptor reflex in young men with hypertension. Cardiovasc Res 16 : 163.

World Health Organization (1978) Arterial hypertension. Technical Report series 628.

Zwillich C, Devlin T, White D, Douglas N, Weil J, Martin R. (1982) Bradycardia during sleep apnea. J Clin Invest 69 : 1286-92.

Résumé

Le syndrome d'apnées du sommeil (SAS) est caractérisé par une brachytachycardie cyclique et est souvent associé à une hypertension artérielle systémique. L'hypertension artérielle essentielle s'accompagne d'une diminution de la sensibilité du baroréflexe à destinée cardiaque. Le but de cette étude a été de déterminer le contrôle baroréflexe de la fréquence cardiaque au cours des apnées en comparant 8 patients normotendus et 6 hypertendus non traités ayant un index d'apnées respectivement de 45 ± 18/heure et 49 ± 18/heure. Le baroréflexe cardiaque a été étudié par l'injection intraveineuse en bolus de 100 μg de phénylephrine à l'éveil, au début des apnées et pendant le sommeil avec pression nasale continue. Les résultats obtenus montrent que la sensibilité du baroréflexe est dans les limites de la normale chez les sujets normotendus à l'éveil et au cours de la pression nasale continue. Elle est abaissée de façon non significative chez les hypertendus pendant les mêmes périodes. Mais surtout la sensibilité du baroréflexe est très augmentée au cours des apnées chez les normotendus (239 % de la valeur d'éveil) alors qu'elle ne varie pas de manière significative chez les hypertendus. Malgré ces différences de sensibilité entre normotendus et hypertendus, il n'y a pas de différence significative entre les variations absolues et relatives de fréquence cardiaque au cours des cycles de bradytachycardie : 28.4 ± 7.8 bpm pour les normotendus et 24.8 ± 11.3 bpm pour les hypertendus. Le baroréflexe cardiaque n'est donc probablement pas le facteur principal de la bradycardie de l'apnée. Cette bradycardie apparaît donc sous la dépendance du chémoréflexe artériel et du réflexe de volume pulmonaire. Chez les hypertendus, la plus grande réactivité pressive à l'injection de phényléphrine témoigne d'une vasoconstriction périphérique plus importante que chez les sujets normaux. Cette vasoconstriction nocturne pourrait participer à la génèse de l'hypertension permanente, mais ceci reste à déterminer.

Effects of CPAP on Cheyne-Stokes respiration and cardiac function in heart failure

T. Douglas Bradley[1][2], Yuji Takasaki[3] and Ruth Rutherford[4]

[1] 212-10 EN, Toronto General Hospital, 200 Elizabeth Street, Toronto, Ontario, M5G 2C4, Canada
[2] Career Scientist of The Ontario Ministry of Health
[3] Second Department of Internal Medicine, Tokai University Hospital, Bohseidai, Isehara, Kanagawa 259-1, Japan
[4] The Sleep Research Laboratory, Queen Elizabeth Hospital and the Department of Medicine, The Toronto Hospital, University of Toronto, Toronto, Ontario, Canada

ABSTRACT

Nine patients with congestive heart failure (CHF) and Cheyne-Stokes respiration (CSR) during sleep were found to have recurrent hypoxic dips associated with apneas. This caused disruption of sleep by recurrent arousals. All patients suffered from symptoms characteristic of sleep apnea syndrome. Application of nasal continuous positive airway pressure (NCPAP) resulted in reversal of CSR and an associated improvement in sleep architecture. The number of apneas and hypopneas per hr. of sleep associated with CSR was reduced from 64 ± 6 to 10 ± 4 ($p<0.001$) and mean nocturnal oxyhemoglobin saturation (SaO_2) increased from 88 ± 1 to 94 ± 1 ($p<0.005$). In addition, the number of arousals per hr. of sleep fell from 58 ± 6 to 19 ± 3 ($p<0.001$). As a result, symptoms of sleep apnea were alleviated. Left ventricular ejection fraction (LVEF) rose from 33 ± 6 to 41 ± 7% ($p<0.005$) one month after starting NCPAP therapy. We conclude that CSR during sleep in patients with CHF can give rise to a sleep apnea syndrome which can be reversed through the application of NCPAP. Furthermore, our findings suggest that nightly application of NCPAP may cause a prolonged improvement in cardiac function in patients with left ventricular heart failure complicated by CSR during sleep.

INTRODUCTION

Cheyne-Stokes respiration (CSR) is a breathing disorder characterized by episodes of crescendo-decrescendo hyperpnea alternating with apneas (Cheyne, 1818, Lange and Hecht, 1962). Apneas can be either central or obstructive, although, in most cases apneas are predominantly central (Dowdell et al., 1990, Takasaki et al., 1989). The pathophysiology of CSR in patients with congestive heart failure (CHF) is thought to involve delay in transmission of arterial blood gas tension changes from the lung to the peripheral and central chemoreceptors (Khoo et al., 1982, Lange and Hecht, 1962). This phase lag destabilizes respiration by causing a tendency for ventilation to overshoot and undershoot the desired level resulting in wide swings in blood gas tensions and ventilation. Other factors that destabilize respiration in patients with CHF would include hypoxemia, low lung volumes and increased collapsability of the upper airway (Longobardo et al., 1966, Younes, 1989).

CSR is seen more frequently during sleep than during wakefulness (Harrison et al., 1934, Younes, 1989). Harrison et al (1934) pointed out that CSR is a cause of paroxysmal nocturnal dyspnea in patients with CHF. Furthermore, recurrent apneas and hypoxic dips related to CSR during sleep could have a detrimental effect on cardiac function both directly (Allen and Orchard, 1987) and indirectly by causing increased sympathetic nervous system activity and catecholamines (Barruzzi et al., 1991, Hedner et al., 1988). Accordingly, CSR during sleep may be of considerable clinical significance and its reversal might be of benefit.

In view of the above, we performed overnight sleep studies in patients with CHF. Among those with CSR during sleep, nasal continuous positive airway pressure (NCPAP) was used to reverse CSR. The rationale for this approach was that NCPAP increases lung volume, reduces upper airway instability and may reduce left ventricular (LV) afterload by increasing intrathoracic pressure (Bradley et al., 1990, Pinsky et al., 1985, Sullivan et al., 1981).

METHODS
Nine patients with CHF observed to have CSR during an exacerbation of CHF were entered into the study. The diagnosis of left ventricular heart failure was based on a history of exertional dyspnea accompanied by an S3 gallop, pulmonary edema and cardiomegally on a chest radiograph. In addition, all had objective evidence of impaired cardiac contractility as indicated by a LV ejection fraction (LVEF) of < 55% determined by gated equilibrium radionuclide angiography (RNA) performed after the patients were in stable medical condition for at least one month. Patients were on standard medical therapy for CHF in all cases. In five patients the underlying cause of CHF was coronary artery disease and, in four, idiopathic dilated cardiomyopathy. Two patients had class IV dyspnea (New York Heart Association criteria), four had class III dyspnea and three had class II dyspnea.

A detailed history revealed that all had a history of restless sleep and daytime fatigue, eight had a history of habitual snoring, five complained of excessive daytime sleepiness and five complained of paroxysmal nocturnal dyspnea. Overnight polysomnography was performed in all patients when they were in stable condition;

standard criteria for sleep staging were used. Rib cage and abdominal motion was recorded using a respiratory inductance plethysmograph (Respitrace, Ambulatory Monitoring Inc., White Plains, New York). Esophageal pressure (Pes) was measured by a balloon catheter system. Arterial oxyhemoglobin saturation was measured by an ear oximeter (Biox II, Boulder, Colorado). Mean nocturnal SaO2 was determined by averaging the high and low SaO2 for each 40 sec. epoch throughout the entire night. Apneas were defined as an absence of a tidal volume (VT) excursion on the inductance plethysmograph for at least 10 sec. Hypopneas were defined as a reduction in VT to < 50% of the baseline value for a period of at least 10 sec. Apneas were defined as either central or obstructive on the basis of the absence or presence of paradoxical chest wall motion and Pes swings, respectively.

Recurrent cycles of apnea-hyperpnea with a crescendo-decrescendo pattern of VT during the ventilatory period, typical of CSR, were observed in all. An example of this pattern during Stage 2 sleep is shown for one patient in Fig. 1. NCPAP was then started and polysomnography repeated. The level of NCPAP was adjusted such that apneas were largely abolished or to the highest pressure that the patient could tolerate (8-12.5 cm H2O). Patients were then sent home on nocturnal NCPAP. One month later, LVEFs were repeated in the daytime off NCPAP. Results of tests performed at baseline and then while on NCPAP were compared by paired Student's t-test analyses. P<0.05 was considered as being statistically significant.

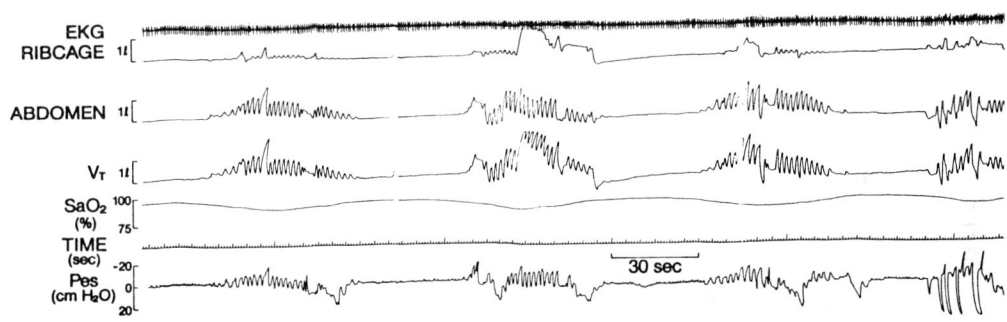

FIG.1. Record of CSR with recurrent apneas during Stage 2 sleep in one subject. The absence of respiratory effort in the abdomen and rib cage channels as well as in the Pes signal indicates the central nature of the apneas. Note also the recurrent dips in SaO2 associated with CSR. EKG = electocardiogram; VT = tidal volume; SaO2 = oxyhemoglobin saturation; Pes = esophageal pressure. (From Takasaki et al., 1989).

RESULTS

All patients had severe sleep apnea associiated with CSR. In eight cases apneas were predominantly central in nature and in one case predominantly obsructive. Results of sleep studies and LVEFs while off then on NCPAP are shown in Table 1.

TABLE 1. EFFECTS OF NCPAP ON SLEEP AND LVEF

	Control	NCPAP	p value
Apneas and hypopneas (#/hr of sleep)	64 ± 6	10 ± 4	<0.001
Mean nocturnal SaO2 (%)	88 ± 1	94 ± 1	<0.005
Slow wave sleep time (min.)	19 ± 5	72 ± 8	<0.005
Rapid eye movement sleep time (min.)	27 ± 7	41 ± 7	<0.025
Arousals (#/hr of sleep)	58 ± 6	19 ± 3	<0.001
Left ventricular ejection fraction (%)	33 ± 6	41 ± 7	<0.005

NCPAP caused a highly significant reduction in the number of apneas and hypopneas irrespective of whether they were central or obstructive. An example of a central apnea associated with CSR is shown for one patient in the upper panel of Fig. 2. In the lower panel of Fig. 2, the same patient is shown while on NCPAP at 10 cm H2O. This figure illustrates that NCPAP reversed central apneas associated with CSR in this patient. Similar findings were observed in all patients. As a result, sleep quality was improved as evidenced by a significant increase in the amount slow wave and rapid eye movement (REM) sleep and a reduction in the number of arousals. In addition, LVEF increased significantly in these patients (Table 1).

These laboratory improvements were associated with clinical improvement as well. Three months after starting NCPAP all patients reported more restfull sleep. Paroxysmal nocturnal dyspnea, daytime fatigue and hypersomnolence were also alleviated. The most remarkable finding, however, was that exercise tolerance improved markedly in all patients. Cardiac functional class improved from IV to II in two patients, from III to II in four patients and from II to I in the remaining three patients. These improvements were seen in the absence of any changes in cardiac medications. Moreover, patients remained free of exacerbations of CHF for prolonged periods. At the last follow up, two patients had been free of overt CHF for 7 and 16 months respectively. However, they both died suddenly of myocardial infarction. The remaining seven patients were free of overt CHF for periods of from 18 to 48 months.

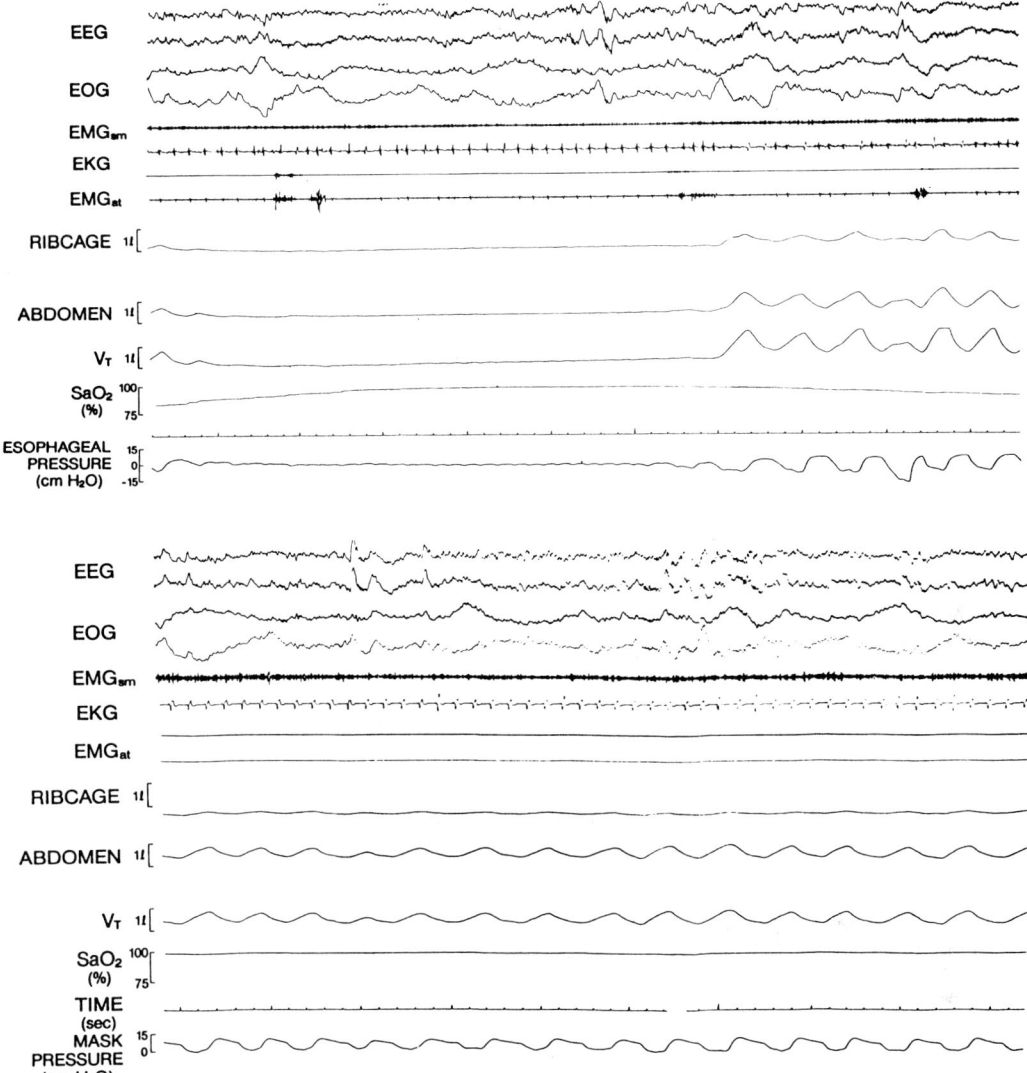

FIG. 2. Upper Panel. Central apnea in one patient during Stage 2 sleep while off NCPAP. **Lower Panel.** Polysomnographic tracing during Stage 2 sleep in the same patient as shown in the upper panel while on NCPAP. Pressure was recorded from the NCPAP mask. Note that breathing has become regular and that SaO2 is maintained above 95%. EEG = electroencephalogram; EOG = electrooculogram; EMGsm = submental EMG; EMGat = anterior tibial EMG. Otherwise abbreviations as for Fig. 1. (From Takasaki et al., 1989).

DISCUSSION

Our data have demonstrated that CSR during sleep in patients with CHF can give rise to disruption of sleep due to recurrent apneas causing hypoxic dips and arousals from sleep. In addition, these pathologic events can give rise to symptoms of sleep apnea such as restless sleep and excessive daytime sleepiness (Takasaki et al., 1989). Of perhaps greater importance, however, was the effect of NCPAP on this breathing disorder and on cardiac function. We have demonstrated that CSR can be reversed using NCPAP whether apneas are central or obstructive in nature. This resulted in alleviation of symptoms associated with sleep apnea. The most intiguing finding was that exertional dyspnea was reduced and that this was associated with a significant improvement in LVEF. Finally, patients remained free of overt CHF for prolonged periods after starting NCPAP. This suggests that NCPAP was having a prolonged beneficial effect on left ventricular (LV) function.

CSR has previously been viewed as a physiologic curiosity with little clinical significance other than as a poor prognostic sign in patients with CHF. Findley et al (1985) reported that patients with CHF and CSR during sleep had a higher mortality rate than patients without CSR adding some credence to this assumption. In addition, Harrison et al (1934) observed that CSR could be associated with frequent awakenings from sleep during the ventilatory phase and that this was often associated with paroxysmal nocturnal dyspnea. These investigators surmised that the consequent disruption of sleep could give rise to fatigue during the daytime. It is noteworthy, therefore, that all our patients complained of severe fatigue and most complained of paroxysmal nocturnal dyspnea and hypersomnolence. Thus it appears that CSR during sleep in patients with CHF can give rise to sleep apnea syndrome.

Although, traditionally, CSR has been viewed as arising from CHF, it seems possible that CSR may give rise to worsening cardiac function. The direct and indirect effects of hypoxia may contribute to such adverse effects (Allen and Orchard, 1987, Hedner et al., 1988, Hedner et al., 1990). Hypoxia probably increases sympathetic nervous system tone and release of catecholamines. This could give rise to increased cardiac irritability and worsen underlying ischemia by increasing myocardial O_2 demand. Furthermore, hypoxia has a direct depressant effect on myocardial contractility. Accordingly, CSR may be part of a vicious cycle in which CHF begets CSR which, in turn, begets worsening cardiac function. Reversal of CSR, therefore, may have beneficial effects not only on symptoms of sleep apnea but on heart function as well (Hanly et al., 1989, Takasaki et al., 1989).

There are several potential mechanisms through which NCPAP could have reversed CSR. NCPAP reduces upper airway resistance (Sullivan et al., 1981). Although instability of the upper airway has not traditionally been thought of as one of the underlying causes of

CSR, recent evidence suggests that it may be a contributing factor (Younes, 1989). All of our patients snored habitually and all were male. The original report of CSR was of an obese alcololic male suffering from both CHF and a cerebrovascular accident (Cheyne, 1818). This description fits very well with that of a typical patient with the Pickwickian syndrome and obstructive sleep apnea (OSA) (Bradley et al., 1985). Patients with idiopathic central sleep apnea have been shown to have increased compliance (i.e. "floppiness") of the upper airway just as have patients with OSA (Bradley et al., 1987, Brown et al., 1985). In addition, Alex et al (1986) demonstrated that patients with CSR could develop upper airway obstruction during the apneic period. Moreover, NCPAP has been shown to reverse some forms of central sleep apnea (Issa et al., 1986). These findings suggest that stabilization of the upper airway may have been one of the means by which NCPAP reversed CSR (Takasaki et al., 1989).

NCPAP raises lung volume and, therefore, could have increased lung O2 and CO2 stores damping oscillations in PO2 and PCO2 (Longobardo et al., 1966). It is also possible that NCPAP may raise PCO2 above the apnea threshold, a possibility consistent with observations in lightly anaesthetized animals (Bishop and Bachofen, 1973). Finally, Bradley et al (1990) have shown that NCPAP can acutely augment cardiac output in patients with CHF. Thus NCPAP may have reduced circulatory delay in the patients described herein.

The finding of potentially greatest importance in our study was the remarkable improvement in cardiac dyspnea and LVEF while on NCPAP. However, since there was no control group, the improvement seen may not have been due to the effects of NCPAP. Nevertheless, all patients reported improvement in exercise tolerance within 1 to 2 weeks after starting NCPAP, providing circumstantial evidence that NCPAP and the concommitent reversal of CSR, was at least partially responsible for this improvement. Although we cannot be certain of the mechanism of this proposed effect, several possibilities can be entertained.

Firstly, NCPAP reduces LV afterload by increaseing intrathoracic pressure (Buda et al., 1979). This reduces the difference between intracardiac and intrathoracic pressure. Furthermore, NCPAP reduces preload by impeding venous return (Grace and Greenbaum, 1982). A reduction in LV end diastolic volume could be beneficial in a dilated heart whose length tension relationship is on the descending portion on the far right of the Starling curve. This could, in turn, cause a secondary decrease in LV wall tension via the Laplace relationship. Secondly, abolition of nocturnal hypoxia by NCPAP could possibly improve myocardial function. However, the degree of nocturnal hypoxia in our patients was not great and it appears unlikely that improved oxygenation would, by itself, result in improved LV function. Thirdly, improved oxygenation with a marked reduction in arousals from sleep could reduce sympathetic nervous tone and catecholamine levels (Baruzzi et al., 1991). If so, potential detrimental effects of chronically elevated chatecholamines could be reversed. Whatever the mechanism, it would seem that application of NCPAP, at night alone, was sufficient to improve cardiac function in the daytime while off NCPAP. This suggests the concept that "resting" the heart at night, through application of NCPAP, may cause beneficial effects that carry over into the daytime (Takasaki et al., 1989).

In conclusion, we have demonstrated that CSR during sleep in patients with CHF may give rise to a sleep apnea syndrome if accompanied by recurrent hypoxia and arousals from sleep. Moreover, our results show that NCPAP can be effective in reversing CSR in these patients causing alleviation in symptoms of sleep apnea. Finally, the data presented herein provides some evidence that application of NCPAP on a nightly basis in patients with CHF, complicated by CSR, could have a sustained beneficial effect on myocardial function. Our findings are not definitive on this point but do indicate the need for further research on the effects of positive airway pressure as a potential adjunctive therapy for certain patients suffering from CHF.

REFERENCES

Alex, C.G., Onal, E., and Lopata, M. (1986). Upper airway occlusion during sleep in patients with Cheyne-Stokes respiration. Am. Rev. Resp. Dis. 133:42-45.

Allen, D.G., and Orchard, C.H. (1977). Myocardial contactile function during ischemia and hypoxia. Circ. Res. 60:153-168.

Baruzzi, A., Riva, R., Cirignotta, F., Zucconi, M., Cappelli, M., and Lugaresi, E. (1991). Atrial natriuretic peptide and catecholamines in obstructive sleep apnea syndrome. Sleep. 14:83-86.

Bishop, B., and Bachofen, H. (1973). Comparative influence of proprioceptors and chemoreceptors in the control of respiratory muscles. Acta. Neurobiol. Exp. 33:381-390.

Bradley, T.D., Rutherford, R., Grossman, R.F., Lue, F., Zamel, N., Moldofsky, H., and Phillipson, E.A. (1985). Role of daytime hypoxemia in the pathogenesis of right heart failure in the obstructive sleep apnea syndrome. Am. Rev. Respir. Dis. 131:835-839.

Bradley, T. D., Brown, I.G., Zamel, N., Phillipson, E.A., and Hoffstein, V. (1987). Differences in pharyngeal properties between snorers with predominantly central sleep apnea and those without sleep apnea. Am. Rev. Respir. Dis. 135:387-391.

Bradley, T.D., Holloway, R., McLaughlin, P., Ross, B, and Liu, P.P. (1990). Hemodynamic effects of CPAP in congestive heart failure. Am. Rev. Respir. Dis. 141 (Supp.):A859.

Brown, I.G., Bradley, T.D., Phillipson, E.A., Zamel, N., and Hoffstein, V. (1985). Pharyngeal compliance in snoring subjects with and without obstructive sleep apnea. Am. Rev. Respir. Dis. 132:211-215.

Buda, A.J., Pinsky, M.R., Ingels, N.B., Daughters, G.T., Stinson, E.B., and Alderman, E.L. (1979). Effect of intrathoracic

pressure on left ventricular performance. N. Engl. J. Med. 303:453-459.
Cheyne, J. (1818). A case of apoplexy in which the fleshy part of the heart was converted to fat. Dublin Hosp. Rev. 2:216-223.
Dowdell, W.T., Javaheri, S., and McGinnis, W. (1990). Cheyne-Stokes respiration presenting as sleep apnea syndrome. Am. Rev. Respir. Dis. 141:871-879.
Findley, L.J., Zwillich, C.W., Ancoli-Israel, S., Kripke, D., Tisi, G., and Moser, K.M. (1985). Cheyne-Stokes respiration during sleep in patients with left ventricular heart failure. S. Med. J. 78:11-15.
Grace, M.P., and Greenbaum, D.M. (1982). Cardiac performance in response to PEEP in patients with cardiac dysfunction. Crit. Care Med. 10:358-360.
Hanly, P.J., Millar, T.W., Steljes, D.G., Baert, R., Frais, M.A., and Kryger, M.H. (1989). The effect of oxygen on respiration and sleep in patients with congestive heart failure. Ann. Int. Med. 111:777-782.
Harrison, T.R., King, C.E., Calhoun, J.A., and Harrison, W.G.Jr. (1934). Congestive heart failure: Cheyne-Stokes respiration as the cause of paroxysmal nocturnal dyspnea at the onset of sleep. Arch. Int. Med. 53:891-910.
Hedner, J., Ejnell, H., Sellgren, J., Hedner, T., and Wallin, G. (1988). Is high and fluctuating muscle nerve sympathetic activity in the sleep apnea syndrome of pathogenetic importance for the development of hypertension? J. Hypertension. 6 Supp. 4:S529-S531.
Hedner, J., Ejnell, H., and Caidahl, K. (1990). Left ventricular hypertrophy independent of hypertension in patients with obstructive sleep apnea. J. Hypertension. 8:941-946.
Issa, F.G., and Sullivan, C.E. (1986). Reversal of central sleep apnea using nasal CPAP. Chest.90:165-171.
Khoo, M.C.K., Kronauer, R.E., Strohl, K.P., and Slutsky, A.S. (1982). Factors inducing periodic breathing in humans: a general model. J. Appl. Physiol. 53:644-659.
Lange, R.L., and Hecht, H.H. (1962). The mechanism of Cheyne-Stokes respiration. J. Clin. Invest. 41:42-52.
Longobardo, G.S., Cherniac, N.S., and Fishman, A.P. (1966). Cheyne-Stokes breathing produced by a model of the human respiratory system. J. Appl. Physiol. 21:1839-1846.
Pinsky, M.R., Matuschak, G.M., and Klain, M. (1985). Determinants of cardiac augmentation by elevations in intrathoracic pressure. J. Appl. Physiol. 58:1189-1198.
Sullivan, C.E., Issa, F.G., Berthon-Jones, M., and Eves, L. (1981). Reversal of obstructive sleep apnea by continuous positive airway pressure applied through the nares. Lancet. 1:862-865.
Takasaki, Y., Orr, D., Popkin, J., Rutherford, R., Liu, P., and Bradley, T.D. (1989). Effect of nasal continuous positive airway pressure on sleep apnea in congestive heart failure. Am. Rev. Respir. Dis. 140:1578-1584.
Younes, M. (1989). The physiologic basis of central apnea and periodic breathing. Current Pulmonology. 10:265-326.

Résumé

Neuf patients porteurs d'une insuffisance cardiaque congestive (ICG) et ayant une respiration de type Cheyne-Stokes (RCS) pendant le sommeil avaient des pics répétés de désaturation associés aux apnées. Ces apnées étaient responsables d'une fragmentation du sommeil par les éveils répétitifs. Tous les patients avaient des symptômes caractéristiques du syndrome d'apnées du sommeil. L'application d'une pression positive nasale continue (PPNC) a eu pour effet la réversibilité de la RSC et l'amélioration associée de l'architecture du sommeil. Le nombre d'apnées et d'hypopnées par heure de sommeil associées à la RSC a diminué de 64 +/- 6 à 10 +/- 4 ($p<0.001$) et la saturation en oxygène moyenne (SaO2) a augmenté de 88 +/- 1 à 94 +/- 1 ($p<0.005$). De plus le nombre de réveil par heure de sommeil a diminué de 58 +/- 6 à 19 +/- 3 ($p<0.001$). En conséquence les symptômes du syndrome d'apnées se sont amendés. La fraction d'éjection ventriculaire gauche a augmenté de 33 +/- 6 à 41 +/- 7% ($p<0.005$) un mois après le début de la PPNC. Nous concluons que la RSC pendant le sommeil chez des patients en ICG peut faire apparaître un syndrome d'apnées qui peuvent être supprimées par la PPNC. De plus nos constatations suggèrent que l'application nocturne de la PPNC peut permettre une amélioration durable de la fonction ventriculaire gauche chez des patients en ICG compliquée par une RSC pendant le sommeil.

Abstracts

Résumés

I. Sleep apnea syndrome : mechanisms

I. Syndrome d'apnées du sommeil : mécanismes

Influence of airway resistance on periodic breathing (PB)

F. Series, I. Series, L. Atton and A. Blouin

Unité de Recherche, Centre de Pneumologie de l'Hôpital et de l'Université Laval, Québec, Canada

We studied the effects of changing airway pressure on the characteristics of PB in 11 spontaneously breathing dogs. PB was induced by abrupt normoxic recovery following a hypoxic stimulus. Airway resistances were modified during recovery by changing the composition of the inspired gas (all with an FiO_2 of 20.9 %) between 4 different trials: trials 1 and 3 with air, trials 2 and 4 with Helium or SF_6 in random order. Minute ventilation, inspiratory flow, supralaryngeal (SL) pressure, and arterial blood gases were recorded at baseline (air), and during the post-hypoxic period. There were no differences in baseline ventilation, SL resistance, and arterial blood gas values preceeding the different trials. The hypoxemic and hypocapnic levels, and the hypoxic-induced hyperventilation reached at the end of the hypoxic tests were identical. The peak flow SLR was significantly higher with SF_6 (21.9 ± 5.5 cm H2O/l/s, Mean ± SEM) than with the other gases (8.8 ± 1.8, and 6.9 ± 1.7 with air, 7.2 ± 2.2 with Helium, $p<0.05$). PB was consistently seen during the post-hypoxic period and was characterized by a strength index value (M) (Waggener, J Appl Physiol 1984; 56: 576-581). M value was significantly higher with SF_6 (3.8 ± 1.1) than with the other gases (1.9 ± 0.5 and 1.8 ± 0.6 with air, 1.6 ± 0.5 with Helium). There was a significant positive relationship between the peak negative SL pressure reached during a ventilatory cycle and the M value of this cycle. We conclude that negative airway pressure influences the stability of the respiratory control system. Supported by The National Center of Excellence of Canada.

Hyperventilation due to experimental asphyxic blood gases is sometimes followed by apnea during sleep but not during wakefulness

K. Gleeson, L.W. Sweer and C.W. Zwillich

Division of Pulmonary/Critical Care, The Pennsylvania State University, Hershey, PA, USA

Experimental airflow obstruction during sleep is followed by hyperventilation which frequently overcorrects arterial blood gases producing ventilatory instability. However, the ventilatory response to experimentally induced asphyxic blood gas changes (hypoxia and hypercapnia) during sleep has not been previously investigated. We therefore studied the ventilatory response to a 50 second stimulation with a 10% O_2, 5% CO_2 gas mixture during wakefulness and non-REM sleep in 5 normal subjects during full night sleep studies. In addition to standard polysomnographic variables, we measured expired ventilation (V_E), end tidal CO_2 ($P_{ET}CO_2$) and O_2 concentrations before, during, and after 50 seconds of stimulation with a 10% O_2 5% CO_2 gas mixture followed by 100% oxygen. Data were collected at least in duplicate for each condition. The inspired gas mixture increased $P_{ET}CO_2$ approximately 7 torr and decreased arterial oxygen saturations to 85-87% in all subjects awake and asleep. During wakefulness this stimulus produced a mean increase in ventilation of 5.6 +/- .4 L/min (90.1 +/- 7.9% increase above baseline). Following this period of stimulated breathing ventilation returned to baseline over an interval of 38.2+/- 20 seconds, with no hypocapnia or hypoventilation relative to baseline occurring. During sleep this same stimulus augmented ventilation by 4.9 +/- .8 L/min (88.4 +/- 12.5% increase above baseline) and was followed by a rapid return to baseline ventilation (15.2+/- 3.0 seconds) again with no hypocapnia occurring. In contrast to wakefulness, however, two of the five subjects developed hypoventilation and apnea (cessation of airflow > 10 seconds) following removal of the asphyxic stimulus. The pattern of ventilation before, during and after this asphyxic stimulation can be seen for a single subject in the figure. We conclude that in some subjects the sleep state alters the ventilatory pattern following asphyxic blood gas stimulation enabling post hyperventilation apnea to occur. This seems to be independent of alveolar hypocapnia and may represent a state related alteration in ventilatory stability following asphyxic hyperventilation.

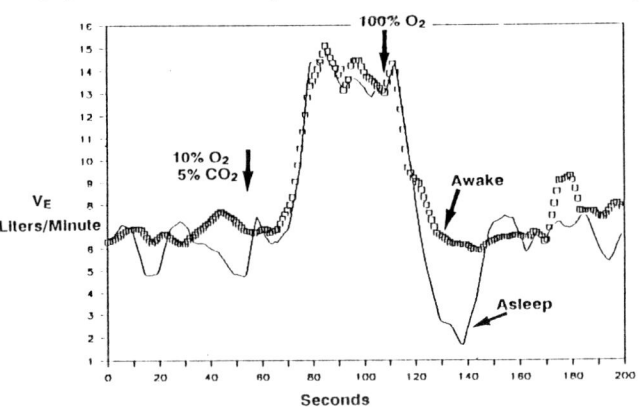

II. SAS : diagnosis and complications
II. SAS : évaluation diagnostique et conséquences

Systolic blood pressure profiles in sleep and breathing disorders

R.J.O. Davies, K.B. Vardi-Visy and J.R. Stradling

Osler Chest Unit, Churchill Hospital, Oxford, UK

The vigorous inspiratory efforts of obstructive sleep apnoea (OSA) and heavy snoring produce falls in systolic blood pressure (SBP) in time with each effort. A rise in SBP occurs concurrently with arousal and apnoea termination. Thus the beat to beat SBP includes information relating to both respiratory effort and sleep disturbance. We report the fluctuations in sleeping systolic blood pressure seen in 9 snorers, 11 untreated OSA patients, and 7 normal controls. EEG, EOGx2, chin EMG, respiration, arterial pulse oximetry, and beat to beat non-invasive blood pressure (Finapres, Ohmeda) were recorded in all subjects. 245 ten minute periods of stable body position, slow wave sleep stage, and respiratory state, were identified. During these periods all falls in SBP occurring over 1.5-7.5 secs were measured. The SBP profile was then smoothed using a moving window mean over five sequential beats to remove the SBP falls due to respiratory effort, and all rises in SBP >18 mmHg, occurring over 4.0-15.0 seconds were counted and expressed as number per hour of sleep.

	SBP falls (mmHg) Respiratory effort	SBP rises (per hr) "Arousals"
normal sleep	6.9 SD2.6	12.9 SD15.8
snoring	10.8 SD4.2	32.5 SD42.2
OSA	12.8 SD4.8	54.2 SD23.0

Sleep and breathing disorders are associated with abnormalities in the pattern of systolic blood pressure over time that reveal information about both respiratory effort and sleep disruption. Thus analysis of these profiles may provide a simple screening test for nocturnal upper airway dysfunction and any related arousals.

Beat-by-beat estimate of right ventricular stroke volume (RVSV) in obstructive sleep apnea (OSA)

M.R. Bonsignore, O. Marrone and S. Romano

Istituto di Fisiopatologia Respiratoria CNR, Via Trabucco 180, 90146 Palermo, Italy

During OSA, either unchanged or decreased cardiac output were reported by thermodilution method (Tilkian et al, Ann Intern Med 1976; 85: 714, and Guilleminault et al, Chest 1986; 89: 331). To further investigate cardiac output behaviour during apneas, 6 OSA patients with normal respiratory function and pulmonary hemodynamics during wakefulness were studied by right heart catheterization during sleep, using a Millar catheter with a flow probe in the main pulmonary artery. The apnea index was 88.3±7.5 (mean±SD). In 69 episodes of OSA, we estimated beat-by-beat right ventricular stroke volume (RVSV) by integrating the area under the flow signal, and heart rate (HR).
With respect to the preapneic values, estimated RVSV tended to increase during apneas (113.8±11.9%) and decreased during the post-apneic period (87.6±6.2%) ($p<0.01$ by ANOVA). HR decreased during apneas to 91.9±6.8% of its preapneic value ($p<0.01$) and returned to baseline in the post-apneic phase (101.7±4.1%). Thus, OSA minimally affected right ventricular output. The slight post-apneic decrease in RVSV not compensated by tachycardia might be due to a mechanical costraint exerted on the heart by the lungs ventilated at high tidal volumes, as it occurs during the post-apneic "big breaths".

Arterial chemoreflex and baroreflex control of heart rate in normotensive and hypertensive sleep apnea patients

V. Le Gros, P. Escourrou, H. Nedelcoux and C. Gaultier

Laboratoire de Physiologie, INSERM CJF 89-09, Hôpital Antoine Béclère 92141 Clamart, France

Introduction : we have previously shown that the baroreflex sensitivity of the control of heart rate (HR) is markedly increased during sleep apnea only in normotensive (NT) patients with sleep apnea syndrome (SAS). Also HR response to hypoxemia is attenuated during wekefulness only in hypertensive (HT) SAS (Hedner et al, Am. Rev. Resp. Dis., 134, 4, A 609, 1991). Aim of the study : to compare chemoreflex and baroreflex control of HR in NT and HT sleep apnea patients. Population : 14 SAS patients, 8 NT (6 men) and 6 untreated HT (all men) of similar age (NT : 52.1 ± 10.9 yrs, HT : 50.7 ± 5.9 yrs) and BMI (NT : 32.6 ± 9.6 kg/m^2, HT : 33.5 ± 4.7 kg/m^2). Method : full night polygraphy with non invasive recording of blood pressure (Finapres 2300) and oxygen saturation (SO$_2$) (Biox 3740). Results: no statistical difference was observed between NT and HT for - changes in HR from apnea to resumption of ventilation : 25.7 ± 11.2 bpm vs. 27.4 ± 12.8 respectively - Chemoreflex control of HR (evaluated by the ratio of changes in HR over changes in SO$_2$) : 2.1 ± 1.2 bpm/% vs. 2.3 ± 1.9 respectively. But the multiple regression of changes in HR vs. changes in SO$_2$ systolic blood pressure (SBP) showed that both variables explain 62 % of the variance in NT and only 29 % in HT according to the following linear models :
- NT : Delta HR = 0.48 x Delta SBP + 0.26 x Delta SO$_2$ - 5.11 (r = 0.79).
- HT : Delta HR = 0.10 x Delta SBP + 0.79 x Delta SO$_2$ + 10.8 (r = 0.53).
Conclusion : The chemoreflex control of HR during apnea is similar in NT and HT. NT patients have an HR control during apnea hightly coupled to SBP and SO$_2$ while HR control by SBP is blunted in HT patient.

Autonomic stress tests in the obstructive sleep apnoea syndrome

D. Veale*, J.L. Pepin, C. Bonnet, J.P. Siché and P. Lévy

*CHRU, Grenoble, France and *Freeman Hospital, Newcastle upon Tyne, UK*

Apneic events in the OSAS are associated with a sequence of cardiovascular responses related to repeated Muller type manouvers and repeated hypoxia. These cardiovascular responses include episodic bradycardia and tachycardia and episodes of hypertension and are mediated through the autonomic nervous system. Patients with autonomic failure have been shown to have OSAS (Schroeder et al: in Guilleminault, Dement eds; Sleep Apnoea Syndromes 1978 p177-196). Thus we have examined autonomic cardiovascular responses (Ewing DJ Ann Int Med 1980; 92:308-11.) in 13 patients (median age 50 yrs) undergoing polysomnography for suspected OSAS. We have, in addition, examined these responses at arousal from sleep in the morning to see if chronic overnight autonomic stimulation leads to impairment of these responses. Tests consisted of heart rate response to Valsalva manoeuvre (a), deep breathing (b), and change from lying to standing (c), and, in addition systolic blood pressure (BP) response to standing (d), and diastolic BP response to sustained handgrip (e). Only one patient had no abnormality and 6 patients had one abnormal test (b in 3 cases). The 5 patients with evidence of OSAS (RDI >15) all had 3 abnormal or marginal tests in the evening. There was no deterioration in response overnight In these patients. Six patients without OSAS had only one abnormality - usually in response to respiratory manoeuvres. We conclude that abnormal autonomic stress responses are common in OSAS and are probably a secondary defect. Control studies are needed to explore the possible mechanisms

Grant from Région Rhone-Alpes.

Cardiovascular reflexes in obstructive sleep apnea syndrome

P. Parchi, E. Sforza, P. Cortelli, G. Pierangeli and E. Lugaresi

Institute of Neurology, University of Bologna, via U. Foscolo 7, 40123 Bologna, Italy

A high incidence of hypertension has been described in OSA patients, probably due to hypoxia-induced sympathetic hyperactivity. Diurnal autonomic function tests were examined in 15 consecutive drug-free male OSA patients without hypertension.
All patients underwent nocturnal polygraphic study and cardiovascular reflex tests including tilt test, Valsalva manoeuver, deep breathing, cold face and isometric handgrip performed using standard criteria. During tests blood pressure (BP) and heart rate (HR) were monitored by a finger arterial pressure device (Finapres) and other parameters by polygraphic recording. Results were compared with a control group of 15 age and sex matched healthy volunteers. The patients presented a BMI of 30.96 $\pm$ 5.06 and a diurnal BP of SBP 130.1, DBP 68.9, both higher than the control group. The severity of OSA syndrome was moderate or severe with an AI ranging from 20.3 to 80.5. The BP and HR responses during the tilt test, isometric effort and cold face test were not significantly different from the control group. The respiratory sinus arrhythmia ($p < 0.01$) and Valsalva ratio ($p < 0.05$) were significantly lower in the OSA group.
The correlations between severity of OSA syndrome and cardiovascular reflex tests were assessed.

Renal excretion of endothelin in obstructive sleep apnea syndrome

K. Ehlenz, P. Herzog, P. von Wichert*, H. Kaffarnik and J.H. Peter*

Department of Endocrinology and Metabolism, Outpatient Clinics*, Medical School, Baldinger Strasse, 3550 Marburg, Germany

The pathogenesis of hypertension in obstructive sleep apnea syndrome (OSAS) is a still unresolved question. Discussing this topic it is important to differentiate fast- and slow-, respectively short- and long-acting processes involved in the control of blood pressure. Besides systemic acting hormones we must also consider local factors involved in the autoregulation of vascular tone. Recently, endothelial derived factors with relaxing and constricting properties were discovered e.g. Endothelin (ET) the most potent vasoconstrictor. ET could be demonstrated in plasma in very low concentrations possibly reflecting a spillover of locally secreted ET. Until now it is not clear whether ET has also systemic effects under physiological conditions. It is suggested that ET may be involved in the pathogenesis of hypertension. ET could also be detected in urine. This might be a simple parameter for the overall ET secretion.

Results: To get first information about endothelin in OSAS we measured the nocturnal excretion rate of Endothelin in 12 patient with severe OSAS before and during nCPAP therapy. Endothelin concentration was determined radioimmunologically after Sep-Pak-extraction. We found a significant reduction of ET excretion rate during nCPAP therapy from 443 ± 35 to 280 ± 33 pg/h ($p < 0.01$).

Dicussion: Increased renal excretion of ET before therapy possibly reflects an overall increased secretion of ET from the vasculature during apnea. Apnea-related hypoxemia may be a trigger for ET secretion in OSAS. We conclude that ET may be involved in the hypertensive reaction during apnea besides an activation of the sympathetic nervous system. On the other hand, ET may play a role in pulmonary vasoconstriction leading to pulmonary hypertension. Nevertheless, further investigations are neded to clarify the pathophysiological significance of these findings and the interaction with other cardiovascular hormones.

Sodium renal excretion in heavy snorers and obstructive sleep apnea syndrome

F. Barbe*, J.J. Kiladjian**, R. Patte**, F. Daniel** and B. Fleury*

*Centre de Traitement des Affections Respiratoires, 74, rue de la Colonie, 75013 Paris, and
** Centre Hospitalier Pasteur Vallery-Radot, 26, rue des Peupliers, 75013 Paris, France

Salt excretion has been shown to increase in obstructive sleep apnea (OSA) patients during the night. In this study nocturnal (N) kidney function was studied in 61 heavy snorers. According to polysomnographic recording the patients were separated into two groups: Group I included 37/61 patients with OSA (AI = 40 ± 23) and group II included 24/61 snorers (AI = 4 ± 3). There was no differences of age (50 ± 11 vs 50 ± 13 years) and BMI (30 ± 7 vs 27 ± 3) between the two groups.

N sodiun fractional excretion (NEFNa%) was compared to diurnal excretion (DEFNa%). NEFNa% and DEFNa% were not significantly different in group I (0.86 ± 0.53 vs 0.78 ± 0.48) and significantly different in group II (0.98 ± 0.53 vs 0.66 ± 0.34 $p<0.05$), but there was not an unique pattern typical for each group: actually 16/37 patients in group I and 9/24 patients in group II increased their NEFNa%.

In conclusion: N sodium urinary excretion was increased in 43% of OSA patients and were increased in 37% of snorers. OSA might not invariably be associated with an unique pattern of circadian salt excretion. A similar pattern might be found in heavy snores.

Breathing frequency in patients with sleep related respiratory disturbances (SRRD)

M. Pradella, D.O. Rodenstein and G. Aubert-Tulkens

Sleep Laboratory, Cliniques Universitaires St Luc, UCL, avenue Hippocrate 10, B-1200 Bruxelles, Belgique

In normal adults, breathing frequency (f) changes little during sleep. In patients with SRRD we occasionally observe a spectacular increase of f during sleep. Out of 650 polysomnographies we found 16 patients (mean ± SD age : 45±13 yrs; body mass index (BMI) : 44±11 kg/m^2) with f > 25 min^{-1} during sleep (tachypneic, T). We performed a one-for-one matching for sex, age and BMI between the T and a control (C) group (age : 45±12 yrs; BMI 44±10 kg/m^2). T patients showed a higher f during wakefulness than C patients (25±8 vs 18±3 min^{-1}; $p<0.02$). C patients showed no significant modification of f in any sleep stage. In T patients, f increased in NREM but not in REM sleep (stages 1 : 31±8; 2 : 32±7; 3 : 31±6; 4 : 30±6; REM 29±4 min^{-1}; all $p<0.02$ except REM). In all stages f was different between T and C patients ($p<0.01$). SaO_2 during sleep and number of desaturations > 4% per h (DI) was similar in T and C patients (mean SaO_2 : 84±8 vs 88±9%; DI : 63±50 vs 58±35). We conclude that some obese patients with SRRD, with a high f during wakefulness, show a significant increase of f during NREM sleep; in most, no clear anthropomorphic, clinical or cardiopulmonary characteristic accounts for this tachypnea.

Respiratory abnormalities during sleep in syringomyelia and syringobulbia

H. Encabo and M. Nogués

Laboratorio de Estudio del Sueño y la Vigilia, Instituto de Investigaciones Neurològicas R. Carrea-Fleni, Ayacucho 2166, 1112 Buenos Aires, Argentina

Despite the recognition of respiratory hazards in syringomyelia-bulbia patients, breathing abnormalities have so far received scant attention, particularly as regards their implication in sudden death.

Two groups were studied one night with polysomnographic methods, one with syringomyelia (8 patients) and the other one with syringomyelia-bulbia (11 patients)

Patients denied excessive daytime sleepiness, repeated nocturnal awakenings, restless sleep, or insomnia. Syringomyelia-bulbia patients showed more severe ventilatory abnormalities than the other group: higher apnea-hypopnea indexes, longer duration of apneas and lower oxigen saturation values were found. There was no brady-tachycardia during the apneas. A two year follow-up study in 8 patients outlined an increment of the absolute number, mean and maximal duration of apneas and hypopneas.

Two patients died during sleep and a third one was resuscitated during a nap. All three cases had severe involvement of the cervical spinal cord as well as the IXth and Xth cranial nerves. Periodic sleep studies may be useful to assess the need of nocturnal assisted mechanical ventilation in syringomyelia-bulbia patients.

III. SAS : effects of treatment
III.   SAS : effets du traitement

Transmural pulmonary artery pressure and oxygen administration in obstructive apneas

O. Marrone, V. Bellia, A. Salvaggio, C. Macaluso and G. Bonsignore

Istituto di Fisiopatologia Respiratoria del CNR, Via Trabucco, 180, 90416 Palermo, Italy

Transmural pulmonary artery pressure (PAP) was monitored during sleep in 6 patients affected by obstructive sleep apnea syndrome. In order to assess the effect of the prevention of hypoxia on PAP behaviour, O_2 was randomly administered via nasal prongs to each patient during one half of the study. In each patient 15 apneas during room air breathing and 15 during O_2 administration were randomly selected in non-REM sleep. On these apneas PAP measurements were taken of highest transmural systolic and diastolic values at the end of apneas (respectively Pstme and Pdtme), lowest values at their beginning, and difference between highest and lowest values (ΔPstm and ΔPdtm). During O_2 administration in all subjects oxyhemoglobin saturation (SaO_2) at the end of the selected apneas was significantly higher, and SaO_2 fall within them was significantly lower, than during room air breathing; in two patients Pstme and Pdtme, and in one patient ΔPdtm, were significantly lower; conversely in another subject Pstme, ΔPstm, and ΔPdtm were significantly higher. No other significant variation in the considered PAP values was detected. In four patients a marked increase in PCO_2 (measured as transcutaneous PCO_2) during O_2 administration, ranging between 4 and 11 mm Hg, could have prevented a decrease in Pstme and Pdtme values. The results suggest that hypoxia during obstructive apnea could determine an increase in transmural PAP values throughout all the event; conversely the variation in PAP within apnea does not seem influenced by the amplitude of the simultaneous SaO_2 variation.

Nasal CPAP and pulmonary haemodynamics in OSA patients

P. Kozev and S. Slavchev

Clinic of Functional Diagnosis, Military Medical Academy, 3 Georgi Sofiiski street, Sofia 1606, Bulgaria

ABSTRACT :

A group of patients with full blown clinical pictures of OSA syndrome were submitted to catheterization of pulmonary artery using Swan-Ganz catheter. Thermodilution method for evaluation of the cardiac output was used. Measurements were done during sleep without and with nasal CPAP application. Changes in pulmonary arterial pressure (PAP) due to the effect of changes in the intrathoracic pressure upon the right ventricule output were recorded. An increased value of systolic PAP during Valsalva maneuvre and reduced value during Müller were consecutively measured in alternating mode. Oxygen desaturation drops do not correlate with PAP increase. Nasal CPAP application abolished obstructive apneas with tendency to normalization of PAP values. A striking effect upon the cardiac output was measured during sleep with nCPAP, reaching in some patients a rise of 64 % above sleep without CPAP and 12 % above the state of wakefulness. Without deniing the widely accepted thesis for the hypoxic vasoconstriction as a reason for the increased level of PAP, our studies suggest that the changes in the intrathoracic pressure during sleep with obstructive apneas play a role of a great importance. All therapeutical methods which reduce the OSA, respectively Müller/Valsalva maneuvres are most appropriate to maintain the normal pulmonary haemodynamics.

Hemodynamic effects of short-term nasal continuous positive airway pressure in obstructive sleep apnea syndrome

E. Sforza and E. Lugaresi

Institute of Neurology, University of Bologna, via U. Foscolo 7, 40123 Bologna, Italy

The nocturnal increase in blood pressure during sleep in Obstructive Sleep Apnea syndrome has been implicated in the pathogenesis of diurnal hypertension. CPAP therapy prevents hypoxemia and apneas and reduces nocturnal and diurnal systemic blood pressure. To determine the effects of acute CPAP therapy, 25 OSAS patients were examined during diagnostic (NCPAP) and CPAP (CPAP) night. The mean value and coefficient of variability of systolic (SBP), diastolic (DBP) pressure and heart rate (HR) were determined at 30 second intervals by a finger arterial pressure device (Finapres) during sleep and awake state. Comparison of the changes during NCPAP and CPAP night showed a significant decrease in SBP ($p<0.005$) and HR ($p<0.03$) during the treated night without significant changes in DBP. The coefficient of variability for all parameters was significantly ($p<0.000$) reduced during CPAP night. From these results we conclude that: 1) the decrease in blood pressure during CPAP night is principally due to a decrease in systolic pressure; 2) the mechanical effects of CPAP may explain the absent changes in diastolic pressure; 3) the cardiovascular parameters during CPAP treatment will only improve with long-term therapy.

Improvement in daytime ventilatory responses to CO_2 with or without inspiratory load after CPAP therapy for obstructive sleep apnea syndrome (OSAS)

T. Perez, A. Didier, C. Puel, M. Tiberge, P. Leophonte and J.P. Besombes

Hôpital Rangueil, 31054 Toulouse, France

Daytime ventilatory response to CO2 is often decreased in patients with OSAS. These patients do not increase their respiratory drive to compensate inspiratory resistive load. The aim of present study was thus to determine whether these alterations were reversible after 2 months of CPAP therapy.
Polysomnography was performed in 10 OSAS patients (age: 55 ± 2.6) before treatment and at 2 months with CPAP therapy. Apnea+ hypopnea index was 38.7 ± 8.5 /hour before therapy and 0.9 ± 0.3 /hour with CPAP. No patient had daytime hypercapnia. Daytime ventilatory response to CO2 was evaluated by Read's method in OSAS patients and in 10 controls (age: 38± 2). Mouth occlusion pressure (P0,1), inspiratory minute ventilation (V) and end tidal PCO2 (PETCO2) were measured during rebreathing. Inspiratory resistance (IR) was constant at 12 cmH2O/ l /sec .

REGRESSION LINE SLOPES (mean ± SEM)

	P0.1/PETCO2	V/PETCO2	
CONTROLS	cmH2O/mmHg	l/min/mmHg	
Baseline	0.31 (0.02)	1.69 (0.14)	
With IR	0.44 (0.03)	1.53 (0.20)	
PATIENTS	*Before CPAP*		
Baseline	0.13 (0.03)***	0.67 (0.18)***	* p < 0.05 vs controls (ANCOVA)
With IR	0.11 (0.03)***	0.50 (0.19)***	** p < 0.01 vs controls
	With CPAP		***p < 0.001 vs controls
Baseline	0.17 (0.03)**	1.10 (0.12)*§	§ p < 0.05 vs before CPAP
With IR	0.21 (0.04)***¶	0.86 (0.09)***§	¶ p < 0.001 vs before CPAP

Before therapy, OSAS patients had significantly decreased responses to CO2, with or without inspiratory load. After CPAP only ventilatory response to nonloaded CO2 rebreathing increased, whereas P0,1 response slope did not change significantly. In contrast, a marked increase in P0,1 response to inspiratory load was found after 2 months of CPAP. However, both ventilation and P0,1 regression slopes remained significantly lower in treated OSAS than in controls. In conclusion CPAP therapy significantly improves ventilatory responses to CO2 and to inspiratory resistive load in OSAS.

Effects of the enhancement of slow wave sleep (SWS) by gamma hydroxybutyrate (γ OH) on obstructive sleep apnea (OSA)

F. Series, I. Series and Y. Cormier

Unité de Recherche, Centre de Pneumologie de l'Hôpital et de l'Université Laval, Québec, Canada

Since respiratory abnormalities are rarely observed in SWS, we studied the effects of a SWS enhancing drug (γOH) in 8 OSA patients. For each patient, 3 conventional polysomnographic studies were done within a week, the first and third recordings were control studies, while γOH was given (2 doses of 30 mg/Kg at 3 hours interval) at the second study. Since the effect of γOH lasts only 3 hours, we analyzed the first six hours of the 3 recordings. SWS was poorly represented at control studies (12.6 ± 1.1 % and 11.0 ± 2.1 % : TST, Mean ± SEM). It significantly increased with γOH (30.7 ± 3.9 % TST) at the expense of stages I - II. SWS and REM sleep latencies decreased significantly with γOH. There was no difference in the apnea and apnea + hypopnea indeces, and the mean apnea duration between the control and γOH studies. Most of the apneic events were observed during stages I-II and REM at controls (92.3 ± 1.9 % and 95.9 ± 2.2), but this % decreased to 77.9 ± 8.9 with γOH. With γOH, Delta waves were often associated with resumption of ventilation following an apnea, while resumption of ventilation corresponded to the transition into a lighter sleep stage at control. We conclude that slow wave sleep is not free of respiratory disturbances and may be implicated in the pathophysiology of OSA. Supported by The National Center of Excellence of Canada.

CPAP effect on EEG spectral analysis in sleep apnea syndrome

M. Rey*, F. Philip-Joet**, M. Reynaud-Gaubert**, C. Delpuech***, M. Saadjian** and A. Arnaud**

*Service de Pneumologie**, d'Explorations Fonctionnelles du Système Nerveux*, CHU Nord, 13015 Marseille. INSERM U280***, 151 Cours Albert Thomas, 69000 Lyon, France*

Automated analysis of sleep EEG Data give access not only to automated sleep staging according to Rechtschaffen and Kales criteria, but also to numerous quantitative data which could lead to the discovery of additional information not detectable by a visual analysis. So we have compared the data of EEG spectral analysis between 2 night running, one with CPAP and the other without CPAP, in 11 subjects with sleep apnea syndrome (SAS). The lewel of CPAP was adjusted to suppress most of the apneas. The spectral analysis of the same EEG channel (C4-A2) for each night was realised by Fast Fourier Transform on 10 seconds epochs with a Respisomnographe (SEFAM). Each night give 2763 ± 30 spectra according to the recording duration. For each night, these spectra were grouped in different category, no more than 254, according to the normalised integral values of the spectre. Each category have one or several spectra, and we have considered as significant each category which have more than 20 spectra. We have analysed the CPAP effect on respiratory and sleep variables, and on the data of spectral analysis. We obsesrved with CPAP a decrease of total apneas from 350 ± 57 to 50 ± 18 ($t(10)= 5,2$; $p<0,001$), an improvement of sleep : the REM duration increased from 20 ± 6 mn to 59 ± 8 mn ($t(10)= 4,1$; $p<0,005$), and the slow wave sleep increased from 15 ± 8 mn to 69 ± 13 mn ($t(10)= 3,7$; $p<0,005$). Theese improvements were associated with a reduction of the number of category of spectra from 231 ± 7 to 207 ± 11 ($t(10)= 2,5$; $p<0,05$), and an increase of number of spectra by category from 41 ± 2 to 46 ± 2 ($t(10)= 2,4$; $p<0,05$). So, a reduction of spectral shapes observed in the night of a subject could account for the better sleep organisation with CPAP treatement.

Appropriated therapy for overlap syndrome (COPD and SAS) : the point at issue

V. Jounieaux, T. Toris and P. Levi-Valensi

Service de Pneumologie, CHU Hôpital Sud, 80054 Amiens Cedex, France

We have retrospectively selected ten patients exhibiting a combination of severe chronic obstructive pulmonary disease ($FEV_1/VC \leq 70\%$ pred) and sleep apnea syndrome (Apnea index ≥ 10). This association was called "overlap syndrome" by D.C. FLENLEY in 1985. In 5 cases, polysomnography was performed looking for obstructive apneas during sleep ("SAS like" patients) and in the other 5 for nocturnal desaturations ("COPD like" patients). The polysomnographic study (room air) assessed two distinct patterns of sleep disorders : desaturation dips related to obstructive apneas (Apnea index : 33.9 ± 12.8) and desaturation dips during REM's (% of TIB spent with a $SaO_2 \leq 90\%$: $63.8 \pm 36.8\%$). We have followed these patients during 26 ± 16 months. 3 benefited of oxygen therapy alone (above 18h per day), 5 of nocturnal CPAP and 2 were lost. No death was noted.

In 1991, six years after its recognition, the overlap syndrome remains an obscure disease. Multicentric studies are obviously required to determine : 1. the incidence of this combination, 2. its clinical and fonctional features and 3. the best therapy (O_2, CPAP, BiPAP, tracheostomy or association ?). At least, it may be emphazised that some groups should be distinguished in the so-called "overlap syndrome" with heavy consequences on therapy.

IV. Sleep and cardio-vascular system (physiology, pathology)

IV. Sommeil et système cardio-vasculaire (physiologie, pathologie)

Effects of minor arousal stimuli on blood pressure in normal sleeping man

R.J.O. Davies, P. Belt, N.J. Ali and J.R. Stradling

Osler Chest Unit, Churchill Hospital, Headington, Oxford, UK

During obstructive sleep apnoea (OSA) transient arousal at the resumption of breathing and normoxia, is co-incident with a substantial but poorly understood rise in blood pressure (BP). To assess the haemodyamic effect of the arousal element alone we have studied arousal stimuli in sleep-deprived normal subjects (5M, 4F, aged 18-29). EEG, EOG x2, chin EMG, and beat to beat BP (Finapres, Ohmeda), were recorded in all subjects. 170 transient arousal stimuli were administered from a vibrating box beneath the pillow. Stimulus length was varied to produce a range of cortical EEG arousals which were graded. Grade 0, no rise in high frequency EEG or EMG. Grade 1, increased high frequency EEG and/or EMG for <10 seconds. Grade 2, increased high frequency EEG and/or EMG >10 seconds. Overall, compared to control, there was a rise in mean systolic (SWS 10.7SD7.2, REM 4.8SD6.8 mmHg) and diastolic (SWS 6.7SD4.6, REM 3.4SD3.0 mmHg) during the 10 seconds after the stimulus (paired t-test, SWS $P<0.0001$, REM $p<0.02$). There was a correlation between this rise and arousal grade in SWS but not REM (analysis of variance).

SWS	Arousal Grade		
	0	1	2
Rise in mean systolic mmHg	7.7SD5.3	10.3SD7.3	15.6SD8.1 $p<0.0001$
Rise in mean diastolic mmHg	3.4SD2.9	7.1SD4.3	10.4SD4.9 $p<0.0001$

Arousal in SWS consistently provoked a BP rise which could explain almost all the BP rise we have seen during OSA. In REM the response is less predictable. During SWS arousal stimuli provoke BP rises even without any EEG change. Thus autonomic features may be a more sensitive marker of arousing stimuli than the cortical EEG.

Influence of sleep state on coronary hemodynamics in young lambs

James E. Fewell, Colleen S. Kondo and Victor Dascalu

Reproductive Medicine Research Group, Departments of Obstetrics-Gynaecology, Medical Physiology and Paediatrics, University of Calgary, Calgary, Alberta, T2N 4N1 Canada

Experiments were done to determine if sleep state influences coronary hemodynamics in 7 lambs. Each lamb was anesthetized and prepared for sleep staging and for measurements of cardiac output (Qp), left circumflex blood flow (Qlcf) and systemic blood pressure (BP). Myocardial oxygen demand was estimated by the product (PRP) of mean systemic blood pressure and heart rate. No sooner than 3 days after surgery, measurements were made in quiet wakefulness (QW), quiet sleep (QS) and active sleep (AS) at an ambient temperature of 25C.

Variable	QW	QS	AS
Qp (ml/min/Kg)	182±33	182±39	166±37*
HR (BPM)	179±26	178±31	161±31*
BP (mmHg)	76±5	75±3	73±5
Qlcf (ml/min/Kg)	3.4±1.3	3.3±1.3	3.1±1.3*
PRP ($\times 10^3$)	13.6±2.7	13.4±2.7	11.7±2.3*

(* $p<0.05$ by MANOVA and Duncans as compared to QW & QS)

Qlcf decreased during AS compared to QW & QS; however, the ratio of Qlcf to Qp did not change. The decrease in coronary blood flow during AS is most likely related to a decrease in myocardial oxygen demand.

Step reduction of alveolar PCO_2 causes ECG abnormalities

Eduardo Dreizzen, Yael Shabtai-Musih and Noam Gavriely

Rappaport Faculty of Medicine and Institute for Research in the Medical Sciences, Technion, Haifa, Israel

In search for mechanisms of sudden death, we evaluated the hypothesis that sudden reduction of alveolar CO_2 concentration either by induction of post-apneic hyperventilation or by step decrease of F_ICO_2 induce cardiac arrhythmias. 20 adult Guinea Pigs were anesthetized, paralyzed, tracheostomized and artificially ventilated. Arterial blood pressure and ECG were recorded. Two experimental protocols were used: In the Group I, 11 Guinea Pigs (weight 770±160 g) were artificially ventilated so that 45 sec. periods of apnea were immediately followed by hyperventilation (3 times normal frequency). A total of 140 runs of apnea-hyperventilation were performed. The values of arterial pH and PCO_2 were 7.37±0.12 and 47±16 mmHg at the end of apnea and 7.55±0.1 and 21±10 mmHg at the end of the hyperventilation period. 2 to 50 sec. after the onset the post-apnea hyperventilation 3 animals developed supraventricular arrhythmias (supraventricular premature beats, sinus arrest) and 2 animals developed a total of 10 ventricular premature beats. No arrhythmia was seen during the period of apnea. In the Group II, 9 Guinea Pigs (weight 510± 30 g) were artificially ventilated at normal rate and tidal volume using 30% F_ICO_2 in oxygen. CO_2 administration was maintained for 30 min. and then suddenly switched to air, without changing the parameters of ventilation. The values of arterial pH and PCO_2 were 6.79±0.06 and 187±11 mmHg during the hypercapnic period and 7.13±0.01 and 61±15, after 2 min. on room air respectively. ECG was normal during the hypercapnic period, except for some occasional ventricular premature beats. During the first 10 min. after switching to air, three kind of ECG alterations were observed: transient T wave changes in 6 animals (hyperkalemia pattern), ventricular premature beats in 4 animals and transient patterns of hyperacute ischemia in 2 animals. We conclude that rapid recovery from apnea could play a significant role in development of cardiac arrhythmias. Further research is needed in order to evaluate the influence of potential contributing factors such as hypoxia and electrolytic disturbances on this phenomenon.

Placebo controlled trial of nocturnal continuous positive airway pressure in chronic heart failure with sleep disordered breathing

R.J.O. Davies, K.J. Harrington and J.R. Stradling

Osler Chest Unit, Churchill Hospital, Headington, Oxford, UK

We have performed a controlled study of nocturnal domiciliary CPAP in five men symptom limited by severe chronic heart failure due to left ventricular dysfunction, (ejection fraction <17%) without symptomatic ischaemia. Full polysomnography (with severity of sleep apnoea quantitated as number of >4% dips in arterial saturation per hour) showed four to have nocturnal Cheyne-Stokes respiration (SaO_2 dip rate 3 to 27 per hr) and one both central and obstructive apnoeas (SaO_2 dip rate 8 per hr). In all subjects fluid retention was adequately controlled (mean frusemide dose 130mg day). Exercise tolerance (bicycle exercise test to exhaustion), and heart failure symptoms (modified Likert questionnaire) were blindly assessed at baseline and after nocturnal domiciliary CPAP at <1.5cm H_2O (placebo) and 7.5cm H_2O (active) each for two weeks in random order. Pulse oximetry was repeated at the end of each period. Two subjects withdrew from the study, both experienced worsening heart failure during active CPAP (7.5 cm H_2O). The three subjects who completed the protocol all improved on placebo, but deteriorated on active therapy when compared to placebo. Changes in nocturnal SaO_2 dip rate were variable.

	Pre-Study	Placebo	Active
Mean Exercise Tolerance (minutes of exercise test completed)	5.08	5.53	4.89
Mean Overall Symptom Score (lower scores are better)	20.3	16.3	19.0

These preliminary results suggest that nocturnal CPAP is not beneficial in severe heart failure with sleep disordered breathing when compared to placebo.

Nocturnal periodic breathing in patients with stable chronic heart failure : effects of oxygen versus placebo

A. Braghiroli, F. De Vito*, C. Sacco, M. Erbetta, V. Ruga, S. Magnaghi*, A. Giordano* and C.F. Donner

Division of Pulmonary Disease and Division of Cardiology*, Clinica del Lavoro Foundation, Medical Center of Rehabilitation, Veruno (NO), Italy

Periodic breathing (PB) induces in pts with chronic heart failure (CHF) severe nocturnal desaturations and disruption of sleep architecture.

The <u>aim</u> of the present ongoing study is to assess the efficacy of supplemental oxygen in preventing nocturnal PB, according to a single blind, cross over, placebo (compressed air) vs. oxygen, random design. The preliminary results concerning 6 pts with clinically stable CHF are reported. Age was 55±9 yrs, weight 65±6 Kg, height 166±5 cm. Lung function was normal (all indices >80% predicted) and diurnal SaO_2 was >90% (93±1.4) in all pts. Ejection fraction was 26±8 (15-35). After an adaptation night, each pt underwent 3 consecutive nocturnal polysomnographies, the first breathing room air, the 2nd and 3rd with a facial Venturi type mask, administering a 28% mixture of oxygen or compressed air.

The main <u>results</u> are reported in the table.

	Basal	P	Oxygen	P	Compressed Air
%of sleep spent in PB	53.1±24.2	(.024)	16.1±14.6	(.035)	49.1±17.1
Avg minimum SaO2%	89.6±3.4	(.042)	92.9±2.8	(.039)	88.6±3.4
Dips SaO2<90%/h	15.8±17.4	(.081)	3.3±5.3	(.168)	12.1±17.2
Obstructive Apneas/h	5.6±7.4	(.576)	4.8±7.5	(.691)	5.1±6.4
Sleep efficiency (%)	76±13.1	(.044)	86.8±6.4	(.101)	79.1±15.4

<u>Conclusions</u>: supplemental oxygen decreases the % of sleep spent in PB, preventing related O2 dips and improves the sleep efficiency. The residual desaturations are determined by obstructive apneas, thus not influenced by oxygentherapy.

Sleep respiratory disorders in patients with stable chronic heart failure: a polysomnographic study

F. De Vito, A. Braghiroli*, C. Sacco*, S. Magnaghi, M. Erbetta*, C.F. Donner* and A. Giordano

Division of Cardiology and Pneumology. Clinica del Lavoro Foundation, Institute of Care and Research, Center of Rehabilitation, Veruno (NO), Italy*

In order to investigate the presence of sleep respiratory disorders and their possible effects on sleep architecture and nocturnal oxyhaemoglobin saturation (SaO2) in patients with chronic heart failure (CHF) 9 pts (8M 1F) clinically stable underwent a formal polysomnography after an adaptation night. Age was 56±9 y. (44-70), weight 68±8 Kg (56-84), height 168±6 cm (158-177). Lung function was normal (all indices > 80% predicted) and diurnal SaO2 was >90%(93.7±2.1)in all pts. Ejection fraction(EF) was 23±7(15-35).Electroencephalogram, electrooculogram, chin and anterior tibialis electromyogram, ECG, oronasal airflow, thoraco-abdominal movements (Respitrace), pulse oximetry were continuously recorded. Periodic breathing (PB) was defined as cyclical sequence of central apneas and /or hypopneas, lasting >10 seconds each, separated by less than 40 sec. of breathing.

PB was found in all pts with a mean duration of 43.7% ±26 of total sleep time (TST). 3 pts showed >5 obstructive apneas/h (10.3±0.4). The respiratory events induced significant dips of nocturnal SaO2(82.1 % ± 8.4) and a disruption of sleep architecture: the TST was only 272±62 min, the sleep efficiency reduced to 71%±17, with predominance of light stages (phase 1: 12.4%±6.8 and phase 2: 61.1%±13.8 of TST). The percentage of sleep spent in PB significantly correlates with sleep efficiency (r=-.68 p<.03) and TST (r=-.55 p<.05).

In conclusion, pts with CHF and depressed EF are at risk for periodic breathing during sleep, with a disruption in sleep architecture and dips of SaO2, potentially inducing severe clinical sequelae.

Sleep apnea and myocardial ischemia

D. Auge

University Clinic, Robert-Koch-Strasse, 40, D-3400 Göttingen, Germany

The occurrence of cardiac arrhythmias in patients with obstructive sleep apnea is well-known. It is not clear wether ST segment changes are associated to the arterial oxygen saturation and the apnea index.
15 male patients with a mean age of 53 years with obstructive sleep apnea and without overt cardiac disease were investigated polysomnographically and underwent 24h-ECG (Reynolds Pathfinder III, Hetford U.K.).
The apnea index of the patients with the obstructive sleep apnea ranged between 10 and 57 and the decrease of the arterial oxygen saturation was at least 4 %. ST segment changes were found in 86 % of the patients. The ST segment changes showed a strong correlation to the apnea index. A negative correlation existed between the arterial oxygen saturation and the ST segment changes.
It has to be suggested that the hypoxemia during the obstructive sleep apnea may be responsible for the ST segment changes.

Sleep apnea syndrome and ischemic heart disease

H.A.M. Middelkoop[1], M. Bootsma, B. Kemp[1], C.A. Swenne, H.A.C. Kamphuisen[1] and A.V.G. Bruschke

Departments of [1]Clinical Neurophysiology and Cardiology, Academic Hospital, PO Box 9600, 2300 RC Leiden, The Netherlands

In the Netherlands, sleep apnea syndrome (SAS), a condition of repetitive, long periods of nocturnal breath cessations has a prevalence of nearly 2% (± 300,000 patients) in mainly elderly male residents. Recently, some reports have pointed at the possibility that there might be a direct causal relationship between nocturnal oxygen desaturation due to apnoeic episodes and cardiovascular diseases, particularly ischemic heart disease. During a nocturnal apnoeic episode, oxygen saturation level can drop to a 50% level, causing a pattern of sinus arrhythmia-bradycardia, eventually followed by abrupt tachycardia. In patients with congestive heart disease, this condition can become life-threatening on account of the appearance of episodes of myocardial ischemia and arrhythmia. However, ischemia and arrhythmia can commonly also be observed in normal sleep, in particular during Rapid-Eye Movement (REM) sleep characterized by increased sympathetic outflow. So, the question arises to what extent can sleep apnea by itself be accounted for the supplementary appearance of nocturnal episodes of ischemia and arrhythmia? In order to elucidate this question and related topics, we have recently started (june 1991) a 4-year project in which we will study extensively at least 20 selected patients suffering from both obstructive SAS and ischemic heart disease. After completion of the selection procedure, subjects will be asked to sleep in our dedicated sleep laboratory for one night. During this night the patients will be subjected to a polysomnographic study. Simultaneous and continuous recording will be done of the ECG, thoraco-abdominal movement by an impedance pneumograph, oronasal airflow by a thermistor, motor activity by a wrist-worn actigraph, and oxygen saturation by a pulse oximeter (Nellcor N-100). Moreover, additional data will be collected by means of questionnaires. In a selected number of patients also muscle sympathetic activity will be recorded. The results of Continuous Positive Airway Pressure treatment in a small number of subjects will be evaluated. Preliminary results of a pilot-study done in one healthy male subject showed that heart-rate as well as oronasal airflow variability was at highest level during REM sleep.

Grant support: Phoenix Foundation, Schiedam, The Netherlands & The Dutch Heart Foundation.

Atrial vulnerability revealed by nasal CPAP

C. Rostykus[1], J.C. Meurice[2], J. Mergy[3], P. Dore[2], J. Paquereau[1] and F. Patte[2]

[1] Laboratoire de Physiologie Générale, CNRS UA 290, Faculté de Médecine, 86034, Poitiers Cedex, France and [2] Service de Pneumologie, [3] Service de Cardiologie A, CHRU de Poitiers, Route de Limoges, 86021, Poitiers Cedex, France

We report a case of supraventricular rhythm disorder occuring as a complication of nasal continuous positive airway pressure (CPAP) in sleep apnea syndrome (SAS) treatment.
A 68 year old man had a confirmed SAS with: predominantly obstructive type of apnea; apnea/hypopnea index=24/hour; deep O_2 desaturations (60%) and sleep architecture perturbations.ECG revealed sinusal rhythm with an intra atrial block (bimodal P wave in D_2). Also few isolated and sporadic premature supraventricular complexes were seen.
During the polysomnographic study done under nasal CPAP (7cm H_2O) we noted the occurence of persistent atrial bigeminy. Five days later, the 24 hours Holter recording showed some sporadic premature supraventricular complexes in the afternoon but a persistent bigeminy immediately after the institution of nasal CPAP (7cm H_2O).
Electrophysiologic investigation and standard right catheterization were performed. They revealed during nasal CPAP (7cm H_2O):
    - an atrial vulnerability with an atrial flutter induced (which disappeared after CPAP was stopped),
    - a decreased cardiac output and a rise in the right atrial pressure.
The patient has been treated with HYDROQUINIDINE which allowed nasal CPAP to be continued.
We believe that this complication associated with nasal CPAP is uncommon and that further studies must be developped to evaluate cardiovascular repercussions of nasal CPAP.

Effects of autonomic blockade on heart rate responses to pyramidal tract stimulation

M. Benachouba and J.C. Roy

Laboratoire de Neurosciences du Comportement, SN4, Université des Sciences et Techniques de Lille Flandres-Artois, 59655 Villeneuve d'Asq Cedex, France

We hypothetized that the pyramidal tract (PT) could directly influence cardiovascular processes, through collaterals, or small fibers reaching the cardiovascular centers at bulbar level. In eighteen cats of either sex, under halothane anaesthesia, a transection of the medulla sparing only the PT was performed, either at high bulbar level (P6) or at low bulbar level (P12). β-adrenergic receptor blockers: propranolol (0,5 mg/kg), atenolol (0,5 mg/kg) and muscarinic receptor blocker: atropine sulfate (0,05 and 0,1 mg/kg) were used. The PT was stimulated stereotaxically, 3 mm rostrally to the plane of transection, before and after the transection. In order to prevent cardiovascular changes resulting from movements elicited by PT stimulations, the animals were paralyzed by gallamine. The results show that either in the intact animal or after a transection at high bulbar level sparing only the PT, or after the adrenergic β-receptor blockade, the PT stimulations evoked increase in heart rate (HR). After a low bulbar transection sparing the PT or after the cholinergic blockade, the stimulations failed to elicit HR variations. We conclude that the PT probably suppressed the vagal cardiac inhibition which consequently induced an increase in HR. During sleep and wakefulness, the PT activity shows phasic variations that influence the bulbar reticular structures (Puizillout et Ternaux, 1974). During movement and during sleep and wakefulness, the motor system influences the bulbar autonomic centers.

V. Sleep and cardiorespiratory adaptations in infants

V. Sommeil et adaptations cardio-respiratoires du nourrisson

Ventilatory pattern, occlusion pressure and sudden infant death syndrome (SIDS)

E. Girin*, M. Bellet*, Y. Grossi*, J. Le Bot**, M.D. Donnou***, C. Cabelguen*** and D. Alix***

Unité d'Explorations Fonctionnelles de l'Enfant et de l'Adulte, Service Lavoisier, Institut Mère et Enfant de Bretagne Occidentale**, Service de Pédiatrie et de Génétique***, CHU de Brest, France*

This is a retrospective study of ventilatory pattern and occlusion pressure (Po.1) performed on sixty eight full term infants with a risk of SIDS (fifty SIDS siblings mean ($\pm$ SD) age 5,0 + 1,4 weeks, eighteen nearmiss for SIDS infants, mean (+ SD) age 14,9 + 4,6 weeks).

Airflow, tidal volume and occlusion pressure were simultaneously recorded during spontaneous quiet sleep. Then, tidal volume (Vt), total respiratory cycle time (Ttot), inspiratory time (Ti), expiratory time (TE) were measured and we calculed frequency (f), minute ventilation (VE), mean inspiratory flow (VT/Ti), respiratory timing (Ti/Ttot) and inspiratory effective impedance (ratio Po.1 over Vt/Ti).

On each infant were also performed a three hour polygraphic electroencephalogram, a twenty four hour cardiorespiratory recording and a twelve hour oesophageal pH metry.

These data were compared to respiratory results. Some children, particularly those who had a severe life-threatening event, showed an increased occlusion pressure with sometimes a decreasing of the ratio Vt/Ti. In their past history, we found a higher frequency of pathological pregacy or perinatal abnormalities. But, the compareason with the other data provided no obvious correspondence with occurence of abnormal respiratory apneas and/or gastroesophageal reflux. More, the observed results for ventilatory pattern and occlusion pressure are in the range of normal values.

Therefore, the ventilatory pattern and occlusion pressure studies, in the hypothesis of an abnormal ventilatory control, should be depend taking in to account the organisation of sleep and circadian rythms of cardiorespiratory control in the infants with risk of SIDS.

Respiratory and cardiac rates in 2-month-old normal infants : nycthemeral changes

M.F. Vecchierini-Blineau and B. Nogues

Laboratoire de Physiologie, Faculté de Médecine, 1, rue Gaston Veil, 44035 Nantes Cedex, France

The aim of this work was to study mean respiratory and cardiac rates during sleep in infants and to analyse these rate variations during daytime and nighttime recordings.
Sleep polygraphic recordings [EEG, EOG, chin EMG, thoracic, abdominal, buccal and nasal respirations, electrocardiogram (lead V2)] were performed in 35 normal 2-month-old infants during the night from 7 p.m. to 6 a.m. and the following day from 9 a.m. to 3 p.m.
Respiratory and cardiac rates were calculated every minute in each quiet (QS) and active (AS) sleep state, excluding episodes with excessive artefacts or frequent respiratory pauses.
RESULTS : - Cardiac and respiratory rates were more elevated ($p < 0.001$) in AS than in QS, regardless of recording time, and during the day than at night, regardless of sleep state. - These mean rates showed great interindividual variability with a very good correlation for each infant as a function of sleep state or time. - Mean respiratory and cardiac rate changes were similar with respect to sleep state and recording time. Mean rates were always highest during the first cycle, then decreased. Apart from this first cycle, mean rates were comparable for all the cycles. Nevertheless, it should be noted that minimal values were found in the middle of the recording period (eighth cycle at night and third cycle during the day). - During sustained sleep episodes, i.e., more than 20 min. for QS and 15 min. for AS, a sharp decrease in both rates was found at the beginning of the episode ; there was then little change in the middle of the state and a slight rise during the last minute. These changes in cardio-respiratory rates were statistically significant during QS but not during AS.
These results suggest that there is a circadian pattern in nycthemeral cardio-respiratory rate changes.

Spontaneous awakenings during sleep in two-month-old infants : influence on respiratory and cardiac rates

B. Nogues and M.F. Vecchierini-Blineau

Laboratoire de Physiologie, Faculté de Médecine, 1, rue Gaston Veil, 44035 Nantes Cedex, France

In infants, numerous spontaneous awakenings were recorded during sleep, including some at feeding time. Respiratory and cardiac rate changes were studied according to the time of awakening (daytime or nighttime) and sleep-state.
Thirty five normal 2-month-old infants were recorded (EEG, EOG, chin EMG, cardiac activity, V2, thoracic, abdominal, buccal and nasal respirations) during the night from 7 p.m. to 6 a.m. and the following day from 9 a.m. to 3 p.m. Spontaneous awakenings of at least ten minutes were classified in 2 groups : with or without feeding. Respiratory and cardiac rates were calculated every minute in each quiet and active sleep state, before and after awakening. Mean cardiac and respiratory rates were always more elevated after than before awakening, regardless of sleep state and recording time. For both sleep states of the cycle, these increased rates persisted after awakening and then decreased progressively. After awakening with feeding, differences in cardiac and respiratory rates were statistically significant ($p < 0.01$ to $p < 0.0001$ when $n > 10$). After awakening without feeding the increased rates were comparable to those after awakening with feeding. However, as rates were generally higher and more variable before awakening without feeding than before awakening with feeding, no statistically significant differences in cardio-respiratory rates could be found.
From these results, it is concluded that : 1 - cardio-respiratory rates always increase after a spontaneous awakening in infants , 2 - feeding has no influence on rates after awakening, and 3 - there is a difference in rate changes before awakening depending on whether feeding occurs or not.

Infants' vagal reactivity disclosed during a standardized ocular compression test and a 12 hours cardiorespiratory monitoring

A. de Broca, A. Mohamedaly, F. Kochert, N. Kalach, M. Vural and B. Risbourg

Centre Régional pour la prévention SIDS, Pédiatrie 2, CHRU, 80054 Amiens Cedex, France

Vagal hypertonia is implicated in a few Near Miss Syndromes as in Sudden Infant Death Syndrom. The aim of our study is to compare infants' vagal reactivity during an ocular compression test (OCT) versus their results during a 12 hours cardio-respiratory monitoring (CRM).
103 infants (44 - 50 weeks post conceptional age) underwent a 12 hours cardio-respiratory monitoring in our unit and a standardized ocular compression test on the morning (1). They were free from neurologic disease and any others treatments. Parental total informed consent was obtained in each case.
During the CRM, vagal reactivity is estimated on the highest variation between two R-R interval within the ten following seconds (Delta Instantaneous Heart Rate in ten seconds divided by 10: Δ IHR). High vagal reactivity is assessed when Δ IHR exceedes 8. We have distinguished in our population, high and normal vagal reactivities (respectively unexpected occurence or not of Δ IHR > 8). Vagal reactivity in OCT is appreciated as precised elsewhere (1) and have distinguished high and normal reactivities with this test (respectively grade 5- 4 and grade 3-2-1-0 (1)). Thus, we have compared the infants'results obtained during OCT versus infants' results obtained during their previous 12 hours CRM.

OCT CRM	high	normal
high	13 (a)	0 (b)
normal	29 (c)	61 (d)

In (a), the two tests are concordant. Thus, the OCT seems useless when CRM presents one or more Δ IHR upper 8. Case (b), the two tests are not concordant. The absence of infant in this situation shows that OCT is really efficient to detect vagal hypertonia. Case (c), the OCT has been more efficient to detect vagal hypertonia than the CRM. This situation justifies to perform one OCT when CRM does not present high Δ IHT. Case (d), the two results are also concordant.

Conclusion : OCT is an excellent test to detect vagal hypertonia and must be performed to detect infant 's vagal reactivity when CRM does not present high Δ IHR .

1   de BROCA et al. (1990) Standardization of oculo cardiac reflex in young infants. Pédiatrie. 45 : 405 - 408.

Atropin test : a new test to appreciate vagal tone in children during sleep

Dagmara Lagarde, Olivier Mouterde and Eric Mallet

Service de Pédiatrie, Centre Hospitalo-Universitaire, 76031 Rouen Cedex, France

The oculocardiac reflex is currently used to diagnose vagal hypertonia. Its realization and interpretation difficult. We attempted to perform a pharmacologic test using atropin : so instead of stimulate vagus activity, we tried to block it : we so explored not vagus reactivity but vagal basal tone. 84 infants aged 3 to 32 weeks were studied, including 26 apparent life threatening events and 58 siblings. The effect of on intraveinous infusion of 0.02 mg/kg of atropin during sleep was studied by cardiac monitoring, and the result compared with those of oculo-cardiac reflex (OCR). Such a dosage is currently used in preanesthesic procedures. It appears a statistic correlation ($p < 0.05$) between the level of heart rate variation and basal heart rate suggesting a real correlation between vagal break and heart rate. We found no correlation between the results of OCR and of atropin test : the explanation of this lack of correlation could be the different mechanism of the two tests. For ethical reasons, we did not realize such a test in controls, so normal values are still to determine. We had to deal with two rashs, and an acute gastric distension. We propose this test as a new mean to appreciate vagal tone in children during-sleep.

Sleep-phase related tc PCO_2 in infants under closed and open loop conditions of the central pH/PCO_2 control system

M.E. Schläfke and T. Schäfer

Department of applied Physiology, Ruhr-University, D-4630 Bochum 1, Germany

The central pH/pCO_2-sensitive homeostatic system of respiration is responsible for the acid-base regulation from birth on. We compared the course of pCO_2 during NREM-sleep as a phase of steady state with the pCO_2 during REM-sleep in healthy infants (H) with intact chemical regulation (closed loop) and in infants with transiently (T) or irreversibly (I) missing CO_2-sensitivity (open loop). Infants with transiently missing CO_2-sensitivity during the first year of life were evaluated as at risk for sudden infant death, one of them became a victim of SIDS, infants with a complete and irreversible loss of CO_2-sensitivity suffered from the Ondine's Curse Syndrome. Means of pCO_2 values from whole night recordings during NREM-sleep were 40.4 mmHg (H), 41.0 mmHg (T), 48 mmHg (SIDS), and 76.1 mmHg (I), during REM-sleep 38.6 mmHg (H), 39.7 mmHg (T), 46.8 mmHg (SIDS), and 47.8 mmHg (I). Although very small the difference of pCO_2-variability during NREM-sleep between H (1.15 mmHg) and T (1.84 mmHg) was highly significant, in SIDS we found 2.25 mmHg, in I 7.5 mmHg or wide variations according to the therapy. We conclude that pCO_2 is principally higher, but more stable during NREM-sleep than during REM-sleep, but NREM-stability is reduced in infants during a transient disturbance of the central homeostatic system.

Heart rate variability in infants at increased risk for sudden infant death syndrome

Mary A. Woo, Marlyn S. Woo, W. Brendle Glomb, Daisy Bautista and Sally L. Davidson Ward

UCLA Medical Center and Childrens Hospital Los Angeles, Los Angeles, CA, USA

Autonomic nervous system (ANS) dysfunction has been described in infants at increased risk for Sudden Infant Death Syndrome (SIDS). A measure of ANS tone is heart rate variability. We analyzed 24-hour Holter recordings on 28 subjects at increased risk for SIDS (12 Apnea of Infancy, 8 subsequent siblings of SIDS, 8 infants of cocaine-abusing mothers) and 7 age-matched controls for standard deviation and Poincaré plots of R-R intervals.
Results: No statistical difference between groups for standard deviation of R-R intervals were found. However, Poincaré plots showed markedly different patterns in 21 (75%) study patients (fig 1) compared to controls who showed consistent patterns (fig 2).

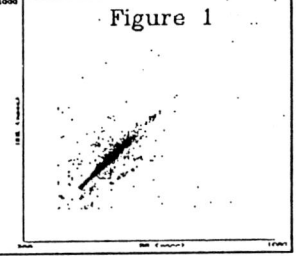

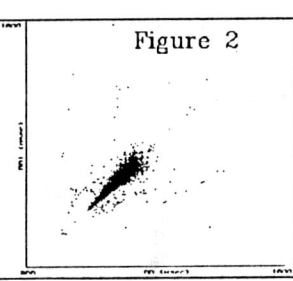

Conclusion: Poincaré plots may be of value in the identification of ANS dysfunction in infants at increased risk for SIDS.

R-R interval Poincaré plots in normal children and in children with congenital central hypoventilation syndrome

Mary A. Woo, Marlyn S. Woo, David Gozal and Thomas G. Keens

UCLA Medical Center and Childrens Hospital Los Angeles, Los Angeles, CA, USA

Children with Congenital Central Hypoventilation Syndrome (CCHS) have abnormal central chemoreceptor function with resultant inappropriate ventilatory responses. Subtle abnormalities in autonomic nervous system (ANS) function also could be present. We analyzed 24-hour Holter recordings in 9 CCHS patients and in 8 age-matched controls for heart rate variability (expressed as standard deviation and Poincaré plots). Results: Standard deviation of heart rate variability was similar in both groups, but CCHS patients demonstrated markedly narrower and more linear patterns in their R-R intervals (fig 1) than controls (fig 2). Conclusion: We speculate that Poincaré plots for CCHS were narrower than controls due to either absence of respiratory sinus arrhythmia or other centrally mediated autonomic dysfunction, and that such plots may be of value in the evaluation of ANS tone.

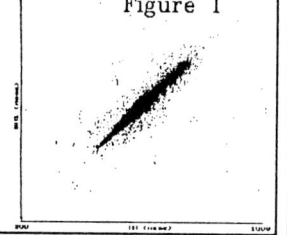

Figure 1

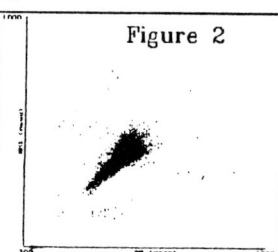

Figure 2

Correlation between event related heart rate changes and mean heart rate in newborns during sleep

*M. Eiselt, **L. Curzi-Dascalova and *U. Zwiener

*Institute of Pathological Physiology, O-6900 Jena, Germany; **INSERM CJF 89-09, Hôpital Antoine Béclère, 92141 Clamart, France

To investigate the relation between mean heart rate and the amplitude of heart rate increase caused by movements or sighs we measured during sleep movement-related heart rate changes in 1 group of normal, full-term newborns (n=28) and sigh-related heart rate changes in 2 groups of normal newborns (full-term, n=13; near-term, n=12) of less than 10 days postnatal age. Heart rate and heart rate changes were measured in beats per minute.

We found that the amplitude of heart rate increase correlates with mean heart rate in all groups ($p < 0.05$). This correlation was more frequently significant during active than during quiet sleep; and in movement-related heart rate changes the calculated slope of regression line was different between active and quiet sleep ($p < 0.05$).

These results imply that amplitude of heart rate changes should be interpreted in relation to mean heart rate and sleep state.

Heart rate variability during sleep in prematures of 39 weeks postconceptional age

*M. Eiselt, **J. Clairambault, **C. Médigue, *C. Leffler and *L. Curzi-Dascalova

*INSERM CJF 89-09, Hôpital Antoine Béclère, 92141 Clamart; **INRIA, 78153 Le Chesnay, France

To investigate the influence of postconceptional age (PCA) and postnatal age on the maturation of the autonomic nervous system, we analysed heart rate (HR) and heart rate variability (HRV) in 3 groups of normal newborns les than 10 days postnatal age (premature, near-term, full-term) and 2 groups of prematures reaching the same PCA as near-term and full-term newborns (28.2+11.2 days postnatal age). HRV was calculated by spectral analysis of interbeat intervals by Short Time Fourier Transform in 3 frequency bands (HF: 1-4 sec., MF: 4-12 sec., LF: 12-50 sec.).

We found that HR in prematures of 39 weeks PCA was higher ($p < 0.001$) and HRV was lower ($p < 0.05$) than in near-term and full-term newborns of the same PCA. HRV in prematures of 39 weeks PCA was similar and HR was higher ($p < 0.05$) than in prematures of less than 36 weeks PCA. Results were similar during active and quiet sleep.

Thus, with respect to HRV, prematures studied at 39 weeks PCA are different from newborns of the same conceptional age, but seem similar to premature infants before 36 weeks PCA. The possible influence of different HR to the value of HRV remains to be investigated.

° Supported by grant RGR62 INSERM-CNAMTS

Heart rate fluctuation analysis in newborns. A review on possibilities, limitations and possibilities of misinterpretation

Matthias Rother, Herbert Witte and Michael Eiselt

Institute of Pathological Physiology, Friedrich Schiller University, O-D-6900 Jena, Germany

The different components of heart rate fluctuations (HRF) are generated by different neuroanatomical structures and are frequently used parameters in cerebral function analysis. A review will be given on methodological influences to these components. These influences are independent of the method of signal processing used and must be considered for all methods of quantitative analysis of HRF.
If mean respiration rate exceeds half of the mean heart rate RESPIRATORY SINUS ARRHYTHMIA (RSA) is not synchronous with respiration, lower frequency ranges are always occupied, called "cardiac aliasing". We could demonstrate that RSA is quantified incorrectly in every 8th newborn by conventional procedures. With increasing mean heart and respiration rate the extent of RSA is reduced. Furthermore, extent of RSA depends on the ratio of mean heart to mean respiration rate, due to aliasing effects of the harmonics of nonsinusoidal signals. This was found both in modelling and physiological studies.
In contrast to the adult NONRESPIRATORY CARDIOVASCULAR HEART RATE FLUCTUATIONS cannot always be detected as a rhythmical event in the neonate due to immaturity or to interferences with other low frequency components of HRF and RSA via "cardiac aliasing".
NEONATAL HEART RATE RESPONSES RELATED TO BODY MOVEMENTS influence the quantification of mean heart rate, nonrespiratory cardiovascular rhythms, RSA and can be used for diagnostic purposes per se. Sleep state related trends may depend more or less on the motor behaviour and the movement-related heart rate reactions. Different approaches were introduced for the use of EVOKED HRF in the neonate We found a decreased threshold to evoke vegetative reactions by acoustic stimulation in babies at risk compared to normals. But before heart rate reactions occur, changes of respiration can be observed.
Several DRUGS such as pancuronium bromide, diazepam and phenobarbital are said to influence HRF in the neonate. But only few controlled studies exist. We found in a pilot study no characteristic changes of HRF after phenobarbital administration. Pathological conditions of short duration like SEIZURES may influence HRF. Changes of HRF may occur simultaneously with epileptogenic EEG discharges. We found different alterations of HRF during neonatal seizures indicating the effect on different vegetative brain stem structures.

Cardiorespirography improves the prognostic value of EEG in neonates

Matthias Rother, Uwe Koschel, Michael Eiselt and *Barbara Clausner

*Institute of Pathological Physiology, *Department of Neonatology of the Childrens Hospital, Friedrich Schiller University Jena, D-O 6900, Germany*

It has been possible to demonstrate the prognostic value of the neonatal EEG since the early 70ies. Analysis of neonatal EEG alone leads to both false positive as well as false negative misclassification Lesions of brain stem structures might be at least partly responsible for neurological sequalae despite a normal EEG. Cardiorespirography (CRG) may reflect neurovegetative brain stem function. Up to now, no direct comparison of the predictive value of EEG and CRG has been performed. Thus, it seems to be useful to examine whether CRG promises to improve the predictive capabilities of neonatal EEG analysis.
Firstly, the prognostic value of the visual analysis of CRG (vCRG) was compared with that of the neonatal EEG in 112 newborns during intensive care (86 newborns with normal and 26 with unfavourable outcome). Conventional clinical data were used as reference. Secondly, the prognostic value of vCRG had to be compared to the computerized (spectral) analysis of CRG (cCRG) and the neonatal EEG in a selected group of 59 neonates (NORMAL n=42, ABNORMAL N=17).
A stepwise variable selection procedure based on the multiple regression was performed to find a model with a small set of significant parameters which contribute significantly to the model.After estimation of the best sets of parameters for the parameter groups these sets were evaluated by discriminant analysis. For part 1 of the study correct predictions by EEG, vCRG, EEG plus vCRG and by the clinical data were computed. For part 2 the correct predictions by EEG, vCRG, EEG plus vCRG, cCRG and cCRG plus EEG were computed.
The analysis showed that EEG is superior to the clinical data for predicting both normal and abnormal outcome. EEG is superior to the cCRG data in predicting normal outcome. cCRG better predicts unfavourable outcome. Combined use of vCRG and EEG improves the predictive value of the EEG parameters to detect normal development. But, best reclassification results were achieved by combined use of cCRG and EEG, especially in detecting abnormal development.

VI. Sleep and altitude
VI. Sommeil et altitude

Heart rate during sleep at high altitude : effect of acclimatization

O. Marrone, S. Romano*, S. Carollo, R. Milazzo and S. Porcu**

*Istituto di Fisiopatologia Respiratoria del CNR, Via Trabucco, 180, 90146 Palermo
**Divisione Aerea Studi Ricerche e Sperimentazioni, Gruppo Neuropsicofisiologia, Pratica di Mare, Roma, Italy

5 normal male subjects, age 24 - 52 years, were subjected to a nocturnal polysomnographic recording, including electroencephalogram, electrooculogram, electromyogram, electrocardiogram and respiratory movements, during the first and third week of stay at high altitude (4940 metres above sea level). Sleep was staged according to standard criteria in 30 seconds epochs. Heart rate (HR) was measured by a computerized method, 15 seconds by 15 seconds. Periodic breathing, that was observed only in NREM sleep, had a variable occurrence among subjects and, within each subject, between nights. On both nights there was a trend to a higher HR during wakefulness than in REM sleep, and in REM sleep than in NREM. In addition, in the second nights a significantly higher HR was detected during wakefulness, NREM and REM sleep in 4 subjects ($p<0.001$). The increase in HR was higher during wakefulness than during sleep. No significant difference between HR in the two nights, either during wakefulness or during sleep, was detected in the fifth subject. The results suggest that HR response to hypoxia increases in most subjects up at least the third week of stay at altitude; in addition, the response seems similarly operating during NREM and REM sleep.

Arterial O_2 saturation during sleep at high altitude in normal and polycythemic highlanders

Hervé Normand*, Janine Bordachar**, Jeanne Raynaud**, Enrique Vargas* and Odile Benoit***

*Faculté de Médecine de Caen, 14000 Caen, **Hôpital Marie Lannelongue, 92350 Le Plessis Robinson, France, *Instituto Boliviano de Biologia de Altura, La Paz, Bolivia, ***CNRS URA 1159, France

Normal highlanders have a lower hypoxic ventilatory response than sea level residents and O2 sensitivity is completely blunted in polycythemic highlanders. Furthermore, at high altitude, the position of SaO2 on the Hb/HbO2 dissociation curve is very sensitive to small changes in PaO2. Therefore the study of SaO2 during sleep in these subjects will provide better insight into the functions of ventilatory metabolic drives during REM and NREM sleep.

We studied 7 normal highlanders (mean age: 41 yrs, mean hematocrit: 51 %) and 14 polycythemic highlanders. (mean age: 48 yrs, mean hematocrit: 68 %) during one night in La Paz, Bolivia (3800 m).

In all subjects, SaO2 decreased as soon as sleep started. At whatever stage of sleep, SaO2 was lower in polycythemic subjects. In normal highlanders and in young polycythemic highlanders, the maximal decrease in SaO2 occured during REM sleep, but in older polycythemic subjects, SaO2 decreased maximally during slow-wave sleep and increased at the start of REM sleep.

This data emphasizes the importance of age on the ventilatory responses of polycythemic highlanders. Their blunted O2 chemosensitivity might account for their deeper desaturation during slow-wave sleep as compared to control subjects, while the increased desaturation during NREM in older polycythemic subjects might be due to the loss of CO2 sensitivity usually observed with age. The sudden rise of SaO2 during REM sleep favors the assumption that ventilatory metabolic drives are of less importance in breathing control during that sleep stage.

Author index
Index des auteurs

Äärimaa T., 169
Ali N.J., 243
Alix D., 255
Andrews D.C., 45
Apprill M., 187
Arnaud A., 238
Atton L., 217
Aubert-Tulkens G., 228
Auge D., 249
Barbe F., 227
Bautista D., 261
Bellet M., 255
Bellia V., 233
Belt P., 243
Benachouba N., 252
Benoit O., 270
Besombes J.P., 236
Blouin A., 217
Bonnet C., 224
Bonsignore G., 233
Bonsignore M.R., 222
Bootsma M., 250
Bordachar J., 270
Bradley T.D., 203
Braghiroli A., 247, 248
Brendle Glomb W., 261
Bruschke A.V.G., 250
Cabelguen C., 255
Carollo S., 269
Casey K.R., 87
Cauchemez B., 105
Cherniack N.S., 15
Clairambault J., 155, 264
Clausner B., 266
Cormier Y., 237
Cortelli P., 225
Curzi-Dascalova L., 155, 263, 264
Daniel F., 227
Dascalu V., 244
Davidson Ward S.L., 261
Davies R.J.O., 221, 243, 246
De Broca A., 258
De Vito F., 247, 248
Dehan M., 145
Delpuech C., 238
Didier A., 236
Donnelly D.F., 35
Donner C.F., 247, 248
Donnou M.D., 255
Dore P., 251
Dreizzen E., 245
Ehlenz K., 226
Eiselt M., 263, 264, 265, 266
Elghozi J.L., 23

Encabo H., 229
Erbetta M., 247, 248
Escourrou P., 193, 223
Feddersen O., 177
Fewell J.E., 244
Fleury B., 227
Gaultier C., 145, 193, 223
Gavriely N., 245
Giordano A., 247, 248
Girard A., 23
Girin E., 255
Gleeson K., 218
Goldman M.D., 87
Gozal D., 262
Grossi Y., 255
Grosswasser J.J., 133
Guilleminault C., 95
Haddad G.G., 35
Harper R.M., 55
Harrington K.J., 246
Herzog P., 226
Jalonen J., 169
Jones C.R., 87
Johnson P., 45
Jounieaux V., 239
Kaffarnik H., 226
Kahn A., 133
Kalach N., 258
Kamphuisen H.A.C., 250
Kauffmann F., 105, 155
Keens T.G., 262
Kemp B., 250
Kiladjian J.J., 227
Kochert F., 258
Kok J., 165
Kondo C.S., 244
Koschel U., 266
Kosev P., 234
Krieger J., 123, 187
Lagarde D., 259
Laguzzi R., 9
Laude D., 23
Le Bot J., 255
Le Gros V., 193, 223
Leffler C., 264
Leophonte P., 236
Levi-Valensi P., 239
Lévy P., 224
Lugaresi E., 225, 235
Maas Y., 165
Magnaghi S., 247, 248
Mahomedaly A., 258
Malacuso C., 233
Mallet E., 259

Marrone O., 222, 233, 269
Médigue C., 155, 264
Mergy J., 251
Meurice J.C., 251
Michel D., 133
Middelkoop H.A.M., 250
Milazzo R., 269
Mirmiran M., 165
Mouterde O., 259
Nedelcoux H., 223
Nogues B., 256, 257
Nogués M., 229
Normand H., 270
Oswald M., 187
Paquereau J., 251
Parchi P., 225
Patte F., 251
Patte R., 227
Peirano P., 155
Penzel T., 79
Pepin J.L., 224
Perez T., 236
Peter J.H., 79, 177, 226
Philip-Joet F., 238
Peirangeli G., 225
Podszus T., 177
Porcu S., 269
Pradella M., 228
Puel C., 236
Ramet J., 145
Raynaud J., 270
Rebuffat E., 133
Rey M., 238
Reynaud-Gaubert M., 238
Risbourg B., 258
Rodenstein D.O., 228
Romano D., 222, 269
Rostykus C., 251
Rother M., 265, 266
Roy T.C., 252
Ruga V., 247
Rutherford R., 203
Saadjian M., 238
Sacco C., 247, 248
Salvaggio A., 233
Schäfer T., 260
Schläfke M.E., 260
Schnittger I., 95
Series F., 217, 237
Series I., 217, 237
Sforza E., 225, 235
Shabtai-Musih Y., 245
Shepard J.W. Jr., 63
Shiomi T., 95

Siché J.P., 224
Slavchev S., 234
Sottiaux M., 133
Spyer K.M., 3
Stoohs R., 95
Stradling J.R., 115, 221, 243, 246
Sweer L.W., 218
Swenne C.A., 250

Takasaki Y., 203
Tiberge M., 236
Toris T., 239
Välimäki I., 169
Vardi-Visy K.B., 221
Vargas E., 270
Veale D., 224
Vecchierini-Blineau M.F., 256, 257

Von Wichert P., 79, 177, 226
Vural M., 258
Wallin B.G., 73
Weitzenblum E., 187
Witte H., 265
Woo A.M., 261, 262
Woo S.M., 261, 262
Zwiener U., 263
Zwillich C.W., 218

Colloques INSERM
ISSN 0768-3154

Other *Colloques* published as co-editions by John Libbey Eurotext and INSERM

153 Hormones and Cell Regulation (11th European Symposium). *Hormones et Régulation Cellulaire (11ᵉ Symposium Européen).*
Edited by J. Nunez and J.E. Dumont.
ISBN : John Libbey Eurotext 0 86196 104 8
INSERM 2 85598 324 X

158 Biochemistry and Physiopathology of Platelet Membrane. *Biochimie et Physiopathologie de la Membrane Plaquettaire.*
Edited by G. Marguerie and R.F.A. Zwaal.
ISBN : John Libbey Eurotext 0 86196 114 5
INSERM 2 85598 345 2

162 The Inhibitors of Hematopoiesis. *Les Inhibiteurs de l'Hématopoïèse.*
Edited by A. Najman, M. Guignon, N.C. Gorin and J.Y. Mary.
ISBN : John Libbey Eurotext 0 86196 125 0
INSERM 2 85598 340 1

164 Liver Cells and Drugs. *Cellules Hépatiques et Médicaments.*
Edited by A. Guillouzo.
ISBN : John Libbey Eurotext 0 86196 128 5
INSERM 2 85598 341 X

165 Hormones and Cell Regulation (12th European Symposium). *Hormones et Régulation Cellulaire (12ᵉ Symposium Européen).*
Edited by J. Nunez, J.E. Dumont and E. Carafoli.
ISBN : John Libbey Eurotext 0 86196 133 1
INSERM 2 85598 347 9

167 Sleep Disorders and Respiration. *Les Evénements Respiratoires du Sommeil.*
Edited by P. Lévi-Valensi and D. Duron.
ISBN : John Libbey Eurotext 0 86196 127 7
INSERM 2 85598 344 4

169 Neo-Adjuvant Chemotherapy. *Chimiothérapie Néo-Adjuvante.*
Edited by C. Jacquillat, M. Weil, D. Khayat.
ISBN : John Libbey Eurotext 0 86196 150 1
INSERM 2 85598 349 5

171 Structure and Functions of the Cytoskeleton. *La Structure et les Fonctions du Cytosquelette.*
Edited by B.A.F. Rousset.
ISBN : John Libbey Eurotext 0 86196 149 8
INSERM 2 85598 351 7

Colloques INSERM
ISSN 0768-3154

172 The Langerhans Cell. *La Cellule de Langerhans.*
Edited by J. Thivolet, D. Schmitt.
ISBN : John Libbey Eurotext 0 86196 181 1
INSERM 2 85598 352 5

173 Cellular and Molecular Aspects of Glucuronidation. *Aspects Cellulaires et Moléculaires de la Glucuronoconjugaison.*
Edited by G. Siest, J. Magdalou, B. Burchell
ISBN : John Libbey Eurotext 0 86196 182 X
INSERM 2 85598 353 3

174 Second Forum on Peptides. *Deuxième Forum Peptides.*
Edited by A. Aubry, M. Marraud, B. Vitoux
ISBN : John Libbey Eurotext 0 86196 151 X
INSERM 2 85598 354 1

176 Hormones and Cell Regulation (13th European Symposium). *Hormones et Régulation Cellulaire (13ᵉ Symposium Européen).*
Edited by J. Nunez, J.E. Dumont, R. Denton
ISBN : John Libbey Eurotext 0 86196 183 8
INSERM 2 85598 356 8

179 Lymphokine Receptors Interactions. *Interactions Lymphokines-récepteurs.*
Edited by D. Fradelizi, J. Bertoglio
ISBN : John Libbey Eurotext 0 86196 148 X
INSERM 2 85598 359 2

191 Anticancer Drugs (1st International Interface of Clinical and Laboratory responses to anticancer drugs). *Médicaments anticancéreux (1ʳᵉ Confrontation internationale des réponses cliniques et expérimentales aux médicaments anticancéreux).*
Edited by H. Tapiero, J. Robert, T.J. Lampidis
ISBN : John Libbey Eurotext 0 86196 223 0
INSERM 2 85598 393 2

193 Living in the Cold (2nd International Symposium). *La Vie au Froid (2ᵉ Symposium International).*
Edited by A. Malan, B. Canguilhem
ISBN : John Libbey Eurotext 0 86196 234 9
INSERM 2 85598 395 9

Colloques INSERM
ISSN 0768-3154

194 Progress in Hepatitis B Immunization. *La Vaccination contre l'épatite B.*
Edited by P. Coursaget, M.J. Tong
ISBN : John Libbey Eurotext 0 86196 249 4
INSERM 2 85598 396 7

196 Treatment Strategy in Hodgkin's Disease. *Stratégie dans la maladie de Hodgkin.*
Edited by P. Sommers, M. Henry-Amar,
J.H. Meezwaldt, P. Carde
ISBN : John Libbey Eurotext 0 86196 226 5
INSERM 2 85598 398 3

198 Hormones and Cell Regulation (14th European Symposium). *Hormones et Régulation Cellulaire (14e Symposium Européen).*
Edited by J. Nunez, J.E. Dumont
ISBN : John Libbey Eurotext 0 86196 229 X
INSERM 2 85598 400 9

199 Placental Communications : Biochemical, Morphological and Cellular Aspects. *Communications placentaires : aspects biochimique, morphologique et cellulaire.*
Edited by L. Cedard, E. Alsat, J.C. Challier,
G. Chaouat, A. Malassiné
ISBN : John Libbey Eurotext 0 86196 227 3
INSERM 2 85598 401 7

204 Pharmacologie Clinique : Actualités et Perspectives. (6e Rencontres Nationales de Pharmacologie clinique).
Edited by J.P. Boissel, C. Caulin, M. Teule
ISBN : John Libbey Eurotext 0 86196 225 7
INSERM 2 85598 454 8

205 Recent Trends in Clinical Pharmacology (6th National Meeting of Clinical Pharmacology).
Edited by J.P. Boissel, C. Caulin, M. Teule
ISBN : John Libbey Eurotext 0 86196 256 7
INSERM 2 85598 455 6

206 Platelet Immunology : Fundamental and Clinical Aspects. *Immunologie plaquettaire : aspects fondamentaux et cliniques.*
Edited by C. Kaplan-Gouet, N. Schlegel,
Ch. Salmon, J. McGregor
ISBN : John Libbey Eurotext 0 86196 285 0
INSERM 2 85598 439 4

Colloques INSERM
ISSN 0768-3154

207 Thyroperoxidase and Thyroid Autoimmunity. *Thyroperoxydase et auto-immunité thyroïdienne.*
Edited by P. Carayon, T. Ruf
ISBN : John Libbey Eurotext 0 86196 277 X
INSERM 2 85598 440 8

208 Vasopressin. *Vasopressine.*
Edited by S. Jard, R. Jamison
ISBN : John Libbey Eurotext 0 86196 288 5
INSERM 2 85598 441 6

210 Hormones and Cell Regulation (15th European Symposium). *Hormones et Régulation Cellulaire (15e Symposium Européen).*
Edited by J.E. Dumont, J. Nunez, R.J.B. King
ISBN : John Libbey Eurotext 0 86196 279 6
INSERM 2 85598 443 2

211 Medullary Thyroid Carcinoma. *Cancer Médullaire de la Thyroïde.*
Edited by C. Calmettes, J.M. Guliana
ISBN : John Libbey Eurotext 0 86196 287 7
INSERM 2 85598 440 0

212 Cellular and Molecular Biology of the Materno-Fetal Relationship. *Biologie cellulaire et moléculaire de la relation materno-fœtale.*
Edited by G. Chaouat, J. Mowbray
ISBN : John Libbey Eurotext 0 86196 909 1
INSERM 2 85598 445 9

215 Aldosterone, Fundamental Aspects. *Aldostérone, aspects fondamentaux.*
Edited by J.P. Bonvalet, N. Farman, M. Lombès, M.E. Rafestin-Oblin
ISBN : John Libbey Eurotext 0 86196 302 4
INSERM 2 85598 482 3

LOUIS-JEAN
avenue d'Embrun, 05003 GAP cedex
Tél. : 92.53.17.00
Dépôt légal : 604 — Juillet 1991
Imprimé en France